BRADY

BTLS: Basic Trauma Life Support

for the EMT-B and First Responder

Third Edition

Edited by

John Emory Campbell
M.D., F.A.C.E.P.

Basic Trauma Life Support International, Inc.

Brady/Prentice Hall Health
Upper Saddle River, New Jersey 07458

Library of Congress Cataloging-in-Publication Data

BTLS : basic trauma life support for the EMT-B and first responder / edited by John Emory Campbell. — 3rd ed.

　　p. cm.

Includes bibliographical references and index.

ISBN 0-13-084581-7 (pbk. : alk. paper)

1. Emergency medicine. 2. Wounds and injuries. 3. First aid in illness and injury. I. Campbell, John E.,1943– II. Title: Basic trauma life support for the EMT-B and first responder

　RC86.7 .C342　2000

　617.1'026—dc21

99-35610
CIP

Publisher: *Julie Alexander*
Acquisitions editor: *Judy Streger*
Director of production and manufacturing: *Bruce Johnson*
Managing production editor: *Patrick Walsh*
Senior production manager: *Ilene Sanford*
Production liaison: *Julie Boddorf*
Production editor: *Barbara J. Barg*
Creative director: *Marianne Frasco*
Interior designer: *Jill Yutkowitz*
Cover designer: *Rob Richman*
Cover photographer: *Mark C. Ide*
Marketing manager: *Tiffany Price*
Marketing coordinator: *Cindy Frederick*
Composition: *Navta Associates, Inc.*
Printing and binding: *Webcrafters*

> *This book is dedicated to Jesus Christ and the principles that he taught. Two thousand years ago his parable of the Good Samaritan set the standards to which we in EMS still strive to meet.*

Printed in the United States of America

10 9 8 7 6 5 4 3 2 1

ISBN 0-13-084581-7

Prentice-Hall International (UK) Limited, *London*
Prentice-Hall of Australia Pty. Limited, *Sydney*
Prentice-Hall Canada Inc., *Toronto*
Prentice-Hall Hispanoamericana, S.A., *Mexico*
Prentice-Hall of India Private Limited, *New Delhi*
Prentice-Hall of Japan, Inc., *Tokyo*
Prentice-Hall Pte. Ltd., *Singapore*
Editora Prentice-Hall do Brasil, Ltda., *Rio de Janeiro*

NOTICE ON CARE PROCEDURES

It is the intent of the authors and publisher that this textbook be used as part of an education program taught by qualified instructors and supervised by a licensed physician. The procedures described in this textbook are based upon consultation with paramedics, nurses, and physicians. The authors and publisher have taken care to make certain that these procedures reflect currently accepted clinical practice; however, they cannot be considered absolute recommendations.

The material in this textbook contains the most current information available at the time of publication. However, federal, state, and local guidelines concerning clinical practices, including, without limitation, those governing infection control and universal precautions, change rapidly. The reader should note, therefore, that new regulations may require changes in some procedures.

It is the responsibility of the reader to familiarize himself or herself with the policies and procedures set by federal, state, and local agencies as well as the institution or agency where the reader is employed. The authors and the publisher of this textbook and the supplements written to accompany it disclaim any liability, loss, or risk resulting directly or indirectly from the suggested procedures and theory, from any undetected errors, or from the reader's misunderstanding of the text. It is the reader's responsibility to stay informed of any new changes or recommendations made by any federal, state, and local agency as well as by his or her employing institution or agency.

NOTICE ON GENDER USAGE

The English language has historically given preference to the male gender. Among many words, the pronouns, "he" and "his" are commonly used to describe both genders. Society evolves faster than language, and the male pronouns still predominate our speech. The authors have made great effort to treat the two genders equally, recognizing that a significant percentage of EMS Providers are female. However, in some instances, male pronouns may be used to describe both males and females solely for the purpose of brevity. This is not intended to offend any readers of the female gender.

CONTENTS

A U T H O R S

Roy L. Alson, M.D., F.A.C.E.P.

Gail V. Anderson Jr., M.D., F.A.C.E.P.
Medical Director
Harbor-UCLA Medical Center
Assistant Dean
UCLA School of Medicine
Los Angeles, California

James J. Augustine, M.D., F.A.C.E.P.
Assistant Clinical Professor
Department of Emergency Medicine
Wright State University
CEO
Premier Health Care Services

Jere F. Baldwin, M.D., F.A.C.E.P., F.A.A.F.P.
Chief, Department of Emergency
Medicine and Ambulatory Services
Mercy Hospital
Port Huron, Michigan

Russell Bieniek, M.D., F.A.C.E.P.
Medical Director of Emergency Services
Saint Vincent Health System
Erie, Pennsylvania

John E. Campbell, M.D., F.A.C.E.P.

James H. Creel Jr., M.D., F.A.C.E.P.

Ann M. Dietrich, M.D., F.A.A.P., F.A.C.E.P.
Attending Physician
Emergency Department
Columbus Children's Hospital
Clinical Assistant Professor
Ohio State University
State Medical Director
Ohio Chapter, BTLS

Raymond L. Fowler, M.D., F.A.C.E.P.
Chairman
Department of Emergency Medicine
Parkway Medical Center
Lithia Springs, Georgia
Medical Director
Douglas County Fire/EMS
Mid Georgia Ambulance Service

Jonathan I. Groner, M.D., F.A.C.S., F.A.A.P.
Trauma Medical Director
Children's Hospital
Columbus, Ohio

Donna Hastings, EMT-P
Grant MacEwan Community College
Edmonton, Alberta, Canada

Leah J. Heimbach, J.D., R.N., NREMT-P
General Counsel
WVU Hospitals, Inc.
Morgantown, West Virginia

Pam Kirkpatrick, R.N.
Program Director
AirMedTeam
Rocky Mountain Helicopters
Redding, California

In Memoriam
Ron W. Lee, M.D., F.A.C.E.P.

Roger J. Lewis, M.D., Ph.D., F.A.C.E.P.
Associate Professor of Medicine
UCLA School of Medicine
Director of Research
Department of Emergency Medicine
Harbor-UCLA Medical Center

David Maatman, NREMT-P/IC
Educator
Cook Research & Education Institute
Spectrum Health
Grand Rapids, Michigan

Richard N. Nelson, M.D., F.A.C.E.P.
Associate Professor of Clinical Emergency Medicine
The Ohio State University
College of Medicine
Medical Director
Emergency Department
The Ohio State University Medical Center

Jonathan G. Newman, M.D., NREMT-P
Emergency Physician
United Hospital Center, Inc.
Clarksburg, West Virginia
Clinical Faculty
West Virginia University
Morgantown, West Virginia

Paul M. Paris, M.D., F.A.C.E.P., L.L.D. (Hon.)

Andrew B. Peitzman, M.D., F.A.C.S.
Director, Trauma Services and
Surgical Critical Care
University of Pittsburgh Medical Center

Paul E. Pepe, M.D., M.P.H., F.A.C.E.P., F.C.C.M.

Jonathan M. Rubin, M.D., F.A.A.E.M.

Corey M. Slovis, M.D, F.A.C.P., F.A.C.E.P.
Professor of Emergency Medicine and Medicine
Chairman, Department of Emergency Medicine
Vanderbilt University Medical Center
Nashville, Tennessee
Associate EMS Medical Director
Nashville Fire/EMS

John T. Stevens, NREMT-P
Douglas County Fire/EMS
Paramedic Instructor
Carroll Technical Institute
Douglasville, Georgia

Ronald D. Stewart, O.C., M.D., F.R.C.P.C., F.A.C.E.P., D.S.C. (Hon.)
Professor of Emergency Medicine
Professor of Community Medicine and
    Epidemiology
Dalhousie University
Halifax, Nova Scotia
Canada

Walt Alan Stoy, Ph.D., EMT-P
Associate Professor and Program Director in
    Emergency Medicine
School of Health and Rehabilitation Sciences
Research Associate Professor of Emergency
    Medicine
School of Medicine
Department of Emergency Medicine
University of Pittsburgh
Director, Office of Education
Director, Office of International Emergency
    Medicine
Center for Emergency Medicine

Richard C. Treat, M.D., F.A.C.S.

Arlo Weltge, M.D., F.A.C.E.P.
Assistant Professor
Emergency Medicine
UT-Houston Medical School
Medical Director
Houston Community College System
Program in EMS
Medical Director
P & S Ambulance Service

Howard Werman, M.D., F.A.C.E.P.
Associate Professor
Department of Emergency Medicine
The Ohio State University
College of Medicine and Public Health
Columbus, Ohio

Janet M. Williams, M.D.
Associate Professor
Department of Emergency Medicine
Director
Center for Rural Emergency Medicine
West Virginia University

Arthur H. Yancy II, M.D., M.P.H., F.A.C.E.P.

INTRODUCTION

The first prehospital trauma course ever developed, *Basic Trauma Life Support,* was introduced for Paramedics and Advanced EMS Providers in August of 1982. BTLS began as a local project of the Alabama Chapter of the American College of Emergency Physicians. Because of a similar need for trauma training for Basic EMTs, Basic Trauma Life Support for Basic EMTs and First Responders was first offered in 1988. This third edition not only updates changes in prehospital trauma care, but also incorporates many suggestions to improve the course itself. The original BTLS course was modeled after the Advanced Trauma Life Support course (for physicians) so that the surgeon, emergency physician, trauma nurse, and EMT would think and act along similar lines. The courses differ in many respects because the prehospital situation differs markedly from the hospital.

Basic Trauma Life Support is endorsed by the American College of Emergency Physicians and the National Association of EMS Physicians. The U.S. National Registry of Emergency Medical Technicians recognizes the course for 16 hours of credit for continuing education for all levels of EMTs. More than just a packaged course, BTLS has become an international organization of instructors of prehospital trauma care. Each local chapter is represented at the international meetings. The purpose of the organization is to foster trauma training worldwide and to maintain up-to-date high standards for the BTLS course.

Basic Trauma Life Support International, with the experience of training thousands of students over the last 17 years, is responsible for the third edition of BTLS for Basic EMTs and First Responders. Authors include distinguished trauma surgeons, emergency physicians, emergency nurses, and paramedics. The authors are balanced between those in academics and "field providers." We have attempted to make changes that make the book more practical and thus more relevant to the real environment of the prehospital situation. Because EMS varies widely over the world, we have added some optional skill stations. There are several new chapters that are not included in the course itself but are pertinent to trauma care.

This course is designed for the EMT-B or First Responder who must initially evaluate and stabilize the trauma patient. Since this is a critical time in the management of these patients, this course is intended to teach the skills necessary for rapid assessment, resuscitation, packaging, and transport. It also stresses those conditions that cannot be stabilized in the field and thus require immediate transport. It is recognized that there is more than one acceptable way to manage most situations, and the procedures described here may be modified by your Medical Director. You should have the physician who provides Medical Direction to your service go over the material and give you advice on how the procedures are done in your area. When teaching this course, the techniques taught here may be modified to correspond to local or regional standards.

The primary objectives of the course are to teach you the correct sequence of evaluation and the techniques of resuscitation and packaging of the patient. You will be given enough practical training to perform these drills rapidly and efficiently, thus giving your patient the greatest chance of arriving at the emergency department in time for definitive care to be lifesaving.

ACKNOWLEDGMENTS

Special thanks to these friends of BTLS who provided invaluable assistance with ideas, reviews, and corrections of the text. This was such a big job, and there were so many people who contributed, that I am sure I have left someone out. My apologies in advance. It is sad to be getting old and forgetful.

Ronald Audette, NREMT-P
Roy Alson, M.D., F.A.C.E.P.
Jere Baldwin, M.D., F.A.C.E.P.
J. David Barrick, B.S., NREMT-P
David Burkland, M.D., F.A.C.E.P.
Jackie Campbell, R.N.
Leon Charpentier, EMT-P
Dennis Cheek, Ph.D., R.N., C.C.R.N.
Jay Cloud
John Commander, EMT-P
David Effron, M.D., F.A.C.E.P.
Daniel Ferreira, M.D.
Cathy Gibson, B.S., EMT-P
K. H. Han, M.D., F.R.C.S., F.F.A.E.M.
Donna Hasting, EMT-P

Leah Heimbach, J.D., R.N., NREMT-P
Eduardo Romero Hicks, M.D.
Christopher D. Jenkins, NREMT-P
Shirley M. Kimble, EMT-P
David Maatman, NREMT-P/IC
Brian Mahoney, M.D., F.A.C.E.P.
Kevin D. Neilson, M.D.
Jonathan Newman, M.D., F.A.C.E.P.
Randy Orsborn, EMT-P
Bill Pheifer III, M.D., F.A.C.S.
John T. Stevens, EMT-P
Ron Stewart, M.D., F.A.C.E.P.
Robert Waddell II, EMT-P
Arlo Weltge, M.D., F.A.C.E.P.
Brian J. Wilson, NREMT-P

Another special thanks goes to the following photographers who donated their work to help illustrate the text.

Roy Alson, M.D., F.A.C.E.P.
Brant Burden, EMT-P
David Effron, M.D., F.A.C.E.P.
Bonnie Meneely, R.N.
Bob Page, NREMT-P
Don Resch

Thanks to Southern Union State Community College EMS Department and Opelika Fire Department for their help in photographing spinal immobilization scenes.

F.F. Kenny Allen
A.O. Keith Burnett, EMT-P
Lt. Lynn Callahan Jr.
Herbie Clark, EMT-P
Buddy Denson, EMT-P
F.F. Steve Miller
Capt. James C. Morgan Jr., EMT-P
Josh Stevens, EMT-P

NOTES FOR TEACHERS

Though suitable as a reference text about prehospital trauma care, this book is designed to be part of an organized hands-on course for Basic EMTs and First Responders. An Instructor's Guide and slides are available to be used in teaching the BTLS course. This course is monitored and certified in each area by the local chapter of Basic Trauma Life Support International, Inc. If you wish to arrange a certified course in your area but do not know the address of your local chapter coordinator, you may write or call:

> Virginia Kennedy Palys
> Executive Director
> Basic Trauma Life Support International, Inc.
> 1 South 280 Summit Avenue
> Court B
> Oakbrook Terrace, Illinois 60181
> Phone: 1-800-495-BTLS

NOTES FOR STUDENTS

The BTLS course is an intensive, demanding experience that requires preparation in advance of the actual course. You should begin studying the book no less than 2 weeks before the course. The actual course is designed not to tell you, but rather to show you and allow you to practice managing trauma patients. If properly prepared, you will find this course to be the most enjoyable you have ever taken.

The first 19 chapters are essential and should be studied thoroughly in the weeks preceding the course. You will be tested on this material. The appendices contain important chapters, but due to time constraints they are not included in the course. You will *not* be tested on the appendices.

Appendix A contains some optional skills. If any optional skills are to be taught in the course, you will be notified in advance so that you may study them.

For information about BTLS or if you would like to place an order for textbooks, call 1-800-495-BTLS.

CHAPTER 1

Scene Size-Up

James H. Creel Jr., M.D., F.A.C.E.P.

(Photo courtesy of Bonnie Meneely, R.N.)

OBJECTIVES

UPON COMPLETION OF THIS CHAPTER, YOU SHOULD BE ABLE TO:

1. Explain the relationship of time to patient survival and explain how this affects your actions at the scene.
2. Discuss the steps of the scene size-up.
3. List the two basic mechanisms of motion injury.
4. Discuss mechanisms and settings for blunt versus penetrating trauma.
5. Identify the three collisions associated with a motor vehicle crash (MVC) and relate potential patient injuries to deformity of the vehicle, interior structures, and body structures.
6. Name the five common forms of MVCs.
7. Describe potential injuries associated with proper and improper use of seat restraints, head rests, and air bags in a head-on collision.
8. Differentiate lateral-impact collision from head-on collision based on the three collisions associated with a MVC.
9. Describe potential injuries from rear-end collisions.
10. Explain why the mortality rate is higher for victims ejected from vehicles in MVCs.
11. Describe the three assessment criteria for falls and relate them to anticipated injuries.
12. Identify the two most common forms of penetration injuries and discuss associated mechanisms and extent of injury.
13. Relate three factors involved in blast injuries to patient assessment.

INTRODUCTION

Trauma, the medical term for injury, continues to be our most expensive health problem. The fourth leading cause of death for all ages, trauma is the leading cause of death for children and adults under the age of 45 years. For every fatality, there are 10 more patients admitted to hospitals and hundreds more treated in emergency departments. The cost of injury is estimated to be over $210 billion annually. This represents a cost twice that of cardiovascular disease and cancer combined. The price of trauma, in both physical and fiscal resources, mandates that we learn more about this disease to treat its effects and decrease its incidence (see Appendix H, Injury Prevention and the Role of the EMS Provider).

PHILOSOPHY OF ASSESSMENT AND MANAGEMENT OF THE TRAUMA PATIENT

For the severely injured patient, survival is time-dependent. The direct relationship between the timing of definitive (surgical) treatment and the survival of trauma patients was first described by Dr. R Adams Cowley of the famous Shock-Trauma Unit in Baltimore, Maryland. He discovered that when seriously injured patients were able to gain access to the operating room within an hour of the time of injury, the highest survival rate was achieved (approximately 85%). He referred to this as the "golden hour."

The golden hour begins at the moment the patient is injured, not at the time you arrive at the scene. Rarely is there much of the hour left when you begin your assessment, so you must be very well-organized in what you do. In the prehospital setting you do not have a golden hour but rather a "platinum ten minutes" in which to identify live patients, make treatment decisions, and begin to move patients to the appropriate medical facility. This means that every action must have a lifesaving purpose. Any action that increases scene time but is not potentially lifesaving must be deleted. Not only must you reduce evaluation and resuscitation to the most efficient and critical steps; you must also develop the habit of assessing and treating every trauma patient in a planned logical and sequential manner so you don't forget critical actions. We have found it best to proceed in a "head-to-toes" manner so that nothing is missed. If you jump around during your assessment, you will inevitably forget to evaluate something important. Teamwork is very important since many actions must be done at the same time.

It has been said that medicine is a profession that was created for obsessive-compulsive people. Nowhere is this more true than in the care of the trauma patient. Often the patient's life depends on how well you manage the details. Not all of the details occur at the scene of the injury. You or a member of your team must:

1. Maintain your ambulance or rescue vehicle so that it is serviced and ready to respond when needed.
2. Know the quickest way to the scene of an injury.
3. Know how to size-up a scene in order to recognize dangers and mechanisms of injury.
4. Know which scenes are safe and if not safe, what to do about it.
5. Know when you can handle a situation and when to call for help.
6. Know when to approach the patient and when to leave with the patient.
7. Be familiar with your equipment and maintain it in working order.
8. Know the most appropriate hospital and the best way to get there.

As if this were not enough, you also have to know:

1. Where to put your hands.
2. Which questions to ask.
3. What interventions to perform.
4. When to perform the interventions.
5. How to perform critical procedures quickly and correctly.

If you think the details are not important, then leave the profession now. Our job is saving lives, a most honorable profession. If we have a bad day, someone will pay for our mistakes with suffering or even death. Since the early beginnings of Emergency Medical Services (EMS), lives have been lost by patients and, unfortunately, even rescuers, for mistakes in every one of the details listed above. Many of us can recall patients that we might have saved if we had been a little smarter, a little faster, or a little better organized. Make no mistake, there is no "high" like saving a life, but you will carry the scars of your failures all of your life. Your mind-set and attitude are very important. You must be concerned but not emotional, alert but not excited, quick but not hasty. Above all, you must continuously strive for what is best for your patient. When your training has not prepared you for a situation, always fall back on the question: What is best for my patient? When you no longer care, burnout has set in and your effectiveness is severely limited. When this happens it is best to seek help (yes, all of us need help when the stress overcomes us) or seek an alternative profession.

Since 1982 the Basic Trauma Life Support (BTLS) organization has been identifying the best methods to get the most out of those few minutes that we have to save the patient's life. We know that not all patients can be saved, but our goal is to never lose a life that could have been saved. The knowledge in this book can help you make a difference. Learn it well.

SCENE SIZE-UP

On-scene trauma assessment begins with certain actions before you approach the patient. Failure to perform these preliminary actions may jeopardize your life as well as the life of your patient. Sizing up the scene is a critical part of trauma assessment. This assessment includes body substance isolation (BSI) review, evaluating the scene for dangers, determining the total number of patients, determining essential equipment needed for this particular scene, and identifying the mechanisms of injuries. Scene size-up actually begins at dispatch when you begin to anticipate what you will find at the scene. You should begin to think about what equipment you will need and whether other resources (more units, special extrication equipment, multiple casualty incident [MCI] protocols) may be needed. While information from dispatch is useful to begin to think about a plan, don't rely on this information too much. Information given to the dispatcher is often exaggerated or even completely wrong. Be prepared to change your plan depending on your own survey of the scene.

STEPS OF THE SCENE SIZE-UP

1. Body substance isolation review
2. Scene safety
3. Initial triage (total number of patients)
4. Essential equipment/additional resources needed on-scene
5. Mechanism of injury

BODY SUBSTANCE ISOLATION REVIEW

Trauma scenes are among the most likely to subject the rescuer to contamination by body fluids. Not only are trauma patients often bloody; they frequently require airway management under adverse conditions. Personal protective equipment (PPE) is always needed at trauma scenes. Protective gloves are always needed, and many situations will require eye protection. It is wise for the rescuer in charge of airway management to have a face shield or eye protection and mask. In highly contaminated situations impervious gowns with mask or face shield may also be needed. Remember to protect your patient from body fluids by changing gloves between patients.

SCENE SAFETY

Begin assessing the scene for hazards as you approach. Your first decision is to determine the nearest safe place to park the ambulance or rescue vehicle. You would like the vehicle as close as possible, and yet it must be far enough away from the scene for you to be safe while you are performing the scene assessment. Next, determine if it is safe to approach the patient(s). Things to consider are:

1. *Crash/rescue scenes:* Is there danger from fire or toxic substances? Is there danger of electrocution? Are there unstable surfaces or structures present such as ice, water, slope, or buildings in danger of collapse? Areas with potential for low oxygen levels or toxic chemical levels (sewers, ships' holds, silos, etc.) should never be entered until you have the proper protective equipment and breathing apparatus. You should never enter a dangerous area without a partner and a safety line attached.
2. *Crime scenes:* There may be danger here even after the crime has been committed. You should have law enforcement personnel at the scene, not only for the safety of you and the victims, but also to help preserve evidence.
3. *Bystanders:* You and the victim(s) may be in danger from bystanders. Are bystanders talking in loud, angry voices? Are people fighting? Are weapons present? Is there evidence of the use of alcohol or illegal drugs? Is this a domestic violence scene? You may not be recognized as a rescuer but rather as a symbol of authority and thus attacked. Are there dangerous animals present? Request law enforcement personnel if there is any sign of danger from violence.

Consider whether the scene poses a continued threat to the patient. If there is danger of fire, water, structure collapse, toxic exposure, etc., the patient may have to be moved immediately. This does not mean that you should expose yourself or your partners to unnecessary danger. You may need to call for special equipment and proper backup from the police, fire department, or power company. If the scene is unsafe you should make it safe or try to remove the patients from the scene without putting yourself in danger. Sometimes there is no immediate good answer to how to do this. Use good judgment. You are there to save lives, not give up your own.

TOTAL NUMBER OF PATIENTS

Determine the total number of patients now. If there are more patients than your team can effectively handle, call for backup. Remember that you usually need one ambulance for each seriously injured patient. If there are many patients, establish medical command and initiate multiple casualty incident (MCI) protocols. Are all patients accounted for? If the patient(s) is unconscious, and there are no witnesses of the incident, look for clues (school books or diaper bag, passenger list in a commercial vehicle) that other patients might be present. Carefully evaluate the scene for other patients. This is especially important at night or if there is poor visibility.

ESSENTIAL EQUIPMENT/ADDITIONAL RESOURCES NEEDED

If possible, carry all essential medical equipment to the scene. This prevents loss of time returning to the vehicle. Remember to change gloves between patients. The following equipment is always needed for trauma patients:

1. Personal protection equipment (See previous discussion.)
2. Long backboard with effective strapping and head immobilization device

3. Appropriately sized cervical spinal immobilization collar (CSIC)
4. Oxygen and airway equipment (Suction and bag-valve mask [BVM] should be included.)
5. Trauma box (bandage material, blood pressure cuff, stethoscope)

If special extrication equipment, more ambulances, or backup personnel are needed, call now! You are less likely to call for help when involved in patient care.

MECHANISM OF INJURY

Once you determine that it is safe to approach the patient, begin to assess for the mechanism of injury. This may be apparent from the scene itself but may require questioning the patient or bystanders. Energy transmission follows the laws of physics; therefore, injuries present in predictable patterns. Knowledge and appreciation of the mechanism of injury allow you to maintain a high index of suspicion to aid in the search for injuries. Missed or overlooked injuries may be catastrophic, especially when they become known only when the compensatory mechanisms are exhausted. Remember that patients who are involved in a high-energy event are at risk for severe injury. *Five to 15 percent of these patients, despite normal vital signs and no apparent anatomic injury on the initial exam, will later exhibit severe injuries that are discovered on repeat examinations.* Therefore, a high-energy event signifies a large release of uncontrolled energy, and you should consider the patient injured until you have proven otherwise. It is important to be aware of whether the mechanism is generalized (MVC, fall from a height, etc.) or focused (stab wound of abdomen, hit in head by hammer). Generalized mechanisms require a rapid trauma survey while focused mechanisms may only require a more limited exam of the affected areas or systems.

Factors to be considered are direction and speed of impact, patient kinetics and physical size, and the signs of energy release (e.g., major vehicle damage). There is a strong correlation between injury severity and automobile velocity changes as measured by the amount of vehicle damage. It is important that you consider these two questions:

1. What happened?
2. How was the patient injured?

Mechanism of injury is also an important triage tool and is information that must always be reported to the emergency physician or trauma surgeon. Severity of vehicle damage has also been suggested as a nonphysiologic triage tool.

Motion (mechanical) injuries are by and large responsible for the majority of the mortality from trauma in the United States. This chapter will review the most common mechanisms of motion injuries and will stress the potential injuries that may be associated with these mechanisms. It is essential to develop an awareness of mechanisms of injury and thus have a high index of suspicion for occult injuries. Always consider the potential injury to be present until it is ruled out in a hospital setting.

There are two basic mechanisms of motion injury, blunt and penetrating. Patients may have injuries from both at the same time.

BASIC MECHANISMS OF MOTION INJURY

1. Blunt injuries
   a. Rapid forward deceleration (collisions)
   b. Rapid vertical deceleration (falls)
   c. Energy transfer from blunt instruments (baseball bat, blackjack)
2. Penetrating injuries
   a. Projectiles
   b. Knives
   c. Falls upon fixed objects

MOTOR VEHICLE COLLISIONS

Various injury patterns will be discussed in the following examples, which include automobiles, motorcycles, all-terrain vehicles (ATVs), and tractors. The important concept to appreciate is that the kinetic energy of motion must be absorbed, and this absorption of energy is the basic component in producing injury. Motion injury may be blunt or penetrating. Generally, blunt trauma is more common in the rural setting, and penetrating trauma is more common in the urban setting. Rapid forward deceleration is usually blunt but may be penetrating. The most common example of rapid forward deceleration is the MVC. You should consider all MVCs to occur as three separate events (see Figure 1-1):

1. The machine collision
2. The body collision
3. The organ collision

Consider approaching a MVC in which an automobile has hit a tree head-on at 40 miles per hour. Appreciation of the rapid forward decelerating mechanism (high-energy event) coupled with a high index of suspicion should make you concerned that the victim may have possible head injury, cervical spine injury, myocardial contusion, any of the "deadly dozen" chest injuries, intra-abdominal injuries, and musculoskeletal injuries (especially fracture or dislocation of the hip). To explain the forces involved here, you must consider Sir Isaac Newton's first law of motion: "a body in motion remains in motion in a straight line unless acted upon by an outside force." Motion is created by force (energy exchange), and therefore force will stop motion. If this energy exchange occurs within the body, damage of the tissues is produced. This law is well exemplified in the automobile crash. The kinetic energy of the vehicle's forward motion is absorbed as each part of the vehicle is brought to a sudden halt by the impact. Remember that the body of the occupant is also traveling at 40 miles per hour until impacted by some structure within the car such as the windshield, steering wheel, or dashboard. With awareness of this mechanism, one can see the multitude of potential injuries that may occur. The following are clues you should be aware of:

1. Deformity of the vehicle (indication of forces involved—energy exchange)
2. Deformity of interior structures (indication of where the patient impacted—energy exchange)
3. Deformity (injury patterns) of the patient (indication of what parts of the body may have been impacted)

MVCs occur in several forms, and each form is associated with certain patterns of injury. The five common forms of MVCs are the following:

1. The head-on collision (frontal)
2. The T-bone or lateral-impact collision (lateral)
3. The rear-impact collision (rear)
4. The rollover collision
5. The rotational collision

HEAD-ON COLLISION

In this type of MVC, an unrestrained body is brought to a sudden halt, and the energy transfer is capable of producing multiple injuries.

Windshield injuries occur in the rapid forward decelerating type of event, in which the unrestrained occupant impacts forcefully with the windshield (see Figure 1-2). The possibility for injuries is great under these conditions. Of utmost concern is the potential for serious airway and cervical spine (C-spine) injury. Remembering the three separate collision events, note the following:

Machine collision: deformed front end
Body collision: spider web pattern of windshield
Organ collision: coup/contracoup brain, soft tissue injury (scalp, face, neck), hyperextension/flexion of C-spine

VEHICLE COLLISION

Collision 1 – Auto hits tree

BODY COLLISION

Collision 2 – Body hits steering wheel, causing broken ribs

Collision 3 – Heart and lungs hit inside of sternum causing myocardial and pulmonary contusions

FIGURE 1-1   The three collisions of a MVC.

From the spider web appearance of the windshield and an appreciation of mechanism of injury, you should maintain a high index of suspicion for possible occult injuries of the C-spine. The head usually strikes the windshield, resulting in direct trauma to the

FIGURE 1-2   In a head-on collision, most injuries are inflicted by the windshield, steering wheel, and dashboard.

face and head. External signs of trauma include cuts, abrasions, and contusions. These may be quite dramatic in appearance; however, the key concern is airway maintenance with C-spine immobilization and evaluation of level of consciousness.

Steering wheel injuries most often occur to an unrestrained driver of a vehicle in a head-on collision. The driver may subsequently also impact with the windshield. The steering wheel is the vehicle's most lethal weapon for the unrestrained driver, and any degree of steering wheel deformity (check under collapsed air bags) must be treated with a high index of suspicion for face, neck, thoracic, or abdominal injury. The two components of this weapon are the ring and column (see Figure 1-3). The ring is a semirigid

FIGURE 1-3   Steering wheel injuries.

plastic-covered metal ring attached to a fixed inflexible post—a twentieth-century battering ram. Utilizing the three-collision concept, check for the presence of the following:

Machine collision: front-end deformity

Body collision: ring fracture/deformity, column normal/displaced

Organ collision: traumatic tattooing of skin

The head-on collision is entirely dependent upon the area of the body that impacts with the steering wheel. These may be readily visible with direct trauma such as lacerations of mouth and chin, contusion/bruises of the anterior neck, traumatic tattoos of the chest wall, and bruising of the abdomen. These external signs may be subtle or dramatic in appearance, but more important, they may represent the tip of the iceberg. Deeper structures and organs may harbor occult injuries due to shearing forces, compression forces, and displacement of kinetic energy. Organs that are susceptible to shearing injuries due to their ligamentous attachments are the aortic arch, liver, spleen, kidneys, and bowel. With the exception of small-bowel tears, these injuries are sources for occult bleeds and hemorrhagic shock. Compression injuries are common with lung, heart, diaphragm, and urinary bladder. An important sign is respiratory distress, which may be due to pulmonary contusions, pneumothorax, diaphragmatic hernia (bowel sounds in chest), or flail chest. Consider a bruised chest wall as a myocardial contusion that requires electrocardiogram monitoring.

In short, the steering wheel is a very lethal weapon that is capable of producing devastating injuries, many of which are occult. Steering wheel deformity is a cause for alarm and must heighten your index of suspicion. You must also relay this information to the receiving physician.

Dashboard injuries occur most often to an unrestrained passenger. The dashboard has the capability of producing a variety of injuries, depending upon the area of the body that strikes the dashboard. Most frequently, injuries involve the face and knees; however, many types of injuries have been described (see Figure 1-4).

Applying the three-event concept of collision, you will note:

Machine collision: deformity of the car

Body collision: fracture/deformity of the dash

Organ collision: facial trauma, coup/contracoup brain, hyperextension/flexion C-spine, knee trauma

Facial, brain, and C-spine injuries have already been discussed. Like chest contusion, knee trauma may represent only the tip of the iceberg. Knees commonly impact with the dashboard. This may range from the simple contusion noted about the patella to the severe compound fracture of the patella. Frank dislocation of the knees can occur. In addition, this kinetic energy may be transmitted proximally and may result in fracture of the femur or fractured/dislocated hip. On occasion the pelvis can impact with the dash, resulting in acetabulum fractures as well as pelvic fractures. These injuries are associated with hemorrhage that may lead to shock. Maintain a high index of suspicion and always palpate the femurs as well as gently squeeze the pelvis and palpate the symphysis pubis.

Miscellaneous weapons involved in MVCs typically include unrestrained objects in the vehicle such as luggage, groceries, books, and, most important, passengers. These objects may become deadly missiles in a rapid forward decelerating type of event.

T-BONE OR LATERAL-IMPACT COLLISION

The mechanism of the T-bone collision is similar to that of the head-on collision, with the addition of lateral energy displacement (see Figure 1-5). Using the three-collision concept, look for the presence of the following:

Machine collision: primary deformity of the car—check the impact side (driver/passenger)

FIGURE 1-4   Dashboard injuries.

Body collision: degree of door deformity (e.g., arm rest bent, outward or inward bowing of door)

Organ collision: cannot be predicted by external exam alone; consider organs underneath areas of external injury

The most common injuries to look for are the following:

Head: coup/contracoup due to lateral displacement

Neck: lateral displacement injuries range from cervical muscle strain to subluxation with neurological deficit

Upper arm and shoulder: injuries on the side of the impact

Thorax/abdomen: injury due to direct force either from inward bowing of door on the side of the impact or from unrestrained passenger being propelled across seat

Pelvis/legs: occupants on the side of the impact are likely to have pelvic, hip, or femur fractures

FIGURE 1-5 In a lateral-impact collision, most injuries are inflicted by intrusion of door, arm rests, side window, or door post.

Injuries of the thorax vary from soft tissue injuries to flail chest, lung contusion, pneumothorax, or hemothorax. Abdominal injuries include those of solid or hollow organs. Pelvic injuries may include fracture/dislocation, bladder rupture, and urethral injuries. Shoulder girdle or lower-extremity injuries are common, depending on the level of the impacting force.

REAR-IMPACT COLLISION

In the most common form of rear-impact collision, a stationary car is struck from the rear by another moving vehicle (see Figure 1-6). Or a slower-moving car may be impacted from the rear by a faster-moving car. The sudden increase in acceleration produces posterior displacement of the occupants and possible hyperextension of the cervical spine if the headrest is not properly adjusted. If the seat back breaks and falls back into the rear seat, there is greater chance of lumbar spine injury. There also may be rapid forward deceleration if the car suddenly strikes something in the front or if the driver applies the brakes suddenly. You should note deformity of the auto anterior and posterior as well as interior deformity and headrest position. The potential for C-spine injuries is great (see Figure 1-7). Also be alert for associated deceleration injuries.

ROLLOVER COLLISION

During a vehicle rollover, the body may be impacted from any direction; thus the potential for injuries is great (see Figure 1-8). The chance for axial loading injuries of the spine is increased in this form of MVC. Rescuers must be alert for clues that imply that the car turned over (e.g., roof dents, scratches, debris, and deformity of roof posts). There are more lethal injuries in this form of accident because there is a greater likelihood of occupants being ejected. Occupants ejected from the car are 25 times as likely to be killed.

FIGURE 1-6　In a rear-impact collision, there is a potential for neck and back injury. *(Photo courtesy of Bonnie Meneely, R.N.)*

ROTATIONAL COLLISION

A rotational mechanism is best described as what occurs when one part of the vehicle stops and the rest of the vehicle remains in motion. A rotational collision usually occurs when a vehicle is struck in the front or rear lateral area. This converts forward motion to a spinning motion. The results are a combination of the frontal-impact and the lateral-impact mechanisms with the same possibilities of injuries of both mechanisms.

OCCUPANT RESTRAINT SYSTEMS

Restrained occupants are much more likely to survive because they are protected from much of the impact inside the auto and are restrained from being ejected from the auto. These occupants are, however, still susceptible to certain injuries. The lap belt is intended to go across the pelvis (iliac crests), not the abdomen. If the belt is in place and the victim is subjected to a frontal deceleration crash, his body tends to fold together like a clasp knife (see Figure 1-9). The head may be thrown forward into the steering wheel or dashboard. Facial, head, or neck injuries are common. Abdominal injuries occur if the lap belt is positioned improperly. The compression forces that are produced when a body is suddenly folded about the waist may injure the abdomen or the lumbar spine.

The three-point restraint or cross-chest lap belt (see Figure 1-10) secures the body much better than does a lap belt alone. The chest and pelvis are restrained, so life-threatening injuries are much less common. The head is not restrained, and therefore the neck is still subjected to stresses that may cause fractures, dislocations, or spinal cord

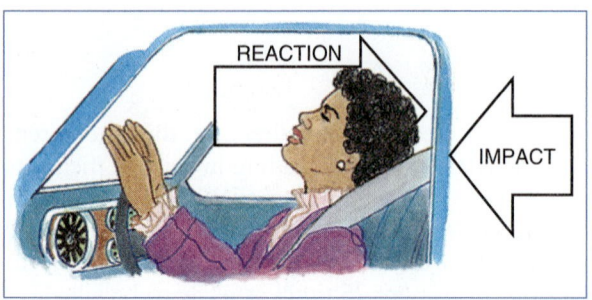

FIGURE 1-7　Mechanism of c-spine injury in rear-impact collision.

FIGURE 1-8   In a rollover collision, there is a high potential for injury. Many mechanisms are involved, and unrestrained victims are frequently ejected. *(Photo courtesy of Bonnie Meneely, R.N.)*

injuries. Clavicular fractures (at the point where the chest strap crosses) are common. Internal organ damage may still occur due to organ movement inside the body.

Like belt restraints, air bags (passive restraints) will reduce injuries in victims of MVCs in *most* but not all situations. Air bags are designed to inflate from the center of the steering wheel and the dashboard to protect the front-seat occupants in case of a frontal deceleration accident. If these function properly, they cushion the head and chest at the instant of impact. This is very effective in decreasing injury to the face, neck, and chest. You should still immobilize the neck until it has been adequately examined. Air bags deflate immediately, so they protect against only one impact. The driver whose car hits more than one object is unprotected after the initial collision. Air bags also do not prevent "down and under" movement, so drivers who are extended (tall drivers and drivers of small low-slung autos) may still impact with their legs and suffer leg, pelvis, or abdominal injuries. It is important for occupants to wear chest and lap belts even when the car is equipped with air bags. Research has recently shown that some drivers who appear uninjured after deceleration accidents have been found to have

CLASP-KNIFE EFFECT

FIGURE 1-9   Clasp-knife effect.

FIGURE 1-10   Air bag and three-point restraint.

AIR BAG AND 3-POINT RESTRAINT
PREVENTS COLLISIONS 2 and 3

serious internal injuries. A clue to which driver may have internal injuries is the condition of the steering wheel. A deformed steering wheel is just as important a clue in an auto equipped with an air bag as in those that are not. This clue may be missed because the deflated air bag covers the steering wheel. Thus a quick "lift and look" under the air bag should be a part of the routine examination of the steering wheel. Some autos are now equipped with side air bags in the doors, some have air bags that come down from the roof to protect the head, and at least one make of auto has air bags under the dash to protect the legs. These obviously give much needed extra protection. There are dangers associated with air bags. Small drivers who bring the seat up close to the steering wheel may sustain serious injuries as the bag inflates. Infants in car seats placed in the front seat may be seriously injured by the air bag.

In summary, when at the scene of a MVC, you must note the type of collision and the clues that imply that high kinetic energy has been spent (e.g., deformities of the vehicle). Maintain a high index of suspicion for occult injuries and thus keep scene time to a minimum. These observations and clues are essential to quality patient care and must be relayed to Medical Direction and the receiving physician.

TRACTOR ACCIDENTS

Another large motorized vehicle with which you must be familiar is the tractor. The U.S. National Safety Council reports that one-third of all farm accident fatalities involve tractors. There are basically two types of tractors: the two-wheel drive and the four-wheel drive. In both, the center of gravity is high, and thus the tractors are easily turned over (see Figure 1-11). The majority of fatal accidents are due to the tractor turning over and crushing the driver. Most overturns (85%) are to the side; these are less likely to pin the driver because he or she has a chance to jump or be thrown clear. Rear overturns, although less frequent, are more likely to entrap and crush the driver because there is almost no opportunity to jump free. The primary mechanism is the crush injury, and the severity depends on the part of the anatomy that is involved. Additional mechanisms are chemical burns from gasoline, diesel fuel, hydraulic fluid, or even battery acid. Thermal burns from hot engine parts or ignited fuel are also common.

Management consists of scene stabilization followed quickly by the primary survey and resuscitation. The following checklist is used in scene stabilization:

1. Engine off?
2. Rear wheels locked?
3. Fuel situation and fire hazard addressed?

FIGURE 1-11 Tractor accidents.

While you are surveying the patient, other rescuers must stabilize the tractor. The center of gravity must be identified before any attempt is made to lift the tractor. The center of gravity of the two-wheel-drive tractor is located approximately 10 inches above and 24 inches in front of the rear axle. The center of gravity of a four-wheel-drive tractor is closer to the midline of the machine. Because tractors usually overturn on soft ground and their centers of gravity are tricky to determine, great care must be taken during lifting to avoid a second crush injury. Because of the weight of the tractor and the length of time (usually prolonged) the driver is pinned, anticipate serious injuries. Often, the patient will go into profound shock as the compressing weight of the tractor is removed—similar to what happens when antishock trousers are suddenly deflated. Rapid, safe management of tractor accidents requires special exercises in lifting heavy machinery as well as good trauma management.

SMALL-VEHICLE CRASHES

Other small vehicles that fall into the motion injury category include the motorcycle, the ATV, the personal watercraft (PWC), and the snowmobile. The operators of these machines are not encased within them, and, of course, there are no restraining devices. When the operator is subjected to the classic head-on, lateral-impact, rear-end, or rollover collisions, his or her only forms of protection are the following:

1. Evasive maneuvering
2. Helmet usage
3. Protective clothing (e.g., leather clothes, helmet, boots)
4. Use of the vehicle to absorb kinetic energy (e.g., bike slide)

MOTORCYCLES: It is extremely important for motorcycle riders to wear helmets. Helmets help prevent head injury (which causes 75% of motorcycle deaths). However, helmets give no protection to the spine. The operator of a motorcycle involved in a crash is much like an ejected automobile occupant. Injuries depend on the part of the anatomy subjected to kinetic energy. Because of the lack of protective encasement, there is a higher frequency of head, neck, and extremity injuries. Important clues include deformity of the motorcycle, distance of skid, and deformity of stationary objects or cars. Again, a high degree of suspicion, appreciation of environmental clues (skid marks, vehicle deformity), identification of load-and-go, and strict BTLS protocols constitute the optimal standard of prehospital care.

ALL-TERRAIN VEHICLES: The ATV was designed as a vehicle to traverse rough terrain. They were used initially by ranchers, hunters, and farmers. Unfortunately, some people view the ATV as a fast toy. Careless misuse has resulted in an ever-increasing morbidity and mortality from accidents—sadly—frequently among the very young. The two basic designs are either three wheeled or four wheeled. The four-wheel design affords reasonable stability and handling, but the three-wheeled ATV has a high center of gravity and is very prone to rollover when turned sharply. Listed below are the three most common mechanisms:

1. Vehicle rollover
2. Fall-off of rider or passenger
3. Forward deceleration of rider from vehicle impact with stationary object

The injuries produced depend upon the mechanism and the part of the anatomy that is impacted. The most frequent injuries are fractures, about half of which are above and half below the diaphragm. The major bony injuries involve the clavicles, sternum, and ribs. Be very suspicious for head or spinal injury.

PERSONAL WATERCRAFT: The use of PWC, such as wave runners, has become very popular in water recreational activities. In 1995 there were approximately 750,000 PWC in operation in the United States. Between 1990 and 1997 there was a 400% increase in the number of injuries from PWC (2,860–12,000). The rate of emergency department-treated injuries related to PWC is about 8.5 times higher than the rate of those from motorboats. These watercrafts are designed to be operated by the driver in a sitting, standing, or kneeling position with one or more passengers located behind the driver in tandem. PWC are able to obtain high speeds very quickly. Mechanism for injury potential is very similar to the ATV. Rollovers impacting with the water at high speeds result in the same potential injury patterns. Collisions with other watercraft produce injury patterns similar to those encountered with motorcycle–auto collisions. Rectal and vaginal trauma may occur when rear-seat passengers or the driver fall off backwards, impacting the water (buttocks first) at high speeds. The likelihood of drowning (even with the use of personal flotation devices) is always a danger. Remember, water is not soft when a body impacts with it at high speeds; therefore you must assess and practice the same index of suspicion as with any high-energy event.

SNOWMOBILES: Snowmobiles are used both as recreational and utility vehicles. The snowmobile has a low clearance and a low center of gravity. The injuries common to this vehicle are very similar to those that occur with the ATV. Turnovers are somewhat more common, and since the vehicle is usually heavier than the ATV, crush injuries are seen more frequently. Again, the injury pattern depends on the part of the anatomy that is directly involved. Be alert for possible coexisting hypothermia. A common injury with the snowmobile is the "hangman" or "clothes line" injury that results from running under wire fences. Be alert for occult c-spine injuries and potential airway compromise.

PEDESTRIAN INJURIES

The pedestrian struck by a car almost always suffers severe internal injuries as well as fractures. This is true even if the vehicle is traveling at low speed. The mass of the auto is so large that high speed is not necessary to impart high-energy transfer. When high speed is involved the results are disastrous. There are two mechanisms of injury. The first is when the bumper of the auto strikes the body, and the second is when the body, accelerated by the transfer of forces, strikes the ground or some other object. An adult usually has bilateral lower leg or knee fractures plus whatever secondary injuries occur when the body strikes the hood of the car and then later the ground. Children are shorter so the bumper is more likely to hit them in the pelvis or torso. They usually land on their heads in the secondary impact. When answering a call to an auto–pedestrian accident, be prepared for broken bones, internal injuries, and head injuries.

FALLS

The mechanism for falls is vertical deceleration. The types of injuries sustained depend upon three factors, listed below, that you must identify and relay to Medical Direction:

1. Distance of fall
2. Anatomic area impacted
3. Surface struck

The primary groups involved in vertical falls are adults and children under the age of 5. In children, the falls most commonly involve males and occur mostly in the summer months in urban high-rise multiple-occupant dwellings. Predisposing factors include poor supervision, defective railings, and the curiosity associated with that age group. Head injuries are common in falls by children because the head is the heaviest part of the body and thus impacts first. Adult falls are generally occupational or due to the influence of alcohol or drugs. It is not uncommon for falls to occur during attempts to escape from fire or criminal activity. Generally, adults attempt to land on their feet; thus their falls are more controlled. In this landing form, the victim usually impacts initially on the feet and then falls backwards landing on the buttocks and outstretched hands. Classically, this "lover's leap" fall may result in the following potential injuries (see Figure 1-12):

1. Fractures of the feet or legs
2. Hip and/or pelvic injuries
3. Axial loading to the lumbar and C-spine
4. Vertical deceleration forces to the organs
5. Colles' fracture of the wrists

The greater the height, the greater the potential for injury. However, do not be deceived into believing that there is little risk for serious injury in a short-distance fall.

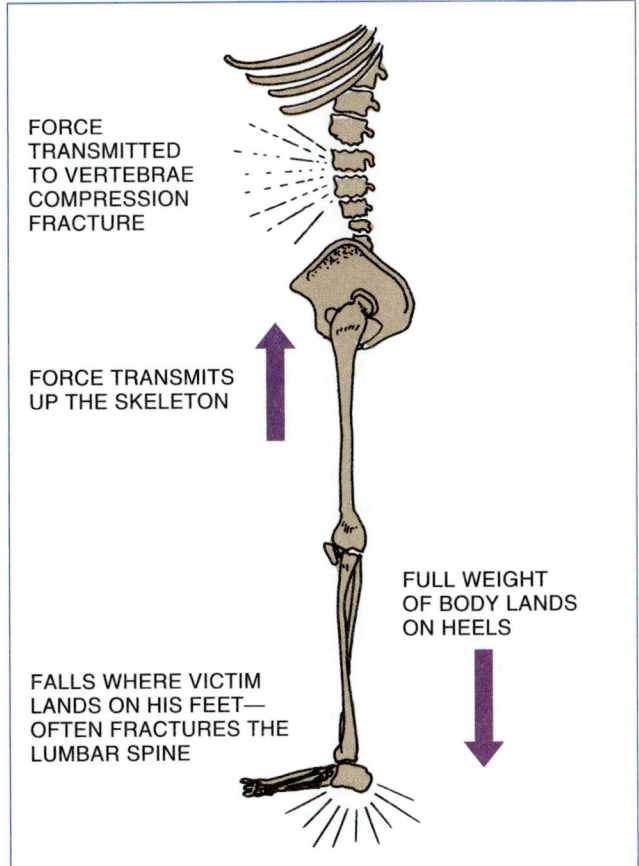

FIGURE 1-12 Axial loading.

FORCE TRANSMITTED TO VERTEBRAE COMPRESSION FRACTURE

FORCE TRANSMITS UP THE SKELETON

FULL WEIGHT OF BODY LANDS ON HEELS

FALLS WHERE VICTIM LANDS ON HIS FEET— OFTEN FRACTURES THE LUMBAR SPINE

Surface density (concrete versus sawdust) and irregularity (gym floor versus staircase) also influence the severity of injury. Relay information about distance fallen and surface struck to Medical Direction with other pertinent information.

PENETRATING INJURIES

Numerous objects are capable of producing penetrating injuries. These range from the industrial saw blade that breaks off at an extremely high rate of speed to the foreign body hurled by a lawn mower. Most high-velocity objects are capable of penetrating the thorax or abdomen. However, the more common forms of penetrating wounds come from the knife and gun.

Knife-wound severity depends on the anatomic area penetrated, the length of the blade, and the angle of penetration (see Figure 1-13). Remember, an upper abdominal stab wound may cause intrathoracic organ injury, and stab wounds below the fourth intercostal space may have penetrated the abdomen. The golden rule with knife wounds that still have the blade inside—do not remove the knife.

Most penetrating wounds inflicted by firearms are due to handguns, rifles, and shotguns. Important factors to obtain, if possible, are the type of weapon and its caliber and the distance from which the weapon was fired.

USEFUL BALLISTIC INFORMATION

Caliber: the internal diameter of the barrel; this corresponds to the ammunition used for the particular weapon.

Rifling: a series of spiral grooves in the interior surface of the barrel of some weapons. Rifling imparts a stabilizing spin to the missile.

Ammunition: case, primer, powder, and slug.

Bullet Construction: usually solid lead alloy; may have a full or partial copper or steel jacket. The shape may be rounded, flat, conical, or pointed. The bullet nose may be soft or hollow (for expansion or fragmentation).

WOUND BALLISTICS

Because the kinetic energy (kinetic energy = $1/2$ mass $\times$ velocity^2) produced by a projectile is mostly dependent upon velocity, weapons are classified as high or low velocity. Weapons with velocities less than 2,000 ft/sec are considered low velocity and include essentially all handguns and some rifles. Injuries from these weapons are much less destructive than those sustained from high-velocity weapons, such as a military rifle. Low-velocity weapons are certainly capable of lethal injuries, depending on the body area struck. All wounds inflicted by high-velocity weapons carry the additional factor of hydrostatic pressure. This factor alone can increase the injury.

Factors that contribute to tissue damage include:

1. *Missile size:* The larger the bullet, the more resistance and the larger the permanent tract.
2. *Missile deformity:* Hollow point and soft nose flatten out on impact, resulting in a larger surface area involved.
3. *Semijacket:* The jacket expands and adds to surface area.
4. *Tumbling:* Tumbling of the missile causes a wider path of destruction.
5. *Yaw:* The missile can oscillate vertically and horizontally (wobble) about its axis, resulting in a larger surface area presenting to the tissue.

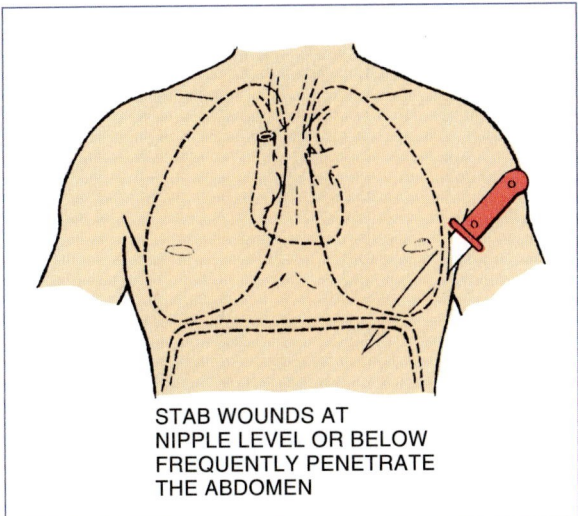

FIGURE 1-13   Stab wounds.

STAB WOUNDS AT
NIPPLE LEVEL OR BELOW
FREQUENTLY PENETRATE
THE ABDOMEN

The wounds consist of three parts:

1. *Entry wound:* Usually smaller than the exit wound; may have darkened, burned edges if bullet is fired from very close range (see Figure 1-14).

2. *Exit wound:* Not all entry wounds will have exit wounds, and on occasion there may be multiple exits due to fragmentation of bone and missile; generally, the exit wound is larger and has ragged edges (see Figure 1-14).

3. *Internal wound:* Low-velocity projectiles inflict damage primarily by damaging tissue that the missile contacts; high-velocity projectiles inflict damage by tissue contact and transfer of kinetic energy to surrounding tissues (see Figure 1-15). Damage is related to the following:
   a. Shock waves
   b. Temporary cavity, which is 30 to 40 times the bullet's diameter and creates immense tissue pressures
   c. Pulsation of the temporary cavity, which creates pressure changes in the adjacent tissue

Generally damage done is proportional to tissue density. Highly dense organs such as bone, muscle, and liver sustain more damage than less-dense organs such as lungs. A key factor to remember is that once a bullet enters a body, its trajectory will not always be in a straight line. Any patient with a missile penetration of the head, thorax, or abdomen should be transported immediately. Personnel who have been shot while

ENTRANCE WOUND (Bullet — Close Range)

EXIT WOUND (Bullet)

FIGURE 1-14   Comparison of entrance and exit wounds.

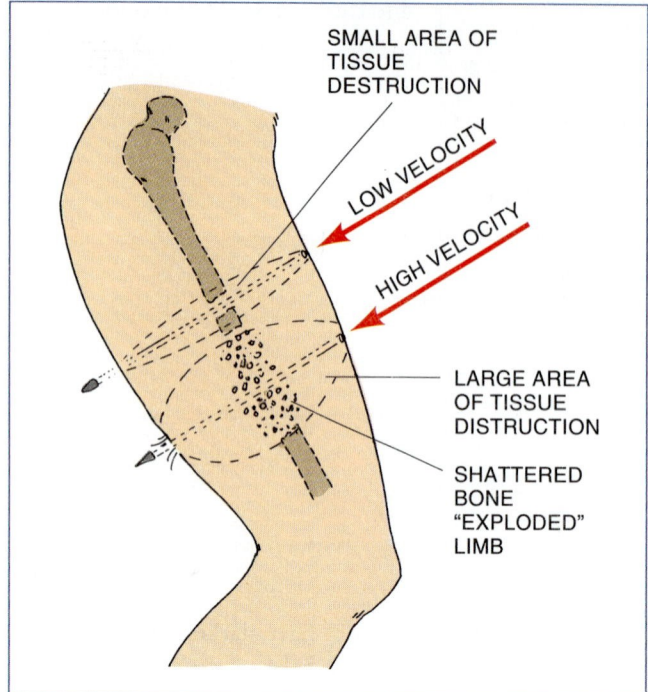

SMALL AREA OF
TISSUE
DESTRUCTION

LOW VELOCITY

HIGH VELOCITY

LARGE AREA
OF TISSUE
DISTRUCTION

SHATTERED
BONE
"EXPLODED"
LIMB

FIGURE 1-15   High-velocity versus low-velocity injury.

wearing a flak vest should be managed with caution; be alert for possible cardiac and other organ contusion.

In shotgun wounds, injury is determined by kinetic energy at impact that is influenced by:

1. Powder
2. Size of pellets
3. Choke of muzzle
4. Distance to target

Velocity and kinetic energy dissipate rapidly as distance is traveled. At 40 yards the velocity is one-half the initial muzzle velocity.

BLAST INJURIES

Blast injuries in this country occur primarily in industrial settings such as grain elevator and gas fume explosions. However, as threat of terrorist activity can no longer be considered remote, blast injury management must be added to BTLS training and knowledge.

The mechanism of injury by blast/explosion is due to three factors:

1. *Primary:* initial air blast
2. *Secondary:* patient being struck by material propelled by the blast force
3. *Tertiary:* body being thrown and impacting on ground or other object

Injuries due to the primary air blast are almost exclusive to the air-containing organs. The auditory system usually involves ruptured tympanic membranes. Lung injuries may include pneumothorax, parenchymal hemorrhage, and, especially, alveolar rupture. Alveolar rupture may cause air embolus that may be manifested by bizarre central nervous system symptoms. Gastrointestinal tract injuries may vary from mild intestinal and stomach contusions to frank rupture (see Figure 1-16). Always suspect lung injuries in a blast victim.

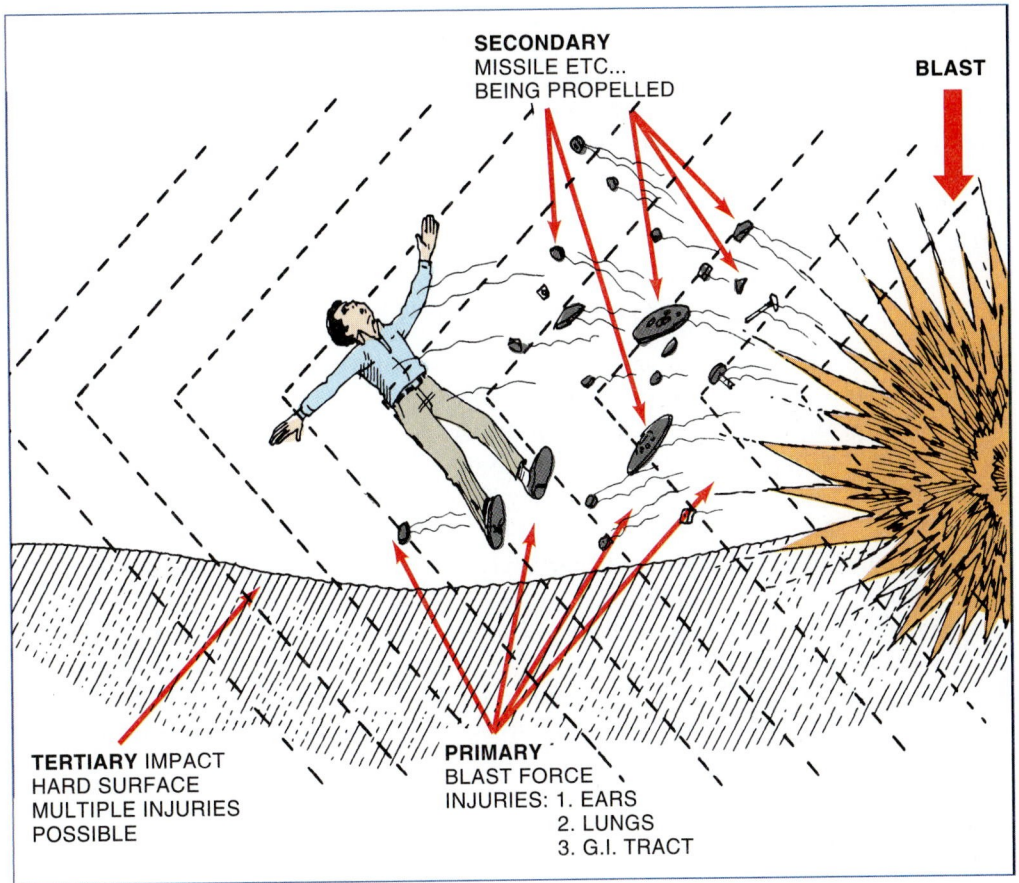

FIGURE 1-16 Blast injury.

Injuries caused by the secondary factors may be penetrating or blunt, and tertiary injuries are much the same as when a person is ejected from an automobile.

SUMMARY

Trauma is the most serious disease affecting young people. Being a rescuer is among the most important professions but requires great dedication and continuous training. Saving patients who have sustained severe trauma requires attention to detail and careful management of time. Teamwork is essential as many actions must occur at the same time.

At the scene of an injury, there are certain important steps to perform before you begin care of the patient. Failure to perform a scene survey will subject you and your patient to danger and may cause you to fail to anticipate serious injuries that your patient may have sustained. You must take proper BSI precautions, assess the scene for dangers, and determine the need for (and call for) special backup or special equipment. Then assess the total number of patients and initiate proper protocols if there are more patients than your team can manage.

You must identify the mechanism of injury and consider it as part of the overall management of the trauma patient. What happened? What type of energy was applied? How much energy was transmitted? What part of the body was affected? If there is a MVC, you must consider the form of the crash as well as survey the vehicle's interior and exterior for damage. Tractor accidents require careful stabilization of the machine to prevent a second injury to the patient. Falls require identification of distance fallen, surface struck, and position of the patient upon impact. Stab wounds require a knowledge of the length of the instrument as well as the angle at which it entered the body.

When evaluating a shooting victim you need to know the weapon, caliber, and distance from which it fired.

Information about the high-energy event (e.g., falls, vehicle damage) is also important to the emergency physician. Be sure to not only record your findings but also give a verbal report to the emergency department physician or trauma surgeon when you arrive. With this knowledge and a high index of suspicion, you can give your patient the greatest chance of survival.

BIBLIOGRAPHY

1. Branche, C. M., J. M. Conn, and J.L. Annest. "Personal Watercraft-Related Injuries." *JAMA,* Vol. 278, No. 8 (August 1997), pp. 663–665.

2. Greenberg, M. I. "Falls from Heights." *Journal of the American College of Emergency Physicians Emergency Procedures,* Vol. 7 (August 1978), pp. 300–301.

3. Huekle, D. F., and J. W. Melvin. "Anatomy, Injury, Frequency, Bio-mechanical Human Tolerance." Society of Automotive Engineers, Technical Paper No. 80098, February 1980.

4. McSwain, N. E. Jr. "Kinematics of Penetrating Trauma." *Journal of Pre-Hospital Care,* Vol. 1 (October 1984), pp. 10–13.

5. McSwain, N. E. Jr. *Pre-Hospital Trauma Life Support,* 2nd ed., pp. 1–40. Akron, OH: Emergency Training, 1990.

6. National Highway Traffic Safety Administration. *Occupant Protection Facts.* Washington, D.C.: National Center for Statistics and Analysis, U.S. Department of Transportation, June 1989.

CHAPTER 2

Assessment and Initial Management of the Trauma Patient

John E. Campbell, M.D., F.A.C.E.P.
Walt Alan Stoy, Ph.D., EMT-P
John T. Stevens, NREMT-P

OBJECTIVES

UPON COMPLETION OF THIS CHAPTER, YOU SHOULD BE ABLE TO:

1. Describe the steps in trauma assessment and management.
2. Describe the Initial Assessment and explain how it relates to the BTLS Rapid Trauma Survey and the Focused Exam.
3. Describe when the Initial Assessment can be interrupted.
4. Describe when critical interventions should be made and where to make them.
5. Identify which patients have critical conditions and how they should be managed.
6. Describe the Detailed Exam.
7. Describe the Ongoing Exam.

TRAUMA ASSESSMENT

The old BTLS Primary and Secondary Trauma Surveys have been adjusted to meet U.S. Department of Transportation patient assessment guidelines. The BTLS Primary Survey has been slightly modified to make it more flexible. Patients with trauma to a focused area (limited to a certain area of the body) or with insignificant mechanisms of injury don't require an exam as comprehensive as the old BTLS Primary Survey. The **new *BTLS Primary Survey*** is a combination of the scene size-up, the Initial Assessment (which is the same for all patients), and the Rapid Trauma Survey *or* the Focused Exam (depending on the situation). This is the only significant change because the Detailed Exam is the same as the old BTLS Secondary Survey and the Ongoing Exam is the same as the old BTLS Reassessment Survey. The Initial Assessment is a very brief exam of level of consciousness (LOC) and the ABCs to prioritize the patient and to determine if immediately life-threatening conditions exist. The purpose of the BTLS Rapid Trauma Survey is to find **all life-threatening injuries** and determine if the patient should have immediate transport. The BTLS Rapid Trauma Survey differs from the Detailed Exam (Secondary Survey) in that the Detailed Exam is an evaluation for **all** injuries, not just **life-threatening** ones.

The patient with the most minor appearing injury will get a brief Initial Assessment before you concentrate on the minor injury. Critical patients will get a much more comprehensive exam, but in each case the exam will begin in the same way (Initial Assessment). The scene size-up will set the stage for how you will perform the rest of the BTLS Primary Survey.

If there is a dangerous **generalized** mechanism of injury (auto crash, fall from a height, etc.) or if the patient is unconscious, you should go from Initial Assessment directly to the BTLS Rapid Trauma Survey. You would then perform interventions, transport, and possibly do a Detailed or Ongoing Exam en route.

If there is a dangerous **focused** mechanism of injury suggesting an isolated injury (bullet wound of thigh, stab wound to the chest, etc.), you would perform the Initial Assessment but the Focused Exam would be limited to the area of injury. The full BTLS Rapid Trauma Survey is not required. You would then perform interventions, transport, and possibly do a Detailed or Ongoing Exam.

If there is no significant life threat in the mechanism of injury (shot off big toe) you would do the Initial Assessment and **if normal,** go directly to a Focused Exam based on the patient's Chief Complaint. *The Detailed Exam would not be necessary.*

To make the most efficient use of time, prehospital assessment and management of the trauma patient is divided into five steps, and each step contains certain priorities (see Figure 2-1). These priorities are the foundation on which trauma care is built.

PATIENT ASSESSMENT USING THE PRIORITY PLAN

SCENE SIZE-UP

On-scene trauma assessment begins with certain actions before you approach the patient. It cannot be stressed too strongly that failure to perform preliminary actions may jeopardize your life as well as the patient's. Perform the scene size-up as described in Chapter 1.

If possible, carry all essential medical equipment to the scene. This saves time by not returning to the vehicle. Remember to change gloves between patients. The following equipment is always needed for trauma patients:

1. Personal protection equipment (See Chapter 1.)
2. Long backboard with effective strapping and head immobilization device
3. Appropriately sized cervical spinal immobilization collar (CSIC)
4. Oxygen and airway equipment (Suction and bag-valve mask should be included.)
5. Trauma box (bandage material, blood pressure cuff, stethoscope)

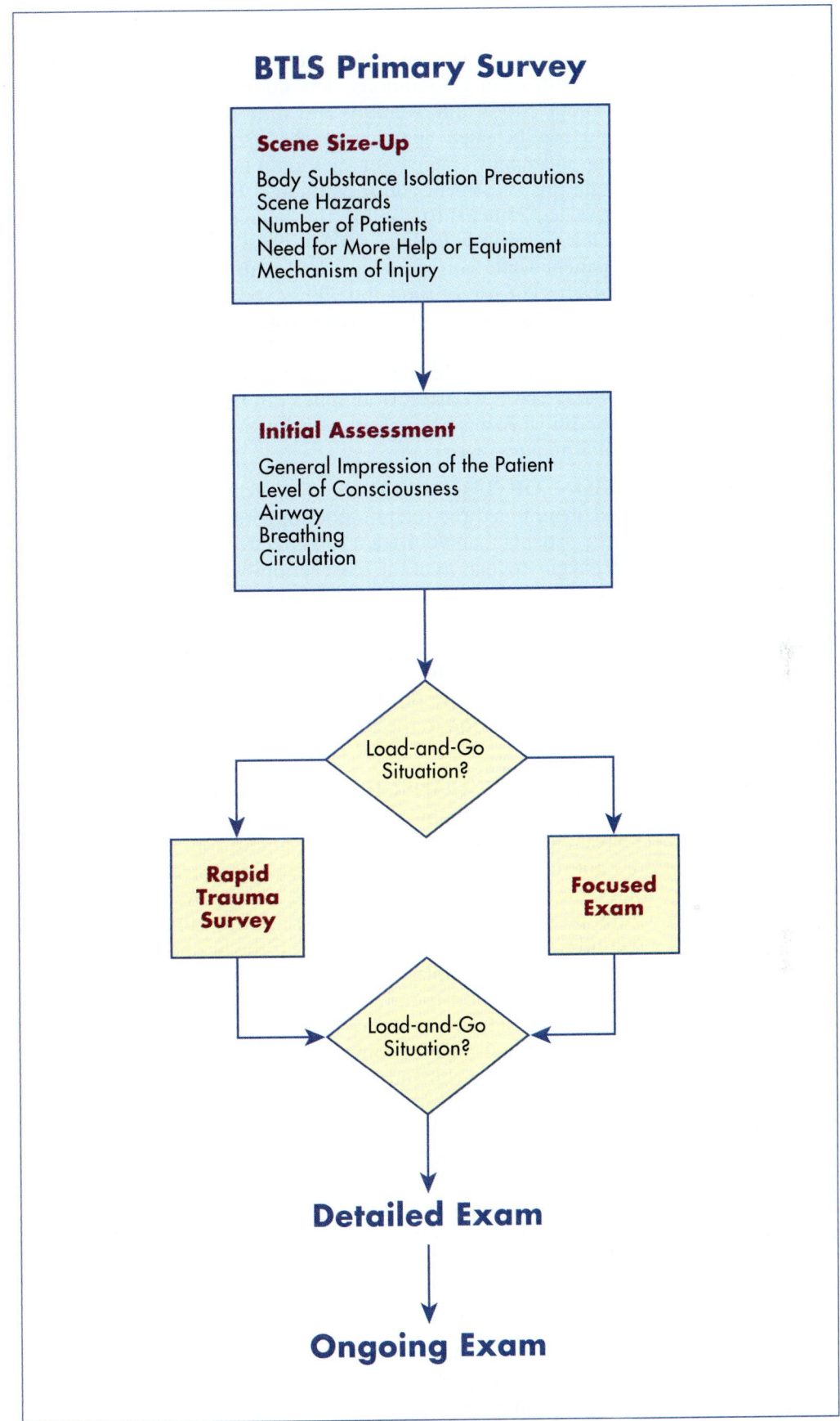

FIGURE 2-1   Steps in the assessment and management of the trauma patient.

INITIAL ASSESSMENT

The purpose of the Initial Assessment is to prioritize the patient and to determine the existence of immediate life-threatening conditions. The information gathered here is used to make decisions about critical interventions and time of transport. Once you determine that the patient may be safely approached, the assessment should proceed quickly (Initial Assessment and Rapid Trauma Survey should take less than 2 minutes) and smoothly. As you begin this assessment you should direct Rescuer #2 (who should have the C-collar and airway equipment) to stabilize the patient's neck (if needed) and to assume responsibility for the airway. Rescuer #3 will place the backboard and the trauma box beside the patient while you are proceeding with your exam. This team approach makes the most efficient use of time and allows you to rapidly perform the Initial Exam without performing airway interventions yourself, which can interrupt your thought process.

Remember, *nothing interrupts the Initial Assessment except treatment of airway obstruction or cardiac arrest* (respiratory arrest or dyspnea can be addressed by Rescuer #2 while you continue the Initial Assessment). For critical patients, the goal should be to have on-scene times of 5 minutes or less.

GENERAL IMPRESSION OF THE PATIENT ON APPROACH: You have already assessed the scene, determined the total number of patients, and initiated MCI protocols if there are more patients than your team can effectively handle (see Chapter 1). Based on initial triage, begin evaluation of the most seriously injured patient first. As you approach, note the patient's approximate age, sex, weight, and general appearance. *The old and the very young are at increased risk.* Female patients may be pregnant. Observe the position of the patient, both his body position and his position in relation to his surroundings. Note his activity (is he aware of his surroundings, anxious, obviously in distress, etc.?). Does he have any obvious major injuries or major bleeding? Your observation of the patient in relation to the scene and the mechanism of injury will help you prioritize the patient.

EVALUATE INITIAL LEVEL OF CONSCIOUSNESS WHILE OBTAINING CERVICAL SPINE CONTROL: Assessment begins immediately, even if the patient is being extricated. The team leader should approach the patient from the front (face to face, so the patient does not turn his head to see you). If there is a mechanism of injury that suggests spinal injury, the second rescuer immediately, and gently, but firmly, stabilizes the neck in a neutral position. The team leader may need to initially stabilize the neck if there is not a second rescuer immediately available. If the head or neck is held in an angulated position and the patient complains of pain on any attempt to straighten it, you should immobilize it in the position found. The same is true of the unconscious patient whose neck is held to one side and does not move when you *gently* attempt to straighten it. You cannot use a cervical collar or commercial head immobilizer in this situation. You must use pads or a blanket roll and careful taping to immobilize the head and neck in the position found. The rescuer stabilizing the neck must not release the neck until he or she is relieved or a suitable stabilization device is applied. The team leader should say to the patient, "My name is _____ . We are here to help you. Can you tell me what happened?" The patient's reply gives immediate information about both the airway and the level of consciousness. If the patient responds **appropriately** to questioning, you can assume that the airway is open and the LOC is normal. If the response is not appropriate (unconscious, or awake but confused), make a mental note of the LOC by the AVPU scale (see Table 2-1). Anything below "A" triggers a systematic search for the causes during the Rapid Trauma Survey.

ASSESS THE AIRWAY: If the patient cannot speak or is unconscious, further evaluation of the airway should follow. Look, listen, and feel for movement of air. The team leader or Rescuer #2 should position the airway as needed. Because of the ever-present danger of spinal injury, *never* extend the neck to open the airway of a trauma patient. If the airway is obstructed (apnea, snoring, gurgling, stridor), use an appropriate method (reposition, sweep, suction) to open it immediately (see Figure 2-2). Failure to provide

Table 2-1   Levels of Mental Status (AVPU).

A—**A**lert (Awake *and* oriented)

V—Responds to **V**erbal stimuli (awake but confused or unconscious but responds in some way to verbal stimuli)

P—Responds to **P**ain (unconscious but responds in some way to painful stimuli)

U—**U**nresponsive (no gag or cough reflex)

SINCE NECK MAY BE INJURED, DO NOT EXTEND THE NECK TO OPEN THE AIRWAY.

USE MODIFIED JAW THRUST

FIGURE 2-2   Opening the airway using the modified jaw thrust. Maintain in-line stabilization while pushing up on the angles of the jaw with your thumbs.

an open airway is one of two reasons to interrupt the Initial Assessment. If simple positioning and suctioning fail to provide an adequate airway, or if the patient has stridor, transport the patient *immediately*.

ASSESS BREATHING: Look, listen, and feel for movement of air. If the patient is unconscious, place your ear over the patient's mouth so you can judge both the rate and depth (tidal volume—see Chapter 4) of ventilations. Look at the movement of the chest (or abdomen), listen to the sound of the air movement, and feel both the movement of air on your cheek and the movement of the chest wall with your hand. Notice if the patient uses accessory muscles in order to breathe. If ventilations are inadequate (less than 12 per minute or too shallow), Rescuer #2 should begin to assist ventilations immediately, using her knees to maintain immobilization of the patient's neck, freeing her hands to apply oxygen or use a bag-valve mask to assist ventilation (see Figure 2-3). When assisting with or providing ventilation, be sure that the patient not only gets an adequate ventilatory rate (see Table 2-2), but also an adequate volume. All patients that are breathing too fast should receive supplemental high-flow oxygen. As a general rule, all patients with multisystem trauma should also receive supplemental high-flow oxygen.

Table 2-2   Normal and Abnormal Respiratory Rates.

	NORMAL	**ABNORMAL**
Adult	12–20	<12 and >24
Small child	15–30	<15 and >35
Infant	25–50	<25 and >60

FIGURE 2-3 Using your knees to maintain immobilization of the neck will free your hands to assist ventilation. *(Photo courtesy of Bob Page, NREMT-P)*

ASSESS CIRCULATION: As soon as you have ensured a patent airway and adequate ventilation, note the rate and quality of the pulses at the wrist (brachial in the infant). Checking the pulse in the neck is not necessary if the patient is awake and alert or if there is a palpable peripheral pulse. Quickly note whether the rate is too slow (<60 in an adult) or too fast (>120), and note also its quality (thready, bounding, weak, irregular). If absent at the neck, immediately start CPR (unless there is massive blunt trauma) and prepare for immediate transport. This is the other reason to interrupt the Initial Assessment. While at the wrist, also note skin color, temperature, and condition (and capillary refill in an infant or small child). Pale, cool, clammy skin, thready radial pulse, and decreased LOC are the best early assessment of decreased perfusion (shock).

Be sure the bleeding has been controlled (direct Rescuer #3 to control). Most bleeding can be stopped by direct pressure or pressure dressings. Air splints or the pneumatic antishock garment (PASG) may be used to tamponade bleeding. Tourniquets may be needed in rare situations. In the past it has been taught that blood-soaked dressings should only have more dressings placed on top of them, but in some cases this only allows more bleeding. If a dressing becomes blood soaked, remove the dressing and redress *once* to be sure direct pressure is being placed on the bleeding area. It is important to report such excessive bleeding to the receiving physician. Do not use clamps to stop bleeders; this may cause injuries to other structures (nerves are present alongside arteries).

RAPID TRAUMA SURVEY OR FOCUSED EXAM

The choice between the Rapid Trauma Survey and the Focused Exam depends on the mechanism of injury and/or the results of the Initial Assessment. If there is a dangerous generalized mechanism of injury (auto crash, fall from a height, etc.) or if the patient is unconscious, you should perform the BTLS Rapid Trauma Survey. If there is a dangerous focused mechanism of injury suggesting an isolated injury (bullet wound of thigh, stab wound to the chest, etc.), you may perform the Focused Exam limited to the area of injury. If there is no significant mechanism of injury (dropped rock on toe) and the Initial

Assessment was normal (alert with no history of loss of consciousness, breathing normally, radial pulse less than 120, not complaining of dyspnea, chest, abdominal, or pelvic pain), you may move directly to the Focused Exam based on the patient's chief complaint.

If you identify a priority patient, you need to find the cause of the abnormal findings and to identify if this is a load-and-go patient.

You have identified a priority patient if there is:

1. A dangerous mechanism of injury.
2. A history that reveals:
   a. Loss of consciousness
   b. Difficulty breathing
   c. Severe pain anywhere
3. An abnormal Initial Assessment:
   a. Altered mental status
   b. Difficulty breathing
   c. Abnormal perfusion
4. Poor general impression

RAPID TRAUMA SURVEY

ASSESSMENT OF THE HEAD, NECK, CHEST, ABDOMEN, PELVIS, AND EXTREMITIES: This is a *brief* exam done to find all life-threats. (A more thorough, detailed exam will follow later if time permits.) Briefly assess (look and feel) the head and neck for injuries and to see if the neck veins are flat or distended and the trachea is in the midline. You may apply a rigid extrication collar at this time. *Note:* If the team leader elected to stabilize the neck, this duty should be transferred to another rescuer at this time.

Now look, feel, and listen to the chest. Look for both asymmetrical and paradoxical movement. Note if the ribs rise with respiration or if there is only diaphragmatic breathing. Look for signs of blunt trauma or open wounds. Feel for tenderness, instability, and crepitation (TIC). Now listen to see if breath sounds are present and equal bilaterally. Listen with the stethoscope over the lateral chest about the fourth interspace in the midaxillary line on both sides. If breath sounds are not equal (decreased or absent on one side), you should percuss the chest to determine whether the patient is just splinting from pain or if a pneumothorax or a hemothorax is present. If abnormalities are found during the chest exam (open chest wound, flail chest, tension pneumothorax, hemothorax), make the appropriate intervention (seal open wound, stabilize flail). Very briefly notice the heart sounds so you will have a baseline for changes such as development of muffled heart sounds.

Rapidly expose and look at the abdomen (distension, contusions, penetrating wounds), and gently palpate the abdomen for tenderness, guarding, and rigidity.

Check the pelvis. Look for deformity or penetrating wounds. Feel for tenderness, instability, and crepitation by *gently* pressing down on the symphysis and *gently* squeezing in on the iliac crests.

Check the extremities. Assess both upper legs, looking for deformity and feeling for TIC. Remember that bilateral femur fractures can produce enough blood loss to be life-threatening. Scan for obvious wounds or deformity of the arms and lower legs. Note whether the patient can move his fingers and toes before transferring to the backboard.

At this point, transfer the patient to a long backboard, *checking the back* as you do this. You have now obtained enough information to determine critical trauma situations that should be treated by immediate transport to the hospital (load-and-go). If a critical situation is present, transport now!

If there is altered mental status, do a brief neurological exam to identify possible increased intracranial pressure (ICP). This exam should include the pupils, Glasgow

Coma Score (GCS), and signs of Cushing's reflex (see Chapter 8). Also look for medical identification devices. Head injury, shock, and hypoxia are not the only things that cause altered mental status. Also think about nontraumatic causes such as hypoglycemia and drug or alcohol overdose.

You should obtain a SAMPLE history (see Table 2-3) and, unless radial pulses are absent, a set of baseline vital signs at this point. You are the only one who gets to see the scene and you may be the only one who gets to take a history. Many patients who are initially alert lose consciousness before arriving at the hospital. You are not only making interventions to deliver a living patient to the hospital; you must be the detective that figures out what happened and why. Pay special attention to the chief complaint and the events prior to the incident (the "S" and "E" of the SAMPLE history). The patient's symptoms may suggest other injuries, and this will affect further examination. It is important to know as much about the mechanism as possible (Was she restrained? How far did she fall? What caused her to fall?). Look for clues to serious injury such as history of LOC, shortness of breath, or pain in the neck, back, chest, abdomen, or pelvis.

Table 2-3 SAMPLE History.

> **S**—symptoms
> **A**—allergies
> **M**—medications
> **P**—past medical history (Other illnesses?)
> **L**—last oral intake (When was the last time there was any solid or liquid intake?)
> **E**—events preceding the incident (Why did it happen?)

FOCUSED EXAM

If the mechanism is limited to a certain area of the body (stab wound of the chest), then you may only need to focus your exam on the affected area (chest and possibly the abdomen), obtain a SAMPLE history (may suggest further exam), and check baseline vital signs (defer until after transport if radial pulse is not present). You would then have enough information to make a decision about urgency of transport and what interventions need to be done immediately.

CRITICAL INTERVENTIONS AND TRANSPORT DECISION

Upon completion of the Initial Assessment and Rapid Trauma Survey, enough information is available to decide if a critical situation is present. *Patients with critical trauma situations are transported immediately.* Most treatment will be done during transport.

To decide whether the patient falls into the load-and-go category, you need to determine whether the patient has any of the following critical injuries or conditions:

1. Initial Assessment reveals:
   a. Altered mental status
   b. Abnormal respiration
   c. Abnormal circulation (shock or uncontrolled bleeding)
2. Signs discovered during the Rapid Trauma Survey that rapidly lead to shock:
   a. Abnormal chest exam (flail chest, open wound, tension pneumothorax, hemothorax)
   b. Tender, distended abdomen
   c. Pelvic instability
   d. Bilateral femur fractures

3. Significant mechanism of injury or poor general impression. As you consider mechanisms, age, general appearance, multiple injuries, etc., you may get a bad feeling about the patient. If so, go with your instincts.

If the patient has one of the critical conditions listed above, immediately load him into an ambulance, and transport rapidly to the nearest *appropriate* emergency facility. When in doubt, transport early. Other than administering high-flow oxygen and providing spinal immobilization, there are only a few procedures that are done at the scene:

1. Initial airway management
2. Assist ventilation
3. Begin CPR
4. Control of major external bleeding
5. Seal sucking chest wounds
6. Stabilize flail chest
7. Stabilize impaled objects

Procedures that are not lifesaving, such as splinting or bandaging must not hold up transport of the critical patient. Be sure to call Medical Direction early so that the hospital is prepared for the patient's arrival.

DETAILED EXAM

This is a more comprehensive exam to pick up additional injuries that might have been missed in the brief BTLS Primary Survey. This assessment also establishes the baseline from which treatment decisions will eventually be made. It is important to record the information discovered in this assessment. *Critical patients should always have this assessment done during transport.* If there is a short transport and you must perform interventions, you may not have time to do the Detailed Exam. If the Primary Survey does not reveal a critical condition, the Detailed Exam may be performed on the scene. Even though the patient appears to be stable, if there is a dangerous mechanism or other dangers (age, poor general health, death of another passenger, etc.), reconsider early transport. "Stable" patients may become unstable quite rapidly. Stable patients with no dangerous mechanism of injury (dropped rock on toe) do not require a Detailed Exam.

You should have obtained most of the pertinent history during the Rapid Trauma Survey, but now you can obtain further information if needed. You should perform your detailed physical exam while you are obtaining the history (if the patient is conscious).

The exam should contain the following elements:

1. *Record vital signs again:* Record pulse, respiration, and blood pressure. Remember, the pulse pressure is as important as the systolic pressure. Many people now consider the pulse oximetry reading one of the vital signs.

2. *Do a neurological exam:* It gives important baseline information that is used in later treatment decisions. This exam should include the following:

   a. Level of consciousness: If the patient is conscious, describe his orientation and emotional status. If he has an altered mental status, record his level of coma (Glasgow Coma Score—see Table 2-4). *If there is altered mental status, you should check the blood glucose and check the oxygen saturation by pulse oximetry.*

   b. Pupils: Are they equal or unequal? Do they respond to light?

   c. Motor: Can the patient move fingers and toes?

   d. Sensation: Can he feel you when you touch his fingers and toes? Does the unconscious patient respond when you pinch his fingers and toes?

3. *Perform a head-to-toes exam in more detail:* Pay particular attention to the patient's complaints and also recheck the injuries that you found previously. The exam should consist of inspection, auscultation, palpation, and sometimes percussion.

Table 2-4 Glasgow Coma Score.

EYE OPENING		VERBAL RESPONSE		MOTOR RESPONSE	
	POINTS		POINTS		POINTS
Spontaneous	4	Oriented	5	Obeys commands	6
To voice	3	Confused	4	Localizes pain	5
To pain	2	Inappropriate words	3	Withdraws	4
None	1	Incomprehensible sounds	2	Abnormal flexion	3*
		Silent	1	Abnormal extension	2**
				No movement	1

*Decorticate posturing to pain
**Decerebrate posturing to pain

a. Begin at the head examining for deformities, contusions, abrasions, penetrations, burns, tenderness, lacerations, or swelling (DCAP-BTLS), raccoon eyes, Battle's sign, and drainage of blood or fluid from the ears or nose. Assess the mouth. Assess the airway again.

b. Check the neck for DCAP-BTLS, distended neck veins, or deviated trachea.

c. Check the chest for DCAP-BTLS. Also check for paradoxical movement of the chest wall and for instability and crepitation of the ribs. Be sure that breath sounds are present and equal on each side. Note rales, wheezing, or "noisy" breath sounds. Notice if heart sounds are as loud as before. (A noticeable decrease in heart sounds may be an early sign of cardiac tamponade.) Recheck seals over open wounds. Be sure flails are well stabilized. If you detect decreased breath sounds, percuss to determine whether the patient has a pneumothorax or hemothorax.

d. Perform an abdominal exam. Look for signs of blunt or penetrating trauma. Feel all four quadrants for tenderness or rigidity. Do not waste time listening for bowel sounds. If the abdomen is painful to gentle pressure during examination, you can expect the patient to be bleeding internally. If the abdomen is both distended and painful, you can expect hemorrhagic shock to occur very quickly.

e. Assess pelvis and extremities. Check for DCAP-BTLS. Be sure to check and record pulse, motor function, and sensation (PMS) on all fractures. Do this before and after straightening any fracture. Angulated fractures of the upper extremities are usually best splinted as found. Most fractures of the lower extremities are *gently* straightened and then stabilized using traction splints or air splints. Critical patients have all splints applied during transport.

Transport immediately if the Detailed Exam reveals the development of any of the critical trauma situations.

When you finish the Detailed Exam, you should finish bandaging and splinting.

ONGOING ASSESSMENT AND MANAGEMENT

This includes the critical procedures performed on scene and during transport, the Ongoing Assessment, and also communication with Medical Direction. The Ongoing Assessment is an abbreviated exam to assess for *changes* in the patient's condition. In some critical cases with short transport times, this exam may take the place of the Detailed Exam.

The Ongoing Assessment should be recorded every 5 minutes in critical patients and every 15 minutes in stable patients. The Ongoing Assessment also should be performed each time the patient is moved, an intervention is performed, or his condition changes. This exam is to find any changes in the patient's condition, so concentrate on reassessing those things that may change.

The Ongoing Assessment should be performed in the following order:

1. Ask the patient about any changes in how he feels.
2. Reassess mental status (LOC and pupils, recheck GCS).
3. Reassess the ABCs.
   a. Reassess the **A**irway.
      (1) Recheck patency.
      (2) If burn patient, assess for signs of inhalation injury.
   b. Reassess **B**reathing and **C**irculation.
      (1) Recheck vital signs.
      (2) Note skin color, condition, temperature.
      (3) Check the neck for jugular venous distention (JVD) and tracheal deviation. (If collar has been applied, remove the front.)
      (4) Recheck the chest. Notice the quality of breath sounds. If breath sounds are unequal, evaluate for splinting, pneumothorax, or hemothorax. Listen to the heart to see if the sounds have become muffled.
4. Reassess the abdomen (if mechanism suggests possible injury). Note the development of tenderness, distention, or rigidity.
5. Check each of the identified injuries (lacerations for bleeding, PMS distal to all injured extremities, flails, pneumothorax, open chest wounds, etc.).
6. Check interventions.
   a. Check oxygen for flow rate.
   b. Check seals on sucking chest wounds.
   c. Check splints and dressings.
   d. Check impaled objects to be sure they are well stabilized.
   e. Check position of pregnant patients.

Accurately record what you see and what you do. Record changes in the patient's condition during transport. Record the time that interventions are performed. Extenuating circumstances or significant details should be recorded in the comments or remarks section of the written report (review documentation in Appendix C).

CONTACTING MEDICAL DIRECTION

When you have a critical patient, it is extremely important to contact Medical Direction as early as possible. It takes time to get the appropriate surgeon and the operating room team in place, and the critical patient has no time to wait. Always notify the receiving facility of your estimated time of arrival (ETA), the condition of the patient, and any special needs on arrival (see Appendix B).

PITFALLS

1. *Approaching the patient before doing a scene size-up:* Foolish haste may subtract a rescuer and add a patient.

2. *Trying to do too much on-scene:* Critical patients are eventually stabilized in the operating room. Their survival may depend on how fast you get them there. Most interventions should be performed in the ambulance during transport.

SUMMARY

Patient assessment is the key to trauma care. The interventions required are not difficult; it is their timing that is often critical. If you know what questions to ask and how to perform the exam, you will know when to perform the lifesaving interventions. This chapter has described a rapid, orderly, and thorough examination of the trauma patient with examination and treatment priorities always in mind. The continuous practice of approaching the patient in the way described here will allow you to concentrate on the patient rather than on what to do next. Optimum speed is achieved by teamwork. Teamwork is achieved by practice. You should plan regular exercises in patient evaluation to perfect each team member's role in the priority plan.

ACRONYMS

ATV—all terrain vehicle

AVPU—**A**lert, responds to **V**erbal stimuli, responds to **P**ainful stimuli, **U**nresponsive

BSI—body substance isolation

BVM—bag-valve mask

CSIC—cervical spine immobilization collar

DCAP-BTLS—deformities, contusions, abrasions, penetrations, burns, tenderness, lacerations, swelling

EMS—emergency medical services

ETA—estimated time of arrival

GSC—Glasgow Coma Score

IPPV—intermittent positive pressure ventilation

LOC—level of consciousness

MCI—multiple casualty incident

MVC—motor vehicle collision

PMS—pulse, motor, sensory

PWC—personal watercraft

SAMPLE—**S**ymptoms, **A**llergies, **M**edicines, **P**ast medical history, **L**ast meal, **E**vents preceding the injury

TIC—tenderness, instability, crepitation

CHAPTER 3

Patient Assessment Skills

Donna Hastings, EMT-P

OBJECTIVES

UPON COMPLETION OF THESE SKILL STATIONS, YOU SHOULD BE ABLE TO:

BTLS Primary Survey

1. Correctly perform the BTLS Primary Survey.
2. Identify within 2 minutes which patients require load-and-go.
3. Describe when to perform critical interventions.

Detailed Exam and Ongoing Exam

1. Correctly perform the Detailed Exam.
2. Describe when to perform critical interventions.
3. Demonstrate proper communications with Medical Direction.
4. Correctly perform the Ongoing (reassessment) Exam.

Assessment and Management of the Trauma Patient

1. Demonstrate the proper sequence of rapid assessment and the management of the multiple-trauma patient.

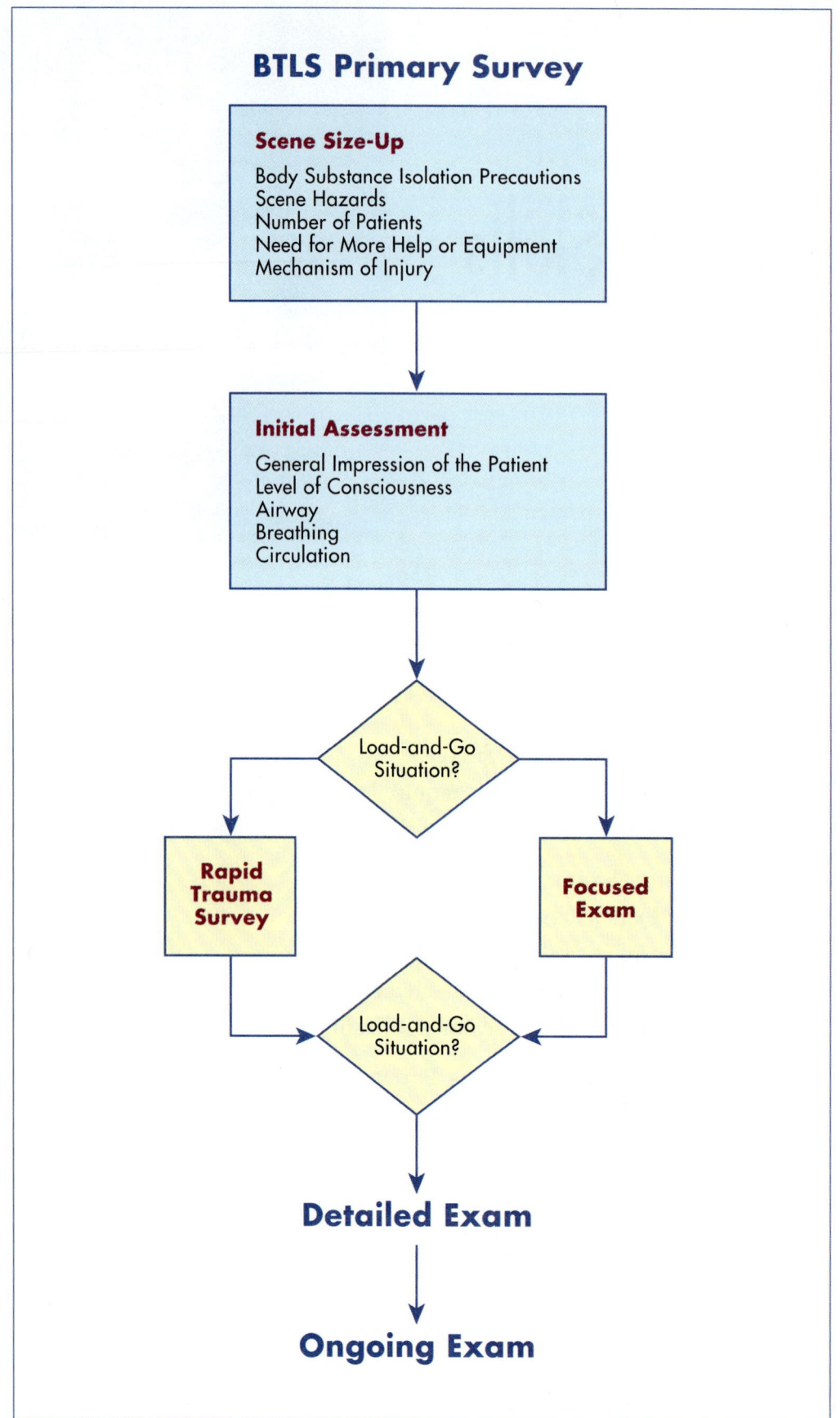

BTLS Primary Survey

Scene Size-Up

Body Substance Isolation Precautions
Scene Hazards
Number of Patients
Need for More Help or Equipment
Mechanism of Injury

Initial Assessment

General Impression of the Patient
Level of Consciousness
Airway
Breathing
Circulation

Load-and-Go Situation?

Rapid Trauma Survey

Focused Exam

Load-and-Go Situation?

Detailed Exam

Ongoing Exam

FIGURE 3-1   Steps in the assessment and management of the trauma patient.

BTLS PRIMARY SURVEY

OBJECTIVES

UPON COMPLETION OF THIS SKILL STATION, YOU SHOULD BE ABLE TO:

1. Correctly perform the BTLS Primary Survey (see Figure 3-1).
2. Identify within 2 minutes which patients require load-and-go.
3. Describe when to perform critical interventions.

PROCEDURE

Short written scenarios will be used along with a model (to act as the patient). You will divide into teams to practice performing the Initial Assessment, critical interventions, and transfer decisions. Each member of the team must practice being team leader at least once and preferably twice. The Critical Information represents the answers you should be seeking at each step of the survey. The Treatment Decision Tree at the end of the chapter represents the actions that should be taken (personally or delegated) in response to your assessment.

CRITICAL INFORMATION—BTLS PRIMARY SURVEY

If you ask the right questions, you will get the information you need to make the critical decisions necessary in the management of your patient. The following questions are presented in the order in which you should ask them to yourself as you perform patient assessment. This is the minimum information that you will need as you perform each step of the Initial Assessment.

SCENE SIZE-UP

Which BSI precautions do I need to take?

Do I see, hear, smell, or sense anything dangerous?

Are there any other patients?

Are additional personnel or resources needed?

Do we need special equipment?

What is the mechanism of injury here?
　　Is it generalized or focused?
　　Is it potentially life-threatening?

INITIAL ASSESSMENT

What is my general impression of the patient as I approach?

Level of Consciousness (AVPU)

Introduce yourself and say: "We are here to help you. Can you tell us what happened?"

Airway

Is the airway open and clear?

Breathing

Is the patient breathing?

What is the rate and quality of respiration?

Ventilation Instructions

Order oxygen for any patient with abnormal respiration, altered mental status, shock, or major injuries.

Delegate assisted ventilation if the patient is hypoventilating (<12 per minute) or if there is inadequate movement of air.

Hyperventilate only those head injury patients who are unresponsive and show signs of cerebral herniation.

Circulation

What is the rate and quality of the pulse at the wrist (and at the neck if not palpable at the wrist)?

Is major external bleeding present?

What is the skin color, condition, and temperature?

Decision

Is this a critical situation?

Are there interventions that I must make now?

RAPID TRAUMA SURVEY

Head and Neck

Are there obvious wounds of the head or neck?

Are the neck veins distended?

Does the trachea look and feel midline or deviated?

Is there deformity or tenderness of the neck?

Chest

Is the chest symmetrical? Is there paradoxical movement? Is there any obvious blunt or penetrating trauma?

Are there any open wounds or paradoxical movement?

Is there TIC of the ribs?

Are the breath sounds present and equal?

   If breath sounds are not equal, is the chest hyperresonant or dull?

Are heart sounds normal or decreased?

Abdomen

Are there obvious wounds?

Is the abdomen soft, rigid, or distended?

Is there tenderness?

Pelvis

Are there obvious wounds or deformity?

Is there TIC?

Upper Legs

Are there obvious wounds, swelling, or deformity?

Is there TIC?

Scan of Lower Legs and Arms

Are there obvious wounds, swelling, or deformity?

Is there TIC?

Can the patient feel/move fingers and toes?

Exam of the Posterior (done during transfer to the backboard)
Is there any deformity, contusions, abrasions, penetrations, burns, tenderness, lacerations, or swelling (DCAP-BTLS) of the patient's posterior side?

Decision
Is there a critical situation?
Are there interventions that I must make now?

History
What is the SAMPLE history? (may have been obtained during the exam)

Vital Signs
Are the vital signs abnormal?

Disability (Perform this exam now if there is altered mental status. Otherwise, postpone this exam until you perform the Detailed Exam.)
Are the pupils equal and reactive?
What is the Glasgow Coma Score?
Are there signs of cerebral herniation (unconscious, dilated pupil(s), hypertension, bradycardia, posturing)?
Does the patient have a medical identification device?

DETAILED EXAM AND ONGOING EXAM

OBJECTIVES

UPON COMPLETION OF THIS SKILL STATION, YOU SHOULD BE ABLE TO:

1. Correctly perform the Detailed Exam.
2. Describe when to perform critical interventions.
3. Demonstrate proper communications with Medical Direction.
4. Correctly perform the Ongoing (reassessment) Exam.

PROCEDURE

Short written scenarios will be used along with a model (to act as the patient). You will divide into teams to practice performing the Detailed Exam, making critical decisions and interventions, and performing the reassessment exam. Each member of the team must practice being team leader at least once and preferably twice. The Critical Information represents the answers you should be seeking at each step of the exam.

CRITICAL INFORMATION—DETAILED EXAM

If you ask the right questions, you will get the information you need to make the critical decisions necessary in the management of your patient. The following questions are presented in the order in which you should ask them to yourself as you perform the Detailed Exam. This is the minimum information that you will need as you perform each step of the exam.

SAMPLE History (complete if not already done)
What is the patient's history?

Vital Signs
What are the vital signs?

Neurological Exam
What is the LOC?
What is the blood glucose (if altered mental status)?
Are the pupils equal? Do they respond to light?
Can the patient move his fingers and toes?
Can the patient feel me touch his fingers and toes?
What is the Glasgow Coma Score (if altered mental status)?

Head
Is there DCAP-BTLS of the face or head?
Is Battle's sign or raccoon eyes present?
Is there blood or fluid draining from the ears or nose?
Is there pallor, cyanosis, or diaphoresis?

Airway
Is the airway open and clear?
If there are burns of the face, are there signs of burns in the mouth or nose?

Breathing
What is the rate and quality of respiration?

Neck
Is there DCAP-BTLS of the neck?
Are the neck veins normal, flat, or distended?
Is the trachea midline or deviated?

Circulation
What is the rate and quality of the pulse?
What is the skin color, condition, and temperature (capillary refill in children)?
Is all external bleeding still controlled?

Chest
Is there DCAP-BTLS of the chest?
Are there any open wounds or paradoxical movement?
Are the breath sounds present and equal?
    If breath sounds are not equal, is the chest hyperresonant or dull?
Are heart sounds normal or decreased?

Abdomen
Is there DCAP-BTLS of the abdomen?
Is the abdomen soft, rigid, or distended?

Pelvis (already examined in the initial assessment—no further exam should be done)

Lower Extremities
Is there DCAP-BTLS of the legs?
Is there normal PMS?
Is range of motion normal? (optional)

Upper Extremities
Is there DCAP-BTLS of the arms?
Is there normal PMS?
Is range of motion normal? (optional)

CRITICAL INFORMATION—ONGOING EXAM

The following questions are presented in the order in which you should ask them to yourself as you perform the Ongoing (reassessment) Exam. This is the minimum information that you will need as you perform each step of the exam.

Subjective Changes
Are you feeling better or worse now?

Mental Status
What is the LOC?
What is pupillary size? Are they equal? Do they react to light?
If altered mental status, what is the Glasgow Coma Score now?

Reassess ABCs
Airway
    Is the airway open and clear?
    If there are burns of the face, are there signs of inhalation injury?

Breathing and Circulation
    What is the rate and quality of respiration?
    What is the rate and quality of the pulse?
    What is the blood pressure?
    What is the skin color, condition, and temperature (capillary refill in children)?

Neck
Is the trachea midline or deviated?
Are the neck veins normal, flat, or distended?
Is there increased swelling of the neck?

Chest
Are the breath sounds present and equal?
    If breath sounds are unequal, is the chest hyperresonant or dull?

Abdomen (if mechanism suggests possible injury)
Is there any tenderness?
Is the abdomen soft, rigid, or distended?

Assessment of Identified Injuries
Have there been any changes in the condition of any of the injuries that I have found?

Check Interventions
Ask the appropriate question for your patient.
    Is the oxygen rate correct?
    Is the oxygen tubing connected?
    Is the open chest wound still sealed?
    Are any of the dressings blood soaked?
    Are the splints in good position?
    Is the impaled object still well stabilized?
    Is the pregnant patient tilted to the left?
    Is the pulse oximeter attached and working?

ASSESSMENT AND MANAGEMENT OF THE TRAUMA PATIENT

OBJECTIVE

UPON COMPLETION OF THIS SKILL STATION, YOU SHOULD BE ABLE TO:

1. Demonstrate the proper sequence of rapid assessment and the management of the multiple-trauma patient.

PROCEDURE

Short written trauma scenarios will be used along with a model (to act as the patient). You will be divided into teams to practice the management of simulated trauma situations using the principles and techniques taught in the course. You will be evaluated in the same manner on the second day of the course. You will be expected to use all the principles and techniques taught in this course while managing these simulated patients. To familiarize yourself with the evaluation procedure, you will be given a copy of a scenario and a grade sheet. Review Chapter 2 and the previous surveys in this chapter.

GROUND RULES FOR TEACHING AND EVALUATION

1. You will be allowed to stay together in three-member groups (different-sized groups are optional) throughout the practice and evaluation stations.
2. You will have three practice scenarios. This allows each member of the team to be team leader once.
3. You will be evaluated as team leader once.
4. You will assist as a member of the rescue team during two scenarios in which another member of your team is being evaluated as team leader. You may assist but all assessments must be done by the team leader. This gives you a total of six scenarios from which to learn: three practices, one evaluation, and two assists while others are evaluated.
5. Wait outside the door until the instructor comes out and gives you your scenario.
6. You will be allowed to look over your equipment before you start your exam.
7. Be sure to ask about scene safety if not provided in the scenario.
8. Be sure to apply your personal protective gear.
9. If you have a live model for a patient, you must talk to that person just as you would a real patient. It is best to explain what you are doing as you examine the patient. Be confident and reassuring.
10. You must ask your instructor for things you cannot find out from your patient. Examples: blood pressure, pulse, breath sounds.
11. Wounds and fractures must be dressed or splinted just as if they were real. Procedures must be done correctly (blood pressure, log-rolling, strapping, splinting, etc.).
12. If you need a piece of equipment that is not available, ask your instructors. They may allow you to simulate the equipment.
13. During practice and evaluation, you may be allowed to go (or may be directed) to any station, but you cannot go to the same station twice.

14. You will be graded on the following:
    a. Assessment of the scene
    b. Assessment of the patient
    c. Management of the patient
    d. Efficient use of time
    e. Leadership
    f. Judgment
    g. Problem-solving ability
    h. Patient interaction
15. When you finish your **testing** scenario, there is to be no discussion of the case. If you have any questions, they will be answered after the faculty meeting at the end of the course.

PATIENT ASSESSMENT PEARLS

1. Do not approach the patient until you have done a scene size-up.
2. Do not interrupt the Initial Assessment except for:
   a. Airway obstruction
   b. Cardiac arrest

   Other critical interventions may be performed by your team members while you complete the Initial Assessment.
3. Give ventilation instructions as soon as you assess the airway and breathing.
4. Prophylactic hyperventilation is no longer recommended for patients with decreased LOC. It is only used for the head injury patient who shows signs of the cerebral herniation syndrome.
5. Assist ventilations for anyone who is hypoventilating (<12 per minute).
6. Give oxygen to all multiple-trauma patients. If in doubt, give oxygen.
7. Transfer the patient to the backboard as soon as the BTLS Primary Survey is completed.
8. When the BTLS Primary Survey is completed, decide if the patient is critical or stable. Critical trauma situations are characterized by any of the following:
   a. Decreased level of consciousness
   b. Difficulty with airway or breathing
   c. Shock
   d. Tender abdomen
   e. Unstable pelvis
   f. Bilateral femur fractures
   g. Poor general impression
9. If the BTLS Primary Survey reveals that the patient has a critical trauma situation, load the patient in the ambulance and transport.
10. If absolutely necessary, certain interventions may have to be done before transport. Remember that you are trading minutes of the patient's golden hour for those procedures. Use good judgment.
11. Critical patients get a Detailed Exam en route to the hospital.
12. Stable patients may get a Detailed Exam at the scene (on the backboard).
13. Transport immediately if your Detailed Exam reveals any of the critical trauma situations.
14. Critical patients should not have traction splints applied at the scene (it takes too long).
15. Call Medical Direction early if you have a critical patient (other physicians may have to be called from home to treat the patient).

16. Repeat the Ongoing Exam:
    a. If the patient's condition changes.
    b. If you make an intervention.
    c. If you move the patient (scene to ambulance, ambulance to emergency room).

17. Unconscious patients with no gag reflex cannot protect their airways.

18. Transport pregnant patients with the backboard tilted slightly to the left. Do not let them roll over onto the floor.

19. Remain calm and think. Your knowledge, training, and concern are the most important tools you carry.

TRAUMA ASSESSMENT—TREATMENT DECISION TREE

INITIAL ASSESSMENT	ACTION
SCENE SIZE-UP	
Safety	Put on gloves, protective clothing. Remove hazards or patient from hazards.
Number of patients	Call for help if needed.
Extrication needed	Call for special equipment if needed.
Mechanisms of injury	Suspect appropriate injuries (e.g., C-spine).
GENERAL IMPRESSION	Begin to establish priorities.
Age, sex, weight	
Position (in surroundings, body position/posture)	
Activity	
Obvious major injuries; major bleeding	
LEVEL OF CONSCIOUSNESS	
Alert/responsive to voice	Maintain C-spine control.
Unresponsive to voice	Modified jaw thrust prn.
AIRWAY	
Snoring	Modified jaw thrust.
Gurgling	Suction.
Stridor	Check for airway obstruction.
Silence	Attempt to ventilate—if unsuccessful: Reposition; extricate immediately. Visualize. Suction. Consider Heimlich maneuver.
BREATHING	
Absent	Ventilate twice (check pulse before continuing ventilation at 12–20 + oxygen).
<12	Assist ventilation at 12–20 + oxygen.
Low tidal volume	Assist ventilation.
Labored	Oxygen by nonrebreather at 15 L/min.
Normal or rapid	Consider oxygen.
RADIAL PULSE	
Absent	Check carotid pulse (see below). Note late shock (consider PASG).
Present	Note rate and quality.
Bradycardia	Consider spinal shock, head injury.
Tachycardia	Attempt to calm to reduce rate; consider shock.

CAROTID PULSE (done if no radial pulse)

Absent	CPR + BVM + oxygen, load-and-go.
Present	Note rate and quality.
Bradycardia	Consider spinal shock, head injury.
Tachycardia	Consider shock.

SKIN

Color and condition

Pale, cool, clammy	Consider shock.
Cyanosis	Give 100% oxygen. Consider ventilation.

MAJOR BLEEDING .... Direct pressure, pressure dressing.

RAPID TRAUMA SURVEY	ACTION

HEAD

Major facial injuries .... Consider airway obstruction.

NECK

Swelling, bruising, retracting	Consider airway obstruction.
Neck vein distention	Consider tamponade, tension pneumothorax.
Tracheal deviation	Consider tension pneumothorax.
Deformity, tenderness	**APPLY C-COLLAR NOW.**

INSPECT/PALPATE CHEST

Symmetrical, stable	Continue exam.
Bruises, crepitus	Consider early cardiac monitoring.
Penetrating wounds	Occlusive dressing.
Paradoxical motion	Stabilize flail.

BREATH SOUNDS

Present and equal	Continue exam.
Unequal	Percuss chest to determine pneumothorax versus hemothorax.

HEART TONES

Present	Note for comparison later.
Muffled with JVD and bilateral breath sounds	Consider pericardial tamponade.

ABDOMEN, PELVIS, UPPER LEGS

If tender abdomen, unstable pelvis, or bilateral femur fractures	Expect development of shock.

MOVEMENT/SENSATION IN EXTREMITIES

Present	Record.
Decreased or absent	Suspect spinal injury.

BACK .... Appropriate management of identified injuries.
Transfer to backboard.
TRANSPORT IMMEDIATELY IF CRITICAL TRAUMA SITUATION IS PRESENT.

SAMPLE HISTORY .... Record.

VITAL SIGNS
Measure pulse, respirations.......................... Record.
Auscultate blood pressure
    Systolic < 80... Consider PASG per local protocol.
    Systolic < 60... Consider PASG inflation en route.

Neurological Exam to Be Done If Patient Has Altered Mental Status

PUPILS
Unequal... Suspect head injury unless patient is
                                              alert, then suspect eye injury. Give
                                              100% oxygen.

GLASGOW COMA SCORE (for decreased LOC)
≤8... Give 100% oxygen.
                                              Consider hyperventilation only if patient
                                              shows signs of cerebral herniation.

ALL PATIENTS WITH
   DECREASED LOC .... Check for medical indentification devices.
                                              Do blood glucose check.

CHAPTER 4

Initial Airway Management

Ronald D. Stewart, M.D., F.A.C.E.P.
John E. Campbell, M.D., F.A.C.E.P.

OBJECTIVES

UPON COMPLETION OF THIS CHAPTER, YOU SHOULD BE ABLE TO:

1. Describe the anatomy and physiology of the respiratory system.
2. Define the following terms:
   a. Hyperventilation
   b. Hypoventilation
   c. Tidal volume
   d. Minute volume
   e. Delivered volume
   f. Compliance
3. Explain the importance of observation as it relates to airway control.
4. Describe methods to deliver supplemental oxygen to the trauma patient.
5. Briefly describe the indications and contraindications and the advantages and disadvantages of the following airway adjuncts:
   a. Nasopharyngeal airways
   b. Oropharyngeal airways
   c. Bag-valve masks
   d. Flow-restricted oxygen-powered ventilation devices
6. Describe the Sellick maneuver.
7. Describe the essential contents of an airway kit.
8. Describe the pitfalls associated with airway management.

Of all the tasks expected of field teams caring for the trauma patient, none is more important than that of airway control. Maintaining an open airway and adequate ventilation in the trauma patient can be a challenge in any setting, but it can be almost impossible in the adverse environment of the field, with its poor lighting, the chaos that often surrounds an accident, the position of the patient, and perhaps hostile onlookers.

Airway control is a task that you must master, since it frequently cannot wait until you get to the hospital. Patients who are cyanotic, or underventilated, or both, are in need of immediate help—help that only you can give them in the initial stages of their care. It falls to you, then, to be fully versed in the basic structure and function of the airway, in how to achieve and maintain an open airway, and in how to oxygenate and ventilate a patient.

Because of the unpredictable nature of the field environment, you will be called on to manage patients' airways in almost every conceivable situation; in wrecked cars, dangling above rivers, in the middle of a shopping center, at the side of a busy highway. You therefore need *options* and alternatives from which to choose. What will help one patient may not work for another. One patient may require a simple jaw thrust to open an airway, while another may require a surgical procedure to prevent impending death.

Whatever the methods required, you must always start with the basics. It is of little value—and in some cases downright dangerous—to apply "advanced" techniques of airway control before beginning basic maneuvers. The discussion of airway control in the trauma patient will be rooted in several fundamental truths: air should go in and out, oxygen is good, and blue is bad. Everything else follows from this.

ANATOMY

The airway begins at the tip of the nose and the lips and ends at the *alveolocapillary membrane,* through which gas exchange takes place between the air sacs of the lung (the *alveoli*) and the lung's capillary network. The airway consists of chambers and pipes that conduct air and its 21% oxygen content to the alveoli during inspiration and carry away the waste *carbon dioxide* that diffuses from the blood into the alveoli.

The beginning of the respiratory tract, the *nasal cavity* and *oropharynx,* perform important functions (see Figure 4-1). Lined with moist *mucous membranes,* these areas serve to warm and filter inhaled gases. They are highly vascular and contain protective lymphoid tissue. Bypassing this portion of the respiratory tract through the use of an endotracheal tube will reduce the natural protection of the vulnerable lung, and you will have to provide some of these protective tasks. That is why suctioning of the airway, as well as the warming and humidification of gases, becomes of such importance in intubated patients.

The lining of the respiratory tract is delicate and highly vascular. It deserves all the respect that you can give it, and that means preventing undue trauma, using liberally lubricated tubes, and avoiding unnecessary poking about. The *nasal cavity* is divided by a very vascular midline *septum,* and on the lateral walls of the nose are "shelves" called the *turbinates.* These projections, which increase the surface area of the mucosa, can get in the way of tubes or other devices that may be necessary to insert into the nostrils. Carefully sliding a well-lubricated tube's bevel along the floor or the septum of the nasal cavity will usually prevent traumatizing the turbinates.

The teeth are the first obstruction we meet in the oral part of the airway. They may be more obstructive in some patients than in others. In any case, the same general principle always applies: **Patients should have the same number and condition of teeth at the end of an airway procedure as they had at the beginning.**

The tongue is a large chunk of muscle and represents the next potential obstruction. These muscles are attached to the jaw anteriorly and through a series of muscles and ligaments to the *hyoid bone,* a wishbone-like structure just under the chin from which the cartilage skeleton (the *larynx*) of the upper airway is suspended. The *epiglottis* is also connected to the hyoid, and elevating the hyoid will lift the epiglottis upward and open the airway further.

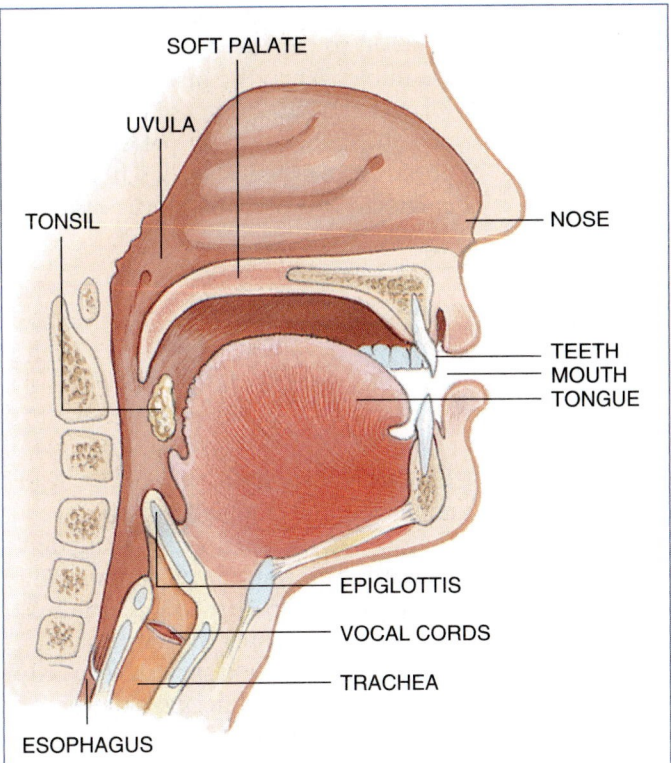

FIGURE 4-1   Anatomy of the upper airway. Note that the tongue, hyoid bone, and epiglottis are attached to the mandible by a series of ligaments. Lifting forward on the jaw will therefore displace all these structures.

The epiglottis is one of the main anatomic landmarks in the airway. You must be familiar with it and be able to identify it by sight and by touch. It looks like a floppy piece of cartilage covered by mucosa—which is exactly what it is—and it feels like the tragus, the cartilage at the opening of the ear canal. Its function is unclear; it may be a "leftover" (i.e., vestigial) piece of anatomy, but it is nonetheless important to you when you must assume control of the airway. The epiglottis is attached to the hyoid and thence to the mandible by a series of ligaments and muscles. In the unconscious patient, the tongue can produce some airway obstruction by falling back against the soft palate and even the posterior pharyngeal wall. However, it is the epiglottis that will produce complete airway obstruction in the supine unconscious patient whose jaw is relaxed and whose head and neck are in the neutral position. In such patients the epiglottis will fall down against the glottic opening and prevent ventilation.

It is essential to understand this crucial fact in the management of the airway. To ensure an open (patent) airway in an unconscious supine patient, you can displace the hyoid anteriorly by lifting forward on the jaw (chin lift, jaw thrust) or by pulling on the tongue. This will lift the tongue out of the way and keep the epiglottis elevated and away from the posterior pharyngeal wall and glottic opening (see Figure 4-2a and b).

The *vocal cords* are protected by the *thyroid cartilage,* a boxlike structure shaped like a "C," with the open part of the "C" representing its posterior wall, which is covered with muscle. When the cords vibrate, sound is produced. In some patients, the cords can close entirely in *laryngospasm,* producing complete airway obstruction. The thyroid cartilage can easily be seen in most people on the anterior surface of the neck as the laryngeal prominence.

Inferior to the thyroid cartilage is another part of the larynx, the *cricoid,* a cartilage shaped like a signet ring with the ring in front and the signet behind. It can be palpated as a small bump on the anterior surface of the neck inferior to the laryngeal prominence. Just behind the posterior wall of the cricoid cartilage lies the esophagus. Pressure on the

FIGURE 4-2A The epiglottis is attached to the hyoid and then to the mandible. When the mandible is relaxed and falls back, the tongue falls upward against the soft palate and the posterior pharyngeal wall, while the epiglottis falls over the glottic opening.

FIGURE 4-2B Extension of the head and lifting the chin will pull the tongue and the epiglottis upward and forward, exposing the glottic opening and ensuring a patent airway. In the trauma patient, only the jaw, or chin and jaw, should be displaced forward, while the head and neck should be kept in alignment.

cricoid at the front of the neck will close off the esophagus to pressures as high as 100 cm H_2O. Use this maneuver (*the Sellick maneuver*) can be used to reduce the risk of gastric regurgitation and to prevent insufflation of air into the stomach during positive pressure ventilation by mouth-to-mouth, bag-valve mask, or flow-restricted oxygen-powered ventilator (see Figures 4-3 and 4-4). If there is any danger of C-spine injury, you must carefully support and stabilize the neck while performing the Sellick maneuver.

The *tracheal rings,* C-shaped cartilaginous supports for the trachea, continue beyond the cricoid cartilage, and the trachea soon divides into the *left* and *right mainstem bronchi.* The open part of the C-shaped rings lies posterior against the esophagus. An impacted swallowed foreign body that remains in the esophagus, or a misplaced esophageal airway or endotracheal tube cuff, can create tracheal obstruction by pressing against the soft posterior tracheal wall and narrowing the lumen. The point at which the trachea divides is called the *carina.* It is important to note that the right mainstem bronchus takes off at an angle that is slightly more in line with the trachea (see Figure 4-5). As a result, tubes or other foreign bodies that are poked or that trickle down the airway usually end up in the right mainstem bronchus.

To help protect the airway from becoming blocked and to reduce the risk of aspiration, the body has developed brisk reflexes that will attempt to expel any offending foreign material from the oropharynx, the glottic opening, or the trachea. These areas are well supplied by sensitive nerves that can activate the swallowing, gag, and cough reflex. Activation of swallowing, gagging, or coughing by stimulation of the upper airway can cause significant cardiovascular stimulation as well as elevation in intracranial pressure.

The *lungs* are the organs through which this gas exchange takes place. They are contained within a "cage" formed by the ribs, and usually fill up the *pleural space*—the *potential space* between the internal chest wall and the lung surface. The lungs have only one opening to the outside, the *glottic opening,* the space between the vocal cords.

FIGURE 4-3   The Sellick maneuver.

Expansion of the chest wall (the cage) and movement of the diaphragm downward cause the lungs to expand (since the pleural space is airtight), and air rushes in through the *glottis*. The air travels down the smaller and smaller tubes to the *alveoli*, where gas exchange (respiration) takes place.

THE PATENT AIRWAY

One of the first maneuvers essential to caring for a patient is ensuring a *patent or open airway*. Without this, all other care is of little use. This must be done quickly, for patients cannot tolerate hypoxia for more than a few minutes. The effect of hypoxia on

FIGURE 4-4A   External view of the anterior neck, showing the surface landmarks for the thyroid cartilage (laryngeal) prominence, the cricothyroid membrane, and the cricoid cartilage.

FIGURE 4-4B   Cut-away view showing the important landmarks of the larynx and upper airway: hyoid, thyroid cartilage, cricothyroid membrane, and cricoid cartilage.

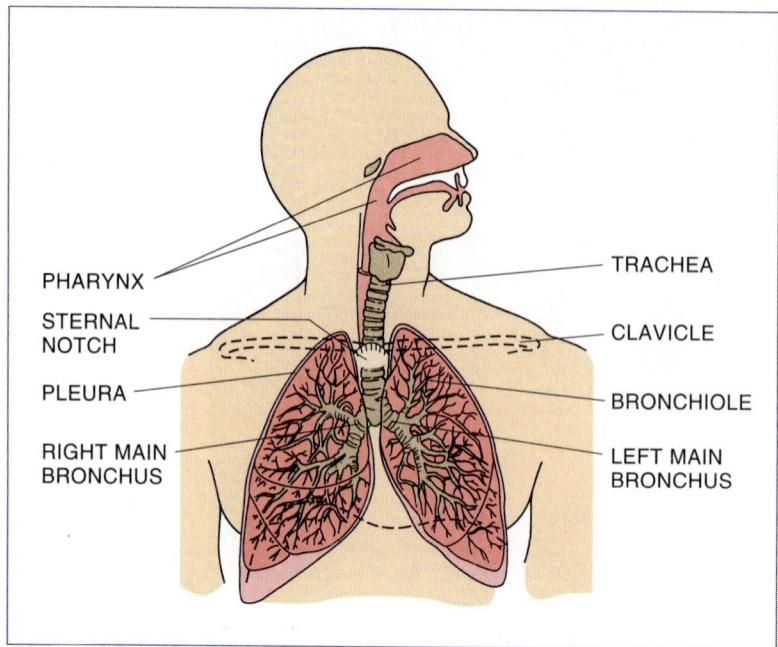

PHARYNX

STERNAL
NOTCH

PLEURA

RIGHT MAIN
BRONCHUS

TRACHEA

CLAVICLE

BRONCHIOLE

LEFT MAIN
BRONCHUS

FIGURE 4-5   The sternal notch, at which point the clavicles join
the sternum, marks the position of the tip of a well-placed endotracheal tube. Note that the right mainstem bronchus curves off at the
carina at an angle slightly more in line with the trachea.

an unconscious injured patient can be devastating, and if hypoxia is compounded by the
absence of adequate perfusion, the patient is in even more difficult straits. Patients suffering from head trauma not only may have hypoxic brain damage from airway compromise but may also build up high levels of carbon dioxide that can increase blood flow to
the injured brain, causing swelling and increased intracranial pressure.

Ensuring an open airway in a patient can be a major challenge in the prehospital
setting. Not only can trauma disrupt the anatomy of the face and airway, but resultant
bleeding can lead to airflow obstruction and can obscure airway landmarks. Add to this
the risk of C-spine injury, and the challenge is readily apparent. You must also remember that some airway maneuvers, including suction and insertion of nasopharyngeal and
oropharyngeal airways, may stimulate a patient's protective reflexes and increase the
likelihood of vomiting and aspiration, cardiovascular stimulation, and increased
intracranial pressure. The first step in providing a patent airway in the unconscious
patient is to ensure that the tongue and epiglottis are lifted forward and maintained in
that position. This is done by either the modified jaw thrust (see Figure 4-6a) or the jaw
lift (see Figure 4-6b). Either of these maneuvers will prevent the tongue from falling
backward against the soft palate or posterior pharyngeal wall and will pull forward on
the hyoid, lifting the epiglottis up out of the way. These are essential maneuvers for
both basic and advanced airway procedures. Done properly, they will open the airway
without tilting the head backward or moving the neck.

Recommending the maneuvers just mentioned assumes that the patient is supine
and that there is an ability on the part of either the patient or the rescuer to clear the airway of blood or secretions. If the patient is unable to control the airway and suction is
not available, place the patient carefully in the *recovery position* or in the left semiprone
position. This can be done with a rigid C-collar in place and with several rescuers to
keep the vertebral column in alignment and to prevent undue movement (Figure 4-7).
In this position secretions can drain, the tongue and epiglottis are displaced forward,
and the airway should remain patent. The risk of C-spine damage is less than the disaster that would occur should the patient vomit while supine. It is important to keep the
head, neck, and vertebral column in alignment, but do not exert traction on head and
neck. Properly trained and equipped rescuers should seldom have to use this position

SINCE NECK MAY BE INJURED, DO NOT EXTEND THE NECK TO OPEN THE AIRWAY.

USE MODIFIED JAW THRUST

FIGURE 4-6A   Opening the airway using modified jaw thrust. Maintain in-line stabilization while pushing up on the angle of the jaw with your thumbs.

FIGURE 4-6B   Jaw lift.

STRAP

because an airway kit with suction is part of the essential equipment to be carried to the scene of any potential trauma patient (see Chapter 1).

In the rare instance where a patient has a foriegn body obstruction of the airway and you are unable to remove it by suction or finger sweeps, you may be forced to do abdominal thrusts or the Heimlich maneuver. In this instance, the concern for C-spine immobilization must come second to the fact that the patient will die within minutes if the airway is not cleared.

Constant vigilance and care are required to maintain a patent airway in your patient. There are several essentials for this task:

1. Continual observation of the patient in order to anticipate problems
2. An adequate suction device with large-bore tubing and attachment
3. Airway adjuncts

OBSERVATION

The patient who is injured is at risk of airway compromise even if completely conscious and awake. This is partially due to the fact that many patients have full stomachs, are anxious, and are prone to vomiting. Some patients will also be bleeding into their oropharynx and thus swallowing blood.

FIGURE 4-7   The *recovery* position. When the patient is suspected of having sustained trauma, and when suction and immobilization devices are not yet available, use this position to prevent aspiration. You should have sufficient personnel available to move the patient carefully, with vertebral column kept in alignment.

In view of these facts, you should constantly observe your patient for airway problems following injury. One team member must be responsible for both airway control and adequate ventilation for any patient who might be at risk of airway compromise.

The general appearance of the patient, the respiratory rate, and any complaints must be noted and addressed. In a patient who is breathing spontaneously, you must check frequently for adequate tidal volume by feeling over the mouth and nose and by observing chest wall movements. Check the supplemental oxygen line periodically to ensure that oxygen is being delivered to the patient at a given flow rate or percentage. Clear blood and secretions. You must be alert for sounds that indicate trouble. Be alert for this danger sign: *noisy breathing is obstructed breathing*. Consider combative patients to be hypoxic until a systematic and rapid evaluation rules this out. Use of pulse oximetry is strongly recommended (see Chapter 5).

SUCTION

All patients who are injured and who have cervical immobilization in place should be considered at high risk for airway compromise. One of the greatest threats to the patent airway is that of vomiting and aspiration, particularly in patients who have recently eaten a large meal washed down with large quantities of alcohol. As a result, portable suction devices should be considered basic equipment for field trauma care and should have the following characteristics (see Figure 4-8):

1. They should be carried in a kit with an oxygen cylinder and other airway equipment; they should not be separated or stored remote from oxygen; otherwise, they represent an "extra" piece of equipment requiring extra hands.
2. They should be hand-powered or battery-powered rather than oxygen-driven. Hand-powered is preferred. You should always have a hand-powered suction as a backup if you use a battery-powered suction.
3. They should generate sufficient pressure and volume displacement to suction pieces of food, blood clots, and thick secretions from the oropharynx.

FIGURE 4-8 Examples of suction apparatus.

4. They should have tubing of sufficient diameter (0.8–1 cm) to handle whatever is suctioned from the patient.

Suction tips of more recent design are of large bore, particularly the new rigid "tonsil-tip" suckers that can handle most clots and bleeding. In some cases the suction tubing itself can be used to withdraw large amounts of blood or gastric contents. Usually Rescuer #2 (see Chapter 2) assumes responsibility for the airway. As the "V.O." (vomit officer), he must be constantly alert to prevent the patient from aspirating.

AIRWAY ADJUNCTS

Equipment to help ensure a patent airway will include various nasopharyngeal, oropharyngeal, and blind insertion airway devices (BIAD). Insertion of these devices must be reserved for patients whose protective reflexes are sufficiently depressed to tolerate them. Care must be taken not to provoke vomiting or gagging, since both occurrences are bad for these patients.

Nasopharyngeal airways should be soft and of appropriate length. They are designed to prevent the tongue and epiglottis from falling against the posterior pharyngeal wall (see Chapter 5 for insertion technique). With gentle insertion there should be few problems with this airway (see Figure 4-9). However, bleeding and trauma to the nasal mucosa are not infrequent. Mild hemorrhage from the nose after insertion of the airway is not an indication to remove it. In fact, it is probably better to keep the nasopharyngeal airway in place so as not to disturb the clot or reactivate the bleeding. The nasopharyngeal airway will be better tolerated than the oropharyngeal one and thus can usually be used in patients who still have a gag reflex.

Oropharyngeal airways are designed to keep the tongue off the posterior pharyngeal wall and thereby help maintain a patent airway (see Figure 4-10; see Chapter 5 for insertion techniques). Special oropharyngeal airways are available. Some are designed as intubator guides while others have proximal ends that protrude from the lips and are designed to be used with balloon masks that seal the mouth and nose.

Esophageal obturator airways, pharyngotracheal airways, esophageal tracheal combitube (Combitube®), and the *laryngeal mask airway* are all blind insertion airway devices.

The esophageal gastric tube airway (EGTA) is designed to be inserted into the esophagus at a level beyond the carina. A cuff is then inflated to reduce the likelihood of gastric distension or regurgitation during bag-valve mask or demand-valve mask

FIGURE 4-9   The nasopharyngeal airway is inserted with the bevel slid along the septum or floor of the nasal cavity.

ventilation. The tube has an opening that allows for the placement of a nasogastric tube for decompression of the stomach (see Appendix A, Optional Skills).

The pharyngotracheal airway is a combination of the EGTA and an endotracheal tube and represents an attempt to solve the problem of possible intratracheal placement of the EGTA and also seeks to provide for tracheal ventilation should blind insertion result in intratracheal positioning. This is an airway device that incorporates two tubes and a balloon that can be inflated to fill the oropharynx (see Appendix A, Optional Skills).

The esophageal tracheal combitube (Combitube®) is a double-lumen tube like the pharyngotracheal airway. It has both a distal balloon to seal the esophagus to help prevent regurgitation and a proximal balloon to seal the pharynx to help prevent air from escaping from the mouth and nose. The pharyngeal balloon can also help prevent blood and other foreign material from being aspirated (see Appendix A, Optional Skills).

SUPPLEMENTAL OXYGEN

Patients who are injured need supplemental oxygen, especially if they are unconscious. It is well recognized that patients suffering from head injury are frequently hypoxic. Supplemental oxygen can be supplied by simple face mask run at 10 to 12 L/min. This will provide the patient with about 40 to 50% oxygen. Nonrebreathing masks with a reservoir bag with oxygen flow rates into the bag of 12 to 15 L/min can provide 60 to 90% oxygen to the patient. These are recommended for all trauma patients requiring supplemental oxygen. Nasal cannulae are well tolerated by most patients, but provide only about 25 to 30% oxygen to the patient. They are recommended for only those patients who refuse to accept an oxygen mask.

Supplemental oxygen must be used to ensure adequate oxygenation when you perform positive pressure ventilation. Oxygenation must be supplemented during mouth-to-mask ventilation by running oxygen at 10 to 12 L/min through the oxygen nipple attached to most masks or by placing the oxygen tubing under the mask and running it at the same rate. Alternatively, you can increase the oxygen percentage delivered during mouth-to-mask breathing by placing a nasal cannula on yourself. This increases the delivered oxygen percentage from 17% to about 30%.

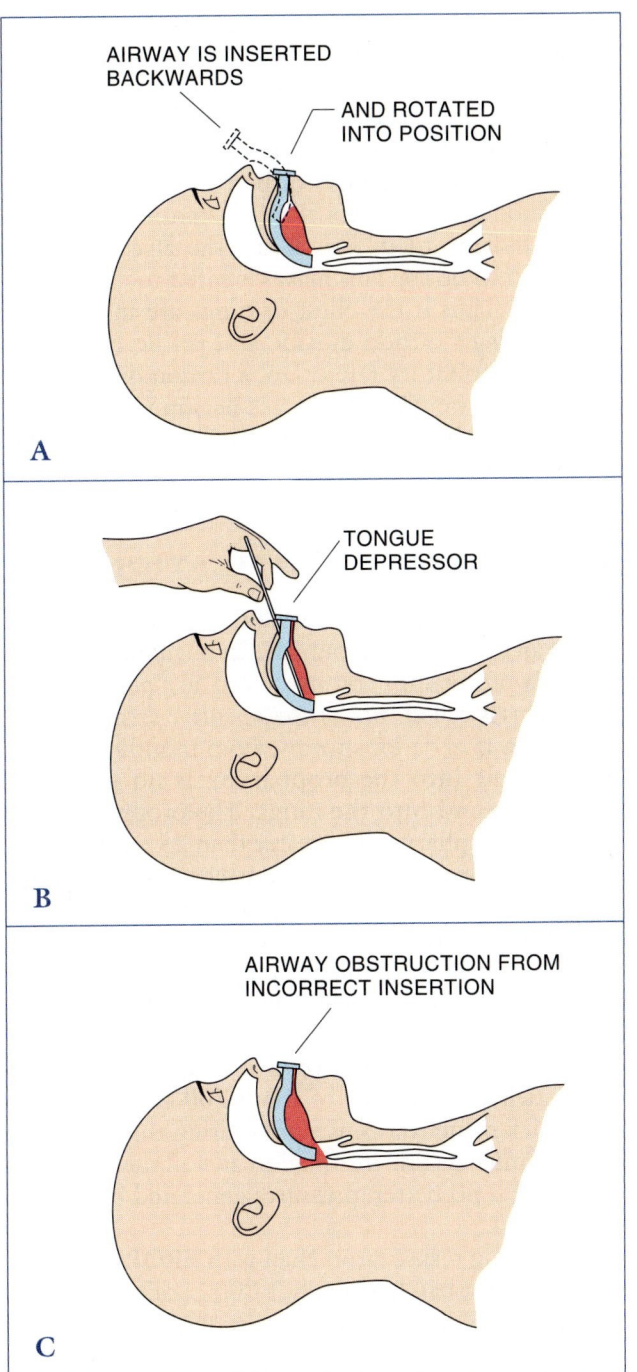

FIGURE 4-10 Insertion of oropharyngeal airway.

Bag-valve mask devices or resuscitator bags with a large (2.5 L) reservoir bag and an oxygen flow rate of 12 to 15 L/min will increase the delivered oxygen from 21% (air) to 90 or 100%. BVMs without the reservoir bag can only deliver 40 to 50% oxygen and thus should not be used.

Flow-restricted oxygen-powered ventilation devices (FROPVD) will provide 100% oxygen at a flow rate of 40 L/min at a maximum pressure of 50 ± 5 cm water.

NORMAL VENTILATION

The movement of air or gases in and out of the lungs is called *ventilation*. At rest, adults normally take in about 400 to 600 cc with each breath. This is called the *tidal volume*.

Multiplying that value by the number of breaths per minute (the respiratory rate) gives the *minute volume,* the amount of air breathed in and out each minute. This is an important value and is normally 5 to 12 L/min. Normal ventilation with normal lungs will produce an oxygen level of about 100 mmHg and a carbon dioxide level of 35 to 40 mmHg. The terms *hypoventilation* and *hyperventilation* do not refer to oxygenation but rather refer to the level of carbon dioxide maintained. A carbon dioxide level below 35 mmHg is called hyperventilation, and values greater than 40 mmHg are called hypoventilation. It is easier for carbon dioxide to diffuse across the alveolocapillary membrane of the lungs than it is for oxygen to do so. This makes it easier to excrete carbon dioxide than to oxygenate the blood. Thus if the chest or lungs are injured, the body may be able to maintain normal levels of carbon dioxide and yet be hypoxic. A patient with a contused lung might have a respiratory rate of 36, a carbon dioxide level of 30 mmHg, and an oxygen level of only 80 mmHg. While this person is *hyperventilating,* he is still *hypoxic.* He does not need to breathe faster; he needs to have supplemental oxygen. When in doubt, give your patient oxygen.

POSITIVE PRESSURE (ARTIFICIAL) VENTILATION

Normal breathing takes place because the negative pressure inside the (potential) pleural space "draws" air in through the upper airway from the outside. In any patient who is unable to do this, or whose airway needs protecting, you may need to "pump" air or oxygen in through the glottic opening. This is called *intermittent positive pressure ventilation* (IPPV). IPPV in trauma patients can take various forms, from mouth-to-mouth to bag-valve-endotracheal tube. **Pumping air into the oropharynx is no guarantee that it will go through the glottic opening and into the lungs.** The oropharynx also leads to the esophagus, and pressure in the oropharynx of greater than 25 cm H_2O will open the esophagus and lead to air being pumped into the stomach (gastric insufflation). Bag-valve masks and FROPVD can produce pressures greater than this. This is why the Sellick maneuver (posterior pressure on the cricoid cartilage) is so very important as a basic airway procedure. When you need to ventilate a patient using IPPV, you should know approximately how much volume you are delivering with each breath you give (*delivered volume*). You can estimate the minute volume by multiplying this volume by the ventilatory rate. A flow-restricted oxygen-powered ventilator that delivers oxygen at the rate of 40 L/min will have a delivered volume of about 700 cc each second that the valve is activated. Unless the Sellick maneuver is used, delivering this volume at a pressure of 50 cm H_2O will almost guarantee gastric insufflation and all the complications resulting from it. Bag-mask breathing is no better; pressures generated by squeezing the bag may equal or exceed 60 cm H_2O.

Delivered volumes are usually less with bag resuscitators than with FROPVD. There are two reasons for this. The average resuscitator bag holds only 1,800 cc of gas, and that is the absolute limit to the volume that could be delivered if you were able to squeeze the bag completely. Using one hand, the best an average adult can squeeze is approximately 1,200 cc. Most people will squeeze only 800 to 1,000 cc with one hand. The other reason for greater delivered volumes with flow-restricted oxygen-powered ventilators is that a FROPVD has a trigger that allows the rescuer to hold a mask on the face with both hands, thus decreasing mask leak. Keep in mind that these volumes, delivered from the ventilating port of these devices, equal the volumes delivered to the patient only if an endotracheal tube is in place. In other words, they do not take into account mask leak. When performing IPPV with a mask, keep the following essentials in mind:

1. Supplemental oxygen must be provided for the patient during IPPV.
2. Suction must be **immediately** available.
3. Ventilation must be done carefully to avoid gastric distension and to reduce the risk of regurgitation and possible aspiration. You can help prevent these complications by using the Sellick maneuver.
4. Careful attention must be paid in estimating the minute volume being delivered to the trauma patient. A minute volume of at least 12 to 15 L should be provided. If an

adult's hand squeezes approximately 800 cc from a bag, "bagging" the patient every 3 or 4 seconds (15 to 20 times per minute) would provide a minute volume of from 12 to 16 L. This should be enough to provide for the patient's increased ventilatory needs. However, in the case of bag-mask breathing, up to 40% mask leak can be expected. Balloon mask designs can reduce this, and a two-person technique, in which one rescuer holds the mask in place with both hands while a second squeezes the bag, may better ensure adequate delivered volumes. During the stress of an emergency situation you will tend to ventilate patients at an increased rate, but delivered volumes are often deficient. Normal rates should be 18 to 24 times per minute. Pay attention to delivered volumes as well, since rate alone cannot compensate for grossly inadequate ventilatory volumes.

COMPLIANCE

When air, or air containing oxygen, is delivered by positive pressure into the lungs of a patient, the "give" or elasticity of the lungs and chest wall will influence how easily it will be for the patient to breathe. If you are performing mask ventilation, a normal elasticity of the lungs and chest wall will allow air to enter the glottic opening and little gastric distension should result. However, if the elasticity is poor, ventilation will be harder to achieve. The ability of the lungs and chest wall to expand and therefore ventilate a patient is known as *compliance*. It is simpler to speak of "good compliance" or "bad compliance" rather than "high" or "low" compliance, since the latter terms can be somewhat confusing.

Compliance is an important concept, since it governs whether you can adequately ventilate a patient. Compliance can become bad (i.e., low) in some disease states of the lung or in patients who have an injury to the chest wall. In cardiac arrest, compliance will also become bad, due to poor circulation to the muscles.

VENTILATION TECHNIQUES

MOUTH-TO-MOUTH

This is a most reliable and effective method of ventilation, with the advantage of requiring no equipment and a minimum of experience and training. In addition, delivered volumes are consistently adequate since mouth seal is effectively and easily maintained. In addition, compliance can be "felt" more accurately, and high oropharyngeal pressures are therefore less likely. This method is almost never used because of the danger of disease transmission. Even though you should rarely have to use mouth-to-mouth ventilation, it is an option.

MOUTH-TO-MASK

Most of the disadvantages of mouth-to-mouth ventilation can be overcome by interposing a face mask between your mouth and that of the patient. Commercially designed pocket masks are particularly suited for the initial ventilation of many types of patients, and some have a side port for supplemental oxygen. Pocket ventilating masks have consistently been shown to deliver larger volumes than bag-mask devices and do so with a greater percentage of oxygen than mouth-to-mouth ventilation. Mouth-to-mask ventilation has significant advantages over other methods, and should be more widely used (see Chapter 5).

FLOW-RESTRICTED OXYGEN-POWERED VENTILATING DEVICE

In the past, the high-pressure, oxygen-powered ventilators (demand valves) were considered too dangerous to use in multiple-trauma patients. Experience with the newer flow-restricted oxygen-powered ventilators (FROPVD) that meet American Heart Association guidelines (oxygen flow rate of 40 L/min at a maximum pressure of 50 ± 5

FIGURE 4-11 The flow-restricted oxygen-powered ventilation device. This valve delivers a set flow of 40 L/min at maximum pressure of 50 ± 5 cm H_2O. Do not use unless it meets these standards and your Medical Director approves.

cm H_2O) suggests that these may now be the equal of bag-valve devices for ventilation (Figure 4-11). They have the advantage of delivering 100% oxygen and allowing use of two hands while using face mask ventilation. FROPVDs are no worse than BVMs at producing gastric distention. However, because it is more difficult to feel lung compliance when ventilating with the FROPVD, there is still some controversy about its use. Follow your Medical Director's advice on the use of a FROPVD.

BAG-VALVE MASK

This descendant of the anesthetic bag is a fixed-volume ventilator with an average delivered volume of about 800 cc. With a two-handed squeeze, over 1 L can be delivered to the patient. They should be used with a reservoir bag or tubing. Plain BVMs without reservoir bag or tubing can only deliver 40 to 50% oxygen and thus should be replaced with reservoir bags.

The most important problem associated with the bag-valve mask devices is the volumes delivered. Mask leak is a serious problem, decreasing the volume delivered to the oropharynx by sometimes 40% or more. In addition, old masks of conventional design have significant dead space beneath them, thus increasing the challenge to provide an adequate volume to the patient. The newer balloon mask has a design that eliminates dead space beneath the mask and provides an improved seal over the nose and mouth. It has been shown in mannequin studies to decrease mask leak and to improve ventilation. It is recommended particularly for trauma patients (see Figure 4-12).

A better seal can sometimes be obtained, and larger volumes delivered, in either the balloon or conventional mask, with the use of an extension tubing attached to the ventilating port of the bag-valve device. This permits the mask to be better seated on the face without a levering effect from the rigid ventilating port connector that tends to unseat the mask. With the extension in place, the bag can be more easily compressed, even against the knee or thigh, thus increasing the delivered volume and overcoming any mask leak (see Figure 4-13).

AIRWAY EQUIPMENT

The most important rule to follow in regard to airway equipment is that it should be in good working order and immediately available. It will do the patient no good if you have to run to get the suction apparatus. In other words, be prepared. This is not difficult. Five basic pieces of equipment are necessary for the initial response to all prehospital trauma calls:

1. Personal protection equipment (see Chapter 1)
2. Long backboard with attached head immobilization device
3. Appropriately sized cervical spinal immobilization collar
4. Airway kit (see below)
5. Trauma box (see Chapter 1)

FIGURE 4-12 The inflated or balloon mask has been shown to reduce mask leak and provide greater volumes during ventilation with bag-mask devices.

The *airway kit* should be completely self-contained and should contain everything needed to secure an airway in any patient. Equipment now available is lightweight and portable. Oxygen cylinders are aluminum, and newer suction devices are less bulky and lighter. It is no longer acceptable to have suction units that are bulky and stored separate from a source of oxygen. Suction units should be contained in a kit with oxygen and other essential airway tools. A lightweight airway kit should consist of the following (see Figure 4-14):

FIGURE 4-13 A ventilating port extension attached to a ventilating bag permits a better mask seal and therefore greater delivered volumes. When the bag is compressed against the thigh, as shown here, delivered volumes may be increased further.

FIGURE 4-14 An airway kit containing the essentials for airway management. Note that portable suction is included in this design. The total weight (with aluminum "D" oxygen cylinder) is approximately 10 kg (22 lb), about the same as a steel "E" oxygen cylinder.

1. Oxygen D cylinder, preferably aluminum
2. Portable battery-powered and hand-powered suction units
3. Oxygen cannulae and masks
4. Bag-valve mask ventilating device (with reservoir bag)
5. Pocket mask with supplemental oxygen intake

The contents of the airway kit are critical; you should check all equipment each shift, and the kit should have a card attached to be initialed by the person checking it.

PITFALLS

All of the following can result in preventable deaths from airway problems:

1. Failure to recognize the need for an airway.

2. Failure to recognize that the patient needs assistance with ventilation.

3. Failure to recognize an airway that is placed incorrectly.

4. Failure to recognize displacement of an airway that was established previously.

5. Aspiration of gastric contents. Suction must be immediately available. Be prepared for equipment failure by having backup equipment available.

SUMMARY

Trauma patients provide the greatest challenge in airway management. To be successful you must have a clear understanding of the anatomy of the airway and be proficient in techniques to open and maintain your patient's airway. You must have the correct equipment organized in a kit that is immediately available when you begin assessment of the trauma patient. To provide adequate ventilation for your patient, you must understand the concepts of tidal volume, minute volume, and lung compliance. Finally, you must become familiar with the various options for control of the airway and develop expertise in performing them.

BIBLIOGRAPHY

1. American Heart Association Committee on Emergency Cardiac Care. "Guidelines for Cardiopulmonary Resuscitation and Emergency Cardiac Care." *Journal of the American Medical Association*, Vol. 268 (1992), p. 2200.

2. Biebuyck, J. F. "Management of the Difficult Adult Airway." *Anesthesiology*, Vol. 75 (1991), pp. 1087–1110.

3. Boidin, M. P. "Airway Patency in the Unconscious Patient." *British Journal of Anaesthesiology,* Vol. 57 (1985), pp. 306–310.

4. Jesudian, M. C. S., R. R. Harrison, R. L. Keenan, and others. "Bag-Valve-Mask Ventilation: Two Rescuers Are Better than One: Preliminary Report." *Critical Care Medicine,* Vol. 14 (1985), pp. 403–406.

5. Martin S. E., G. Ochsner, and others. "Laryngeal Mask Airway in Air Transport When Intubation Fails: Case Report." *The Journal of Trauma: Injury, Infection, and Critical Care,* Vol. 42, No. 2 (1997), pp. 333–336.

6. Mosesso V. N., K. Kukitsch, and others. "Comparison of Delivered Volumes and Airway Pressures when Ventilating Through an Endotracheal Tube with Bag-Valve Versus Demand-Valve." *Prehospital and Disaster Medicine,* Vol. 9, No. 1 (1994), pp. 24–28.

7. Ravussin P., and J. Freeman. "A New Transtracheal Catheter for Ventilation and Resuscitation." *Canadian Anaesthesiology Society Journal,* Vol. 32 (1985), pp. 60–64.

8. Salem M. R., A. Y. Wong, M. Mani, and others. "Efficacy of Cricoid Pressure in Preventing Gastric Inflation During Bag-Mask Ventilation in Pediatric Patients." *Anesthesiology,* Vol. 40 (1974), pp. 96–98.

9. Stewart R. D., R. M. Kaplan, B. Pennock, and others. "Influence of Mask Design on Bag-Mask Ventilation." *Annals of Emergency Medicine,* Vol. 14 (1985), pp. 403–406.

10. White, S. J., R. M. Kaplan, and R. D. Stewart. "Manual Detection of Decreased Lung Compliance as a Sign of Tension Pneumothorax" (abstr). *Annals of Emergency Medicine,* Vol. 16 (1987), p. 518.

11. Youngberg, J. A., G. Graybar, and D. Hutchings. "Comparison of Intravenous and Topical Lidocaine in Attenuating the Cardiovascular Responses to Endotracheal Intubation." *Southern Medical Journal,* Vol. 76 (1983), pp. 1122–1124.

CHAPTER 5

Airway Management Skills

Donna Hastings, EMT-P

OBJECTIVES

UPON COMPLETION OF THIS CHAPTER, YOU SHOULD BE ABLE TO:

1. Suction the airway.
2. Insert a nasopharyngeal and oropharyngeal airway.
3. Use the pocket mask.
4. Use the bag-valve mask.
5. Use the pulse oximeter.
6. Describe the preparations necessary to perform endotracheal intubation.
7. Assist with orotracheal laryngoscopic intubation.
8. Assist with nasotracheal intubation.
9. Confirm correct tube placement.
10. Anchor the endotracheal tube.

BASIC AIRWAY MANAGEMENT

PROCEDURES

SUCTIONING THE AIRWAY

Use of the hand-powered suction device also should be taught at this time.

1. Attach the suction connecting tubing to the portable suction machine.
2. Turn the device on and test it.
3. Insert the suction tip through the nose (soft or whistle tip) or mouth (soft or rigid) without activating the suction.
4. Activate the suction and withdraw the suction tube.
5. Repeat the procedure as necessary.

   Note: Although the intent is to suction foreign matter, air and oxygen are also being suctioned out of the patient. Never suction for greater than 15 seconds. After suctioning, reoxygenate the patient as soon as possible.

INSERTING NASOPHARYNGEAL AIRWAYS

1. Choose the appropriate size. It should be as large as possible but still fit easily through the patient's external nares. The size of the patient's little finger can be used as a rough guide.
2. Lubricate the tube with a water-based lubricant.
3. Insert it straight back through the right nostril with the beveled edge of the airway toward the septum.
4. Gently pass into the posterior pharynx with a slight rotating motion until the flange rests against the nares.
5. To insert in the left nostril, turn the airway upside down so that the bevel is toward the septum; then insert straight back through the nostril until you reach the posterior pharynx. At this point, turn the airway over 180 degrees and insert it down the pharynx.

   Note: If the tongue is occluding the airway, a jaw thrust or chin lift must be done to allow the nasopharyngeal airway to go *under* the tongue

INSERTING OROPHARYNGEAL AIRWAYS

1. Choose the appropriate size. The distance from the corner of the mouth to the lower part of the external ear is a good estimate.
2. Open the airway:
   a. Scissor maneuver
   b. Jaw lift
   c. Tongue blade
3. Insert the airway gently without pushing the tongue back into the pharynx.
   a. Insert the airway under direct vision using a tongue blade. This is the preferred method and is safe for adults or children.
   b. Insert the airway upside down or sideways and rotate into place. This method should not be used for children.
4. If the oropharyngeal airway causes gagging, remove and replace with a nasopharyngeal airway.

USING A POCKET MASK WITH SUPPLEMENTAL OXYGEN

1. Stabilize the patient's head in a neutral position.
2. Connect the oxygen tubing to the oxygen cylinder and the mask.
3. Open the oxygen cylinder and set the flow rate at 12 L/min.

4. Open the airway.

5. Insert the oral or nasal airway.

6. Place the mask on the face and establish a good seal.

7. Ventilate mouth-to-mask with enough volume (about 800–1,000 cc oxygen) to cause adequate chest rise. The inspiratory phase should last 1.5 to 2.0 seconds. Let the patient exhale for 1.5 to 4.0 seconds.

USING THE BAG-VALVE MASK

1. Stabilize the patient's head in a neutral position.

2. Connect the oxygen connecting tubing to the bag-valve system and oxygen cylinder.

3. Attach the oxygen reservoir to the bag-valve mask.

4. Open the oxygen cylinder and set the flow rate at 12 L/min.

5. Select the proper size mask and attach it to the bag-valve device.

6. Open the airway.

7. Insert the oral airway (insert the nasal airway if the patient has a gag reflex).

8. Place the mask on the face and have your partner establish and maintain a good seal.

9. Using both hands, ventilate with about 800 to 1,000 cc oxygen.

10. If you are forced to ventilate without a partner, use one hand to maintain a face seal and the other hand to squeeze the bag. This decreases the volume of ventilation because less volume is produced by only one hand squeezing the bag.

USING THE PULSE OXIMETER

A pulse oximeter is a noninvasive photoelectric device that measures the arterial oxygen saturation and pulse rate in the peripheral circulation. It consists of a portable monitor and a sensing probe that clips onto the patient's finger, toe, or earlobe (see Figure 5-1). The device displays the pulse rate and the arterial oxygen saturation in a percentage value ($\%SaO_2$). This is a very useful device that should be used on all patients with any type of respiratory compromise. The pulse oximeter is useful to assess the patient's respiratory status, the effectiveness of oxygen therapy, and the effectiveness of BVM or FROPVD ventilation.

FIGURE 5-1   Portable pulse oximeter. *(Courtesy of David Effron, M.D., FACEP)*

Remember that the device measures %SaO_2, not the arterial partial pressure of oxygen (PaO_2). The hemoglobin molecule is so efficient at carrying oxygen that it is 90% saturated (90%SaO_2) when the partial pressure of oxygen is only 60 mmHg (100 is normal). If you are used to thinking about PaO_2 (where 90–100 mmHg is normal), then you may be fooled into thinking that a SaO_2 reading (pulse oximeter) of 90% is normal when it is actually critically low. As a general rule, any pulse oximeter reading below 92% is cause for concern and requires some sort of intervention (open airway, suction, oxygen, assisted ventilation, intubation, decompression of tension pneumothorax, etc.). A pulse oximeter reading below 90% is critical and requires *immediate* intervention to maintain adequate tissue oxygenation. Try to maintain a pulse oximeter reading of 95% or higher. However, do not withhold oxygen from a patient with a pulse oximeter reading above 95% who also shows signs and symptoms of hypoxia or difficulty breathing.

The following are conditions that make the pulse oximeter reading unreliable:

1. Poor peripheral perfusion (shock, vasoconstriction, hypotension). Do not attach the sensing probe onto an injured extremity. Try not to use the sensing probe on the same arm that you are using to monitor the blood pressure. Be aware that the pulse oximeter reading will go down while the blood pressure cuff is inflated.
2. Severe anemia.
3. Carbon monoxide poisoning. This will give falsely high readings because the sensing probe cannot distinguish between oxyhemoglobin and carboxyhemoglobin.
4. Hypothermia.
5. Excessive patient movement.
6. High ambient light (bright sunlight, high-intensity light on area of the sensing probe).
7. Nail polish or a dirty fingernail if you are using a finger probe. Use acetone to clean the nail before attaching the probe.

To use the pulse oximeter, turn on the device, clean the area that you are to monitor (earlobe, fingernail, or toenail), and attach the sensing clip to the area.

Remember that while very useful, the pulse oximeter is just another tool to help you assess the patient. Like all tools, it has limitations and should not replace careful physical assessment.

ASSISTING WITH ADVANCED AIRWAY MANAGEMENT

PREPARATIONS

Whatever the method of intubation used, both patients and rescuers should be prepared for the procedure. The following equipment is considered basic to all intubation procedures (see Figure 5-2):

1. *Gloves:* Rubber examining (not necessarily sterile) gloves should be worn for all intubation procedures.
2. *Eye Protection:* Goggles or face shield.
3. *Oxygenation:* All patients should be ventilated or should breathe high-flow oxygen (12 L/min) for several minutes prior to the attempt.
4. *Equipment:* Check all equipment, and keep at hand in an organized kit. For laryngoscopic intubation, the endotracheal tube should be held in a "field hockey stick" or open "J" shape by a malleable stylet that is first lubricated and inserted until the distal end is just *proximal* to the side hole of the endotracheal tube. Check the cuff of the endotracheal tube by inflating it with 10 cc of air. *Completely* remove the air and leave the syringe filled with air attached to the pilot tube. Lubricate the cuff and distal end of the tube.

FIGURE 5-2 An "intubation wrap" contains the essentials for carrying out endotracheal intubation. The kit folds on itself and is compact and portable. When opened, it provides a clean working surface.

5. *Suction:* Suction must be immediately at hand.

6. *Assistant:* You should assist with the procedure. Apply the Sellick maneuver during ventilation and the subsequent intubation attempt. You may also help hold the head and neck immobile and count aloud to 30.

INTUBATION TECHNIQUES

LARYNGOSCOPIC OROTRACHEAL INTUBATION: In this method, the upper airway and the glottic opening are visualized, and the tube is slipped gently through the cords. The advantages of this method include the ability to see obstructions and to visualize the accurate placement of the tube. It has the disadvantage of requiring a relatively relaxed patient without anatomic distortion and with minimal bleeding or secretions.

EQUIPMENT

1. A straight (Miller) or curved (Macintosh) blade and laryngoscope handle.
2. A transparent endotracheal tube, 28 to 33 cm in length and 7.0, 7.5, or 8.0 mm in internal diameter for the adult patient.
3. A stylet to help mold the tube into a field hockey stick shape.
4. A water-soluble lubricant—there is no need for it to contain a local anesthetic.
5. A 10 or 12 cc syringe.
6. Magill forceps.
7. Tape and tincture of benzoin or endotracheal tube holder.
8. Suction equipment in good working order.

PROCEDURE

1. Following ventilation and initial preparations, you should hold the head, perform the Sellick maneuver, and count slowly *aloud* to 30 as the ALS provider performs the intubation.
2. When the tube is inserted, you or the ALS provider should check the tube for placement by the confirmation protocol below.

NASOTRACHEAL INTUBATION: The nasotracheal route of endotracheal intubation in a prehospital setting may be justified when you cannot open the adult patient's mouth because of clenched jaws and when you cannot ventilate the patient by other means. The greatest disadvantage of this method is its relative difficulty, depending as it does upon the appreciation of the intensity of the breath sounds of spontaneously breathing patients. It is a blind procedure and as such requires extra effort to demonstrate proper intratracheal placement.

The success of this method will also depend upon an anterior curve to the tube that will prevent its passing into the esophagus. Prepare two tubes prior to carrying out the intubation attempt. Insert the distal end of the 7-mm tube into its proximal opening, thus molding it into a formed circle. Preparing two tubes permits the immediate use of the second, more rigid tube should the first plastic tube become warm with body temperature, thus losing its anterior curve. You may assit by lifting the tongue and jaw forward, since this maneuver lifts the epiglottis anteriorly out of the way of the advancing tube.

PROCEDURE

1. Perform routine preparation procedures.
2. Hold the head, perform the Sellick maneuver, and count slowly *aloud* to 30 as the ALS provider performs the intubation.
3. Confirm tube placement using the confirmation protocol below.

CONFIRMATION OF TUBE PLACEMENT: One of the greatest challenges of intubation is ensuring the correct intratracheal placement of endotracheal tubes. An unrecognized esophageal intubation is a lethal complication of this lifesaving procedure. Even in the context of prehospital care, it is inexcusable. Every effort must be made to avoid this catastrophe, and a strict protocol must be followed to reduce the risk.

A simple yet effective protocol for tube confirmation is possible and practical. Such a protocol should recognize the unreliable nature of auscultation as the sole method of confirming intratracheal placement. Correct intratracheal placement should be suspected from the following initial signs:

1. An anterior displacement of the laryngeal prominence as the tube is passed distally.
2. Coughing, bucking, or straining on the part of the patient. *Note:* Phonation—any noise made with the vocal cords—is absolute evidence that the tube is in the esophagus, and the tube should be removed immediately.
3. Breath condensation on the tube with each ventilation—not 100% reliable, but very suggestive of intratracheal placement.
4. Normal compliance with bag ventilation—the bag does not suddenly "collapse," but rather there is some resilience to it and resistance to lung inflation.
5. No cuff leak after inflation—persistent leak indicates esophageal intubation until proven otherwise.
6. Adequate chest rise with each ventilation.

The following procedure should then be carried out *immediately* to prove correct placement:

1. Auscultate three sites as shown in Figure 5-3:
   a. The epigastrium—the most important; it should be silent, with no sounds heard.
   b. Right and left midaxillary lines.
2. Inspect for full movement of the chest with ventilation.

Watch for any change in the patient's color or in the pulse oximeter reading. Also observe the EKG monitor for changes.

Commercial suction bulbs are available for confirming tube placement. They are more reliable than CO_2 detectors. Squeeze the bulb and insert the end into the 15-mm

FIGURE 5-3   Sites to auscultate when *initially* checking placement of the endotracheal tube.

adapter on the endotracheal tube. Release the bulb. If the tube is in the trachea the bulb will expand immediately. If the tube is in the esophagus, the bulb will remain collapsed.

Commercial CO_2 detectors are also available to attach in-line between the ET tube and the BVM or FROPVD. These indicate by a color change that there is CO_2 in the expired air and thus indicate that the tube is in the trachea rather than the esophagus. They help monitor that the tube is maintained in place, especially in the case of helicopter transport where there is too much noise to monitor breath sounds.

Apply the protocol for confirmation of tube placement immediately following intubation and again after several minutes of ventilation. Thereafter, repeat the protocol after movement of the patient from the floor to the stretcher, after loading onto the ambulance, each time you perform the reassessment survey, and immediately prior to arrival at the hospital.

When you perform the Detailed Exam, or when there is a question of correct tube placement after the above confirmation protocol, you should:

1. Auscultate six sites as shown in Figure 5-4:
    a. The epigastrium; it should be silent with no sounds heard.
    b. Right and left apex.
    c. Right and left midaxillary lines.
    d. The sternal notch—"tracheal" sounds should be readily heard here.
2. Inspect the chest for full movement of the chest with ventilation.
3. Gently palpate the tube cuff in the sternal notch while compressing the pilot balloon between the index finger and thumb; a pressure wave should be felt in the sternal notch.
4. Use adjuncts such as a suction bulb or CO_2 detectors to help confirm.

Any time placement is still in doubt in spite of the above protocol, the ALS provider must visualize directly or remove the tube. Never assume that the tube is in the right place—always be sure and record that the protocol has been carefully followed.

ANCHORING THE TUBE: This can be a frustrating exercise. Not only does it require some fine movements of the hands when we appear to be all thumbs, but it is difficult to perform this task when ventilation, movement, or extrication is being carried out. There is one thing to keep in mind: **There is no substitute for the human anchor.** That is, one person should be held responsible for ensuring that the tube is held fast and that it does not migrate in or out of the airway. To lose a tube can be a catastrophe, especially if the patient is rather inaccessible or the intubation was a difficult one to begin with.

Fixing the endotracheal tube in place is important for several reasons. First, movement of the tube in the trachea will produce more mucosal damage and may increase the risk of postintubation complications. In addition, movement of the tube will stimu-

FIGURE 5-4 Sites to auscultate when performing the Detailed Exam or if there is doubt about the placement of the endotracheal tube.

late the patient to cough, strain, or both, leading to cardiovascular and intracranial pressure changes that could be detrimental. Most important, there is a greater risk in the prehospital setting of dislodging a tube and losing control of the airway if it is not anchored solidly in place.

The endotracheal tube can be secured in place by either tape or a commercially available holder. While taping a tube in place is convenient and relatively easily done, it is not always effective. There is often a problem with the tape sticking to skin wet with rain, blood, airway secretions, or vomitus. If you are using tape, several principles should be followed:

1. Insert an oropharyngeal airway to prevent the patient from biting down on the tube.
2. Dry the patient's face and apply tincture of benzoin to better ensure proper adhesion of the tape.
3. Carry the tape right around the patient's neck when anchoring the tube. Do not move the neck. Do not tie it so tight that it occludes the external jugular veins.
4. Anchor the tube at the corner of the mouth, not in the midline.

Because of the difficulty of fixing the tube in place with tape, it may be better to use a commercial endotracheal tube holder that uses a strap to fix the tube in a plastic holder that also acts as a bite block (see Figure 5-5). Since flexion or extension of the patient's head can move the tube in or out of the airway by 2 or 3 cm, it is a good practice to restrict head and neck movement of any patient who has an endotracheal tube in place. If the patient is immobilized because of the risk of C-spine injury, flexion and extension should not be a concern.

FIGURE 5-5 A commercial endotracheal tube holder.

CHAPTER 6

Thoracic Trauma

Andrew B. Peitzman, M.D., F.A.C.S.
Paul Paris, M.D., F.A.C.E.P.

OBJECTIVES

UPON COMPLETION OF THIS CHAPTER, YOU SHOULD BE ABLE TO:

1. Identify the major symptoms of thoracic trauma.
2. Describe the signs of thoracic trauma.
3. State the immediate life-threatening thoracic injuries.
4. Explain the pathophysiology and management of an open pneumothorax.
5. Describe the clinical signs of a tension pneumothorax in conjunction with appropriate management.
6. Explain the pathophysiology and management in massive hemothorax.
7. Define flail chest in relation to associated physical findings and management.
8. Identify the triad of physical findings in the diagnosis of cardiac tamponade.
9. Explain the cardiac involvement and management associated with blunt injury to the chest.
10. Summarize other injuries and their appropriate management.

INTRODUCTION

Twenty-five percent of trauma deaths are due entirely to thoracic injuries, and half of trauma patients with multiple injuries have an associated chest injury. Two-thirds of these patients with fatal thoracic trauma are alive when they reach the emergency department and only 15% require surgery. Thus, these are salvageable trauma patients. The goal of this chapter is to enable you to recognize signs and symptoms of major thoracic injury and provide appropriate care. Major thoracic injury may result from MVCs, falls, gunshot wounds, crush injuries, stab wounds, or other mechanisms.

ANATOMY

The thorax is a bony cavity that is formed by 12 pairs of ribs that join posteriorly with the thoracic spine and anteriorly with the sternum. The intercostal neurovascular bundle runs along the inferior surface of each rib (see Figure 6-1).

The inner side of the thoracic cavity and the lung itself are lined with a thin layer of tissue, the pleura. The space between the two pleural layers is normally only a potential space. However, this space may be occupied by air, forming a pneumothorax, or blood, forming a hemothorax. This potential space can hold 3 liters of fluid on each side in an adult.

As shown in Figure 6-2, one lung occupies each thoracic cavity. Between the two chest cavities is the mediastinum, which contains the heart, aorta, superior and inferior vena cava, trachea, major bronchi, and esophagus. The spinal cord is protected by the vertebral column. The diaphragm separates the thoracic organs from the abdominal cavity. The upper abdominal organs, including the spleen, liver, kidneys, pancreas, and stomach, are protected by the lower rib cage (see Figure 6-3). Any patient with a penetrating thoracic wound at the level of the nipples (fourth intercostal space) or lower should be assumed to have an abdominal injury as well as a thoracic injury. Similarly, blunt deceleration injuries such as steering wheel injuries often injure both thoracic and abdominal structures.

Penetrating wounds that traverse the mediastinum have a particularly high potential for life-threatening injury because of the vital cardiovascular and tracheobronchial structures within this area.

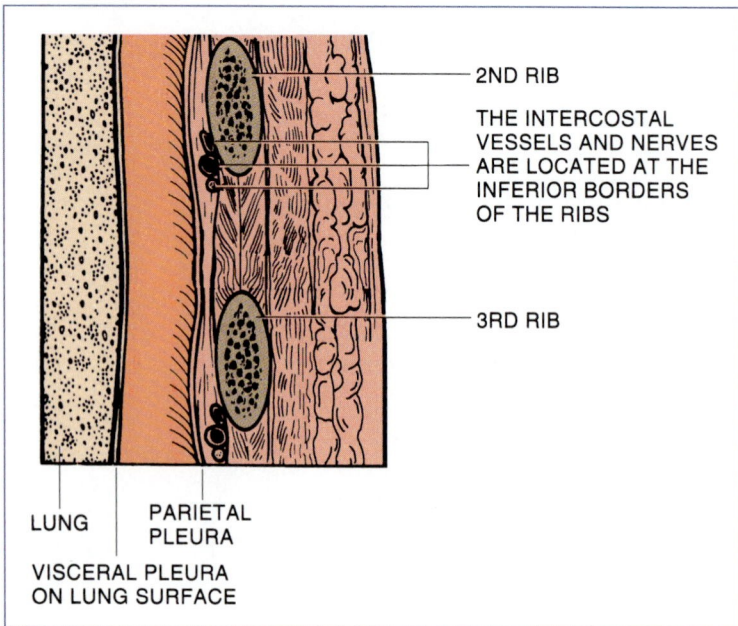

FIGURE 6-1   Rib with intercostal vessels and nerve.

FIGURE 6-2 Thorax.

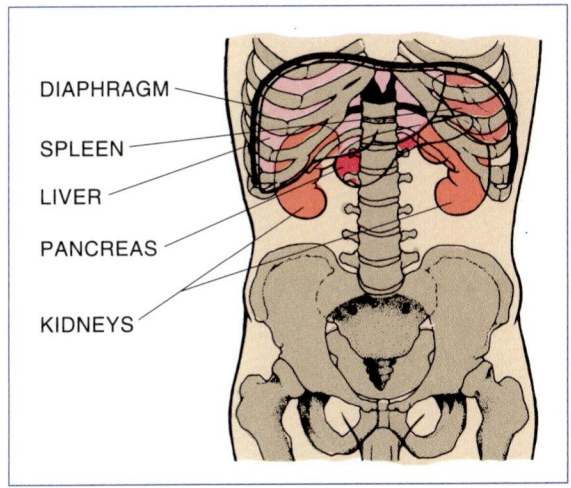

FIGURE 6-3 Intrathoracic abdomen.

PATHOPHYSIOLOGY

When evaluating a patient with probable thoracic trauma, always follow the BTLS assessment priorities (Chapter 2) to avoid missing life-threatening injuries. During the BTLS primary survey, search for the most dangerous injuries first to give your patient the best chance for survival. As with any trauma patient, the mechanism of injury is very important in caring for the thoracic trauma patient. Thoracic injuries may be the result of blunt or penetrating trauma. With blunt trauma, the force is distributed over a large area, and visceral injuries occur from deceleration, sheering forces, compression, or bursting. Penetrating injuries, usually gunshot wounds or stab wounds, distribute the forces of injury over a smaller area. However, the trajectory of a bullet is often unpredictable, and all thoracic structures are at risk.

The common end point in thoracic injury is tissue hypoxia. Tissue hypoxia may result from the following:

1. Inadequate oxygen delivery to the tissues secondary to airway obstruction
2. Hypovolemia from blood loss
3. Ventilation/perfusion mismatch from lung parenchymal injury
4. Changes in pleural pressures from tension pneumothorax
5. Pump failure from severe myocardial injury

ASSESSMENT

The major symptoms of chest injury include shortness of breath, chest pain, and respiratory distress. The signs indicative of chest injury include shock, hemoptysis, cyanosis, chest wall contusion, flail chest, open wounds, distended neck veins, tracheal deviation, or subcutaneous emphysema. Check the lung fields for the presence and equality of breath sounds. Life-threatening thoracic injuries should be identified immediately. Major thoracic injuries to identify may be remembered as the "deadly dozen."

The following injuries must be detected and treated during the BTLS Primary Survey:

1. Airway obstruction
2. Open pneumothorax
3. Tension pneumothorax
4. Massive hemothorax
5. Flail chest
6. Cardiac tamponade

Life-threatening injuries that are more likely to be detected during the Detailed Exam or during hospital evaluation are the following:

7. Traumatic aortic rupture
8. Tracheal or bronchial tree injury
9. Myocardial contusion
10. Diaphragmatic tears
11. Esophageal injury
12. Pulmonary contusion

AIRWAY OBSTRUCTION

Airway management remains a major challenge in the care of any multiple-trauma patient. This has been discussed in Chapter 4. Always assume that there is an associated C-spine injury when securing the airway.

OPEN PNEUMOTHORAX

This is caused by a penetrating thoracic injury and may present as a sucking chest wound. The signs and symptoms are usually proportional to the size of the chest wall defect (see Figure 6-4).

Normal ventilation involves a negative pressure being generated inside the chest by diaphragmatic contraction. As air is drawn through the upper airway, the lungs expand. With a large open wound of the chest, the path of least resistance for airflow is through

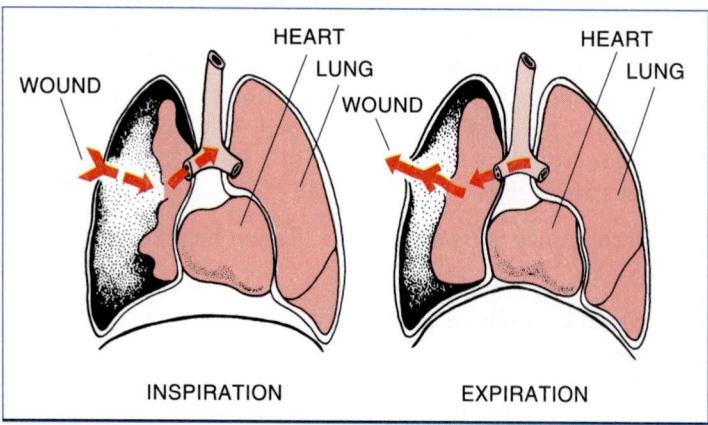

FIGURE 6-4 Open pneumothorax.

the chest wall defect. This air will only enter the pleural space. It will not enter the lung and therefore will not contribute to oxygenation of the blood. Ventilation is impaired and hypoxia results.

MANAGEMENT OF OPEN PNEUMOTHORAX

1. Ensure an airway.
2. Promptly close the chest wall defect by any available means. You may accomplish this with a defibrillation pad, Vaseline gauze, a rubber glove, or plastic dressing. Placing an occlusive dressing carries the risk of a tension pneumothorax. To circumvent this problem, tape the occlusive dressing on three sides to produce a flutter valve: air can escape from the chest but will not enter (see Figure 6-5). A commercial chest seal (Asherman chest seal) with a one-way valve is now available. A chest tube will be needed ultimately, followed by operative closure of the chest wall defect.
3. Administer oxygen.
4. Monitor the heart if you have monitoring equipment.
5. Transport rapidly to the appropriate hospital.

FIGURE 6-5   Treatment of sucking chest wound.

Tension Pneumothorax

This injury occurs when a one-way valve is created from either blunt or penetrating trauma. Air can enter but not leave the pleural space (see Figure 6-6). This causes collapse of the affected lung and will then push the mediastinum in the opposite direction with resultant kinking of the superior and inferior vena cava, and loss of venous return to the heart. A shift of the trachea and mediastinum away from the side of the tension pneumothorax will also compromise ventilation of the other lung, although this is a late phenomenon.

Clinical signs of a tension pneumothorax include dyspnea, anxiety, tachypnea, diminished breath sounds and hyperresonance to percussion on the affected side, hypotension, and distended neck veins. Tracheal deviation is a late finding and its absence does not rule out the presence of a tension pneumothorax. In a review of 108 field patients diagnosed with tension pneumothorax and requiring needle decompression, none were recorded as having a deviated trachea.

Management of Tension Pneumothorax

1. Establish an open airway.
2. Administer high-concentration oxygen.
3. Rapidly transport to the appropriate hospital.
4. Notify Medical Direction.

Massive Hemothorax

Blood in the pleural space is a hemothorax (see Figure 6-7). A *massive hemothorax* occurs as a result of at least 1,500-cc blood loss into the thoracic cavity. Each thoracic cavity may contain up to 3,000 cc of blood. Massive hemothorax is more often due to penetrating than blunt trauma, but either injury may disrupt a major pulmonary or systemic vessel. As blood accumulates within the pleural space, the lung on the affected side is compressed. If enough blood accumulates (rare), the mediastinum will be shifted away from the hemothorax. The inferior and superior vena cava and the contralateral lung are compressed. Thus the ongoing blood loss is complicated by hypoxemia.

Signs and symptoms of massive hemothorax are produced by both hypovolemia and respiratory compromise. The patient may be hypotensive from blood loss and compression of the heart or great veins. Anxiety and confusion are produced by hypov-

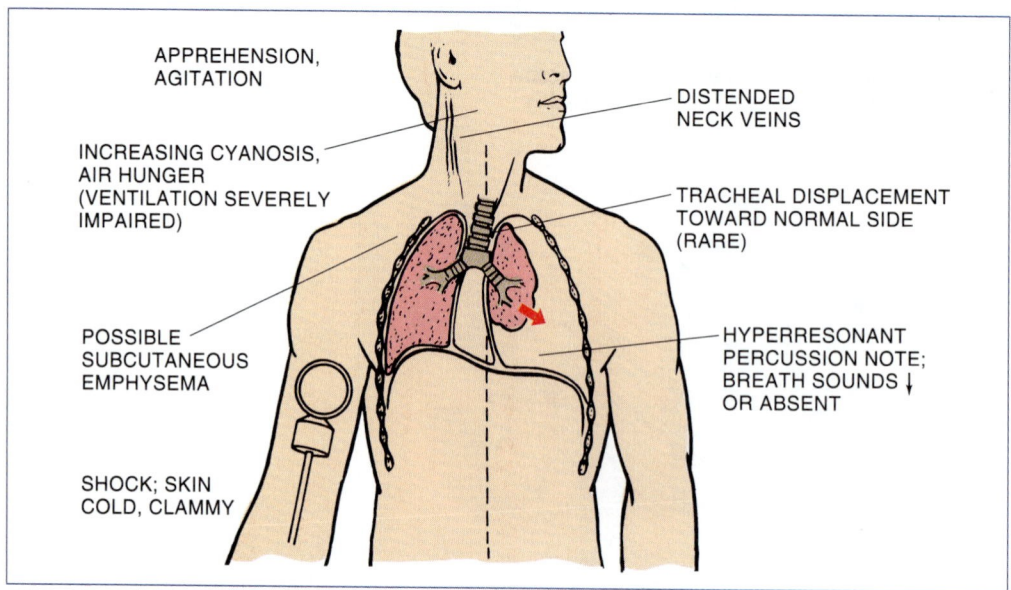

Figure 6-6 Physical findings of tension pneumothorax.

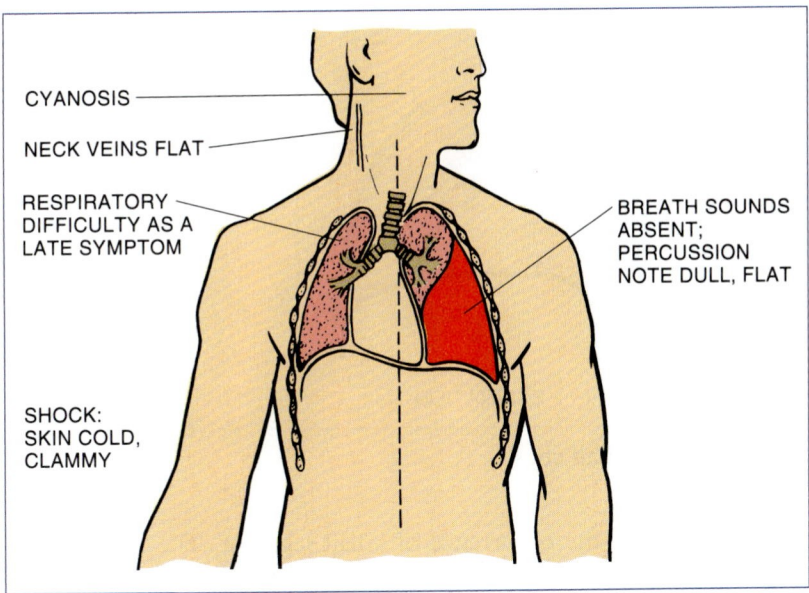

FIGURE 6-7 Physical findings of massive hemothorax.

olemia and hypoxemia. Clinical signs of hypovolemic shock may be apparent. The neck veins are usually flat secondary to profound hypovolemia, but may *rarely* be distended due to mediastinal compression. Other signs of hemothorax include decreased breath sounds and dullness to percussion on the affected side. See Table 6-1 for comparison of tension pneumothorax and massive hemothorax.

MANAGEMENT OF MASSIVE HEMOTHORAX

1. Secure an airway.
2. Apply high-flow oxygen.
3. Rapidly transport to the appropriate hospital.
4. Notify Medical Direction.

Table 6-1   Comparison of Tension Pneumothorax and Hemothorax.

	TENSION PNEUMOTHORAX	HEMOTHORAX
Primary presenting symptom	Difficulty breathing, then shock	Shock, then difficulty breathing
Neck veins	Usually distended	Usually flat
Breath sounds	Decreased or absent on side of injury	Decreased or absent on side of injury
Percussion of chest	Hyperresonant	Dull
Tracheal deviation away from the side of the injury	Rarely present as a late sign	Usually not present

FLAIL CHEST

This occurs when three or more adjacent ribs are fractured in at least two places. The result is a segment of the chest wall that is not in continuity with the thorax. A lateral flail chest or anterior flail chest (sternal separation) may result. With posterior rib fractures, the

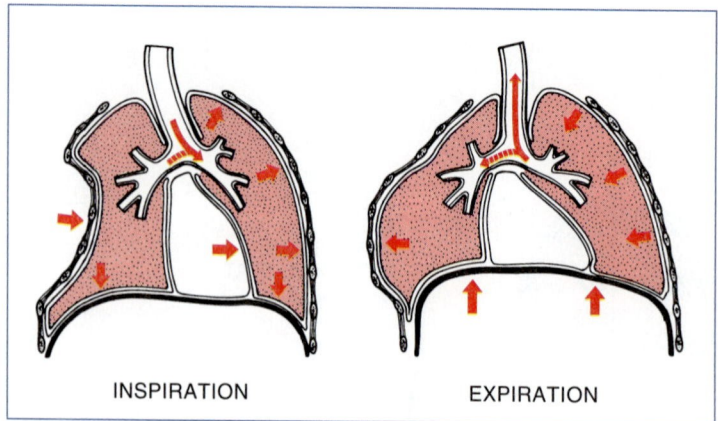

INSPIRATION EXPIRATION

Figure 6-8 Pathophysiology of flail chest.

heavy musculature usually prevents the occurrence of a flail segment. The flail segment moves with paradoxical motion relative to the rest of the chest wall (see Figures 6-8 and 6-9). The force necessary to produce this injury also bruises the underlying lung tissue, and this pulmonary contusion also will contribute to the hypoxia. The patient is at risk for the development of a hemothorax or pneumothorax. With a large flail segment, the patient may be in marked respiratory distress. Pain from the chest wall injury exacerbates the already impaired respiration from paradoxical motion and the underlying lung contusion. Palpation of the chest wall may reveal crepitus in addition to the abnormal respiratory motion.

Management of Flail Chest

1. Ensure an airway.
2. Administer oxygen.
3. Assist ventilation if required. Remember that pneumothorax is commonly associated with a flail chest.
4. Rapidly transport to the appropriate hospital.
5. Stabilize the flail segment with manual pressure then with bulky dressings taped to the chest wall (see Figure 6-10). This is usually not necessary until the patient is sta-

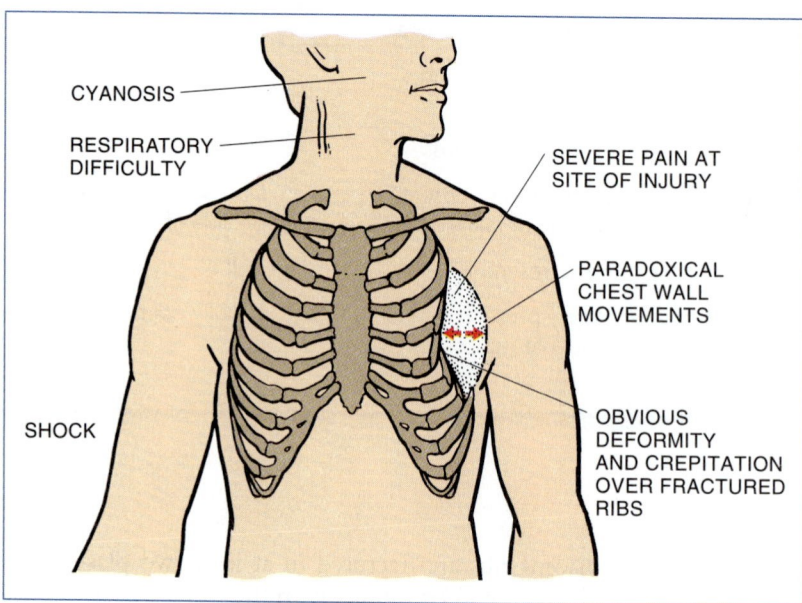

CYANOSIS

RESPIRATORY DIFFICULTY

SEVERE PAIN AT SITE OF INJURY

PARADOXICAL CHEST WALL MOVEMENTS

SHOCK

OBVIOUS DEFORMITY AND CREPITATION OVER FRACTURED RIBS

Figure 6-9 Physical findings of flail chest.

TAPE PAD IN PLACE, EXTENDING
TAPE TO BOTH SIDES OF CHEST

INTUBATION AND POSITIVE PRESSURE
VENTILATION IS THE BEST STABILIZATION

FIGURE 6-10 Stabilizing flail chest.

bilized on a backboard. Trying to maintain manual pressure on a flail segment while performing log-rolling may be dangerous to maintaining a stable spine.

6. Notify Medical Direction.

7. Monitor the heart if you have monitoring equipment. Associated myocardial trauma is frequent.

CARDIAC TAMPONADE

This injury is usually due to penetrating injury. The pericardial sac is an inelastic membrane that surrounds the heart. If blood collects rapidly between the heart and pericardium from a cardiac injury, the ventricles of the heart will be compressed. A small amount of pericardial blood may compromise cardiac filling. As the compression of the ventricles increases, the heart is less able to refill and cardiac output falls.

Diagnosis of cardiac tamponade classically relies upon the triad of hypotension, distended neck veins, and muffled heart sounds (Beck's triad). Muffled heart sounds may be very difficult to appreciate in the prehospital setting. The patient may have a paradoxical pulse. If the patient loses his peripheral pulse during inspiration, this is suggestive of a paradoxical pulse and the presence of cardiac tamponade. The major differential diagnosis in the field is tension pneumothorax. With cardiac tamponade, the patient will be in shock with a midline trachea and equal breath sounds (see Figure 6-11) unless there is an associated pneumothorax or hemothorax.

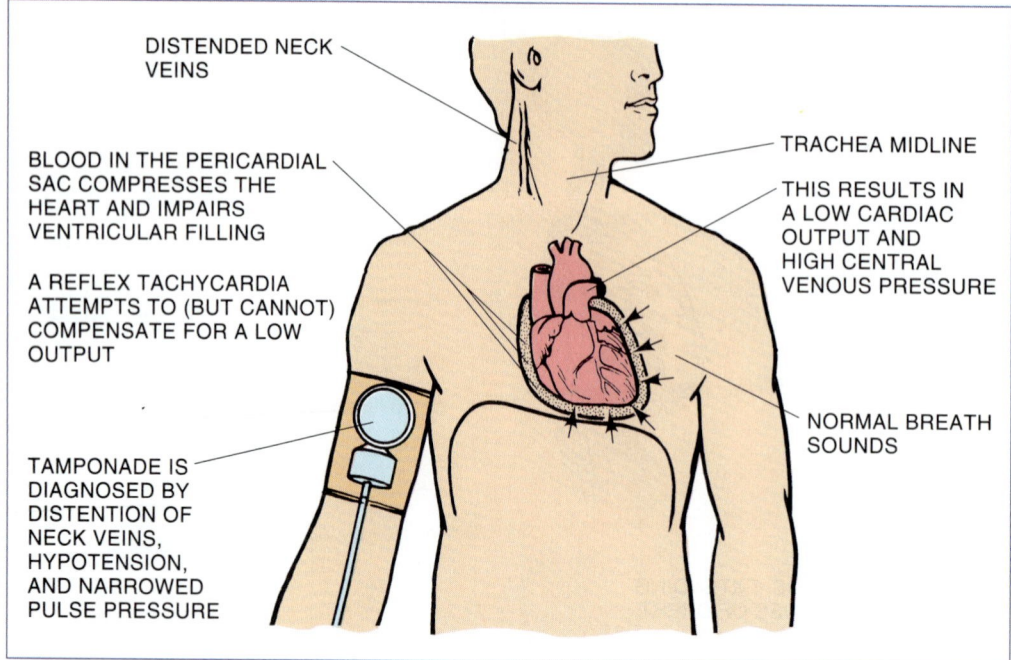

DISTENDED NECK VEINS

BLOOD IN THE PERICARDIAL SAC COMPRESSES THE HEART AND IMPAIRS VENTRICULAR FILLING

A REFLEX TACHYCARDIA ATTEMPTS TO (BUT CANNOT) COMPENSATE FOR A LOW OUTPUT

TAMPONADE IS DIAGNOSED BY DISTENTION OF NECK VEINS, HYPOTENSION, AND NARROWED PULSE PRESSURE

TRACHEA MIDLINE

THIS RESULTS IN A LOW CARDIAC OUTPUT AND HIGH CENTRAL VENOUS PRESSURE

NORMAL BREATH SOUNDS

FIGURE 6-11   Pathophysiology and physical findings of cardiac tamponade.

MANAGEMENT OF CARDIAC TAMPONADE

1. Ensure an airway and administer oxygen.
2. This lesion is rapidly fatal and cannot be readily treated in the field. Load the patient and proceed rapidly to the appropriate hospital.
3. Notify Medical Direction.
4. Monitor the heart if you have monitoring equipment.

TRAUMATIC AORTIC RUPTURE

This is the most common cause of immediate death in motor vehicle accidents or falls from heights. Ninety percent of these patients die immediately. For the survivors, salvage is feasible with prompt diagnosis and surgery. Traumatic thoracic aortic tears usually are due to deceleration injury with the heart and aortic arch moving suddenly anteriorly, transecting the aorta where it is fixed at the ligamentum arteriosum. In the 10% who do not exsanguinate promptly, the aortic tear will be contained temporarily by surrounding tissues and the adventitia. However, this is temporary and will usually rupture unless surgically repaired.

The diagnosis of a contained thoracic aortic laceration is impossible in the field and may be missed even in the hospital. The history from the scene is critically important since many of these patients have no obvious signs of chest trauma. Information about damage to the car or steering wheel with a deceleration injury or the height from which the patient fell are vital. Infrequently, the patient may present with upper extremity hypertension and diminished lower extremity pulses.

MANAGEMENT OF POTENTIAL AORTIC TEARS

1. Ensure an airway.
2. Administer oxygen.
3. Rapidly transport to the appropriate hospital.
4. Notify Medical Direction.

TRACHEAL OR BRONCHIAL TREE INJURY

These injuries may be the result of penetrating or blunt trauma. Penetrating upper airway injuries often have associated major vascular injuries and extensive tissue destruction. Blunt trauma may present with subtle findings. Blunt injury usually ruptures the trachea or mainstem bronchus near the carina. Presenting signs of blunt or penetrating injury include subcutaneous emphysema of the chest, face, or neck or an associated pneumothorax or hemothorax. Give 100% oxygen and transport immediately.

MYOCARDIAL CONTUSION

This is a potentially lethal lesion resulting from blunt chest injury. Blunt injury to the anterior chest is transmitted via the sternum to the heart, which lies immediately posterior to it (see Figure 6-12). Cardiac injuries from this mechanism may include valvular rupture, pericardial tamponade, or cardiac rupture, but myocardial contusion most commonly occurs. This bruising of the heart is basically the same injury as an acute myocardial infarction and likewise presents with chest pain, dysrhythmia, or cardiogenic shock (rare). In the field, cardiogenic shock cannot be distinguished from cardiac tamponade. The chest pain may be difficult to differentiate from the associated musculoskeletal discomfort that the patient also suffers as a result of the injury. All patients with blunt anterior chest trauma should be presumed to have a myocardial contusion.

MANAGEMENT OF MYOCARDIAL CONTUSION

1. Administer oxygen.
2. Transport the patient to the appropriate hospital.
3. Monitor the heart if you have monitoring equipment.

DIAPHRAGMATIC TEARS

Tears in the diaphragm may result from a severe blow to the abdomen. A sudden increase in intra-abdominal pressure, such as a seat belt injury or kick to the abdomen, may tear the diaphragm and allow herniation of the abdominal organs into the thoracic cavity. This occurs more commonly on the left than the right, since the liver protects the right hemidiaphragm. Blunt trauma produces large radial tears in the diaphragm. Penetrating trauma may also produce holes in the diaphragm, but these tend to be small.

Traumatic diaphragmatic hernia is difficult to diagnose even in the hospital. The herniation of abdominal contents into the thoracic cavity may cause marked respiratory distress. On examination, the breath sounds may be diminished, and infrequently bowel sounds may be heard when the chest is auscultated. The abdomen may appear scaphoid if a large quantity of abdominal contents are in the chest.

FIGURE 6-12 Pathophysiology of myocardial contusion.

MANAGEMENT OF DIAPHRAGMATIC RUPTURE

1. Ensure an airway.
2. Administer oxygen.
3. Transport the patient to the appropriate hospital.
4. Notify Medical Direction.

ESOPHAGEAL INJURY

This injury is usually produced by penetrating trauma. Management of associated trauma including airway or vascular injuries is generally more pressing than the esophageal injury. However, esophageal injury is lethal if unrecognized in the hospital. Operative repair is required.

PULMONARY CONTUSION

This very common chest injury results from blunt trauma. Contusion of the lung may produce marked hypoxemia. Management consists of assisted ventilation if indicated, oxygen administration, and transport.

OTHER CHEST INJURIES

Impalement injuries of the chest may be caused by any penetrating object, usually a knife. As in other areas of the body, the object should not be removed in the field. Stabilize the object, ensure an airway, and transport the patient.

Traumatic asphyxia is an important set of physical findings. The term is a misnomer since the condition is not caused by asphyxia. The syndrome results from a severe compression injury to the chest, such as from a steering wheel, a conveyor belt, or a heavy object. The sudden compression of the heart and mediastinum transmits this force to the capillaries of the neck and head. The patients appear similar to those of strangulation with cyanosis and swelling of the head and neck. The tongue and lips are swollen, and conjunctival hemorrhage is evident. The skin below the level of the crush injury to the chest will be pink unless there are other problems.

Traumatic asphyxia indicates that the patient has suffered a severe blunt thoracic injury, and major thoracic injuries are likely to be present. Management includes airway maintenance, treating other injuries, and rapid transport.

Similarly, *sternal fractures* indicate that the patient has suffered marked blunt trauma to the anterior chest. These patients should be presumed to have a myocardial contusion. Diagnosis can be made by palpation.

Scapular fractures, and *first or second rib fractures* require a significant force. The incidence of associated major thoracic vascular injury is high, and these patients should be promptly transported.

Simple pneumothorax may result from blunt or penetrating trauma. Fractured ribs are the usual cause in blunt trauma. This is caused by accumulation of air within the potential space between the visceral and parietal pleura. The lung may be totally or partially collapsed as the air continues to accrue in the thoracic cavity. In a healthy patient this should not acutely compromise ventilation, if a tension pneumothorax does not evolve. Patients with less respiratory reserve may not tolerate even a simple pneumothorax.

Diagnosis of a pneumothorax is based on pleuritic chest pain, dyspnea, decreased breath sounds on the affected side, and hypertympany to percussion. Close observation is required in anticipation of the patient developing a tension pneumothorax.

Simple rib fracture is the most frequent injury to the chest. If the patient does not have an associated pneumothorax or hemothorax, the major problem is pain. This pain will prohibit the patient from breathing adequately. On palpation, the area of rib fracture will be tender and may be unstable. Give oxygen and monitor for pneumothorax or hemothorax while encouraging the patient to breathe deeply.

PITFALLS

1. *Jumping to the conclusion that you have a tension pneumothorax because there are decreased breath sounds on one side of the chest:* The diagnosis of tension pneumothorax requires several other findings. Patients with simple rib fractures but no pneumothorax will have decreased breath sounds on the affected side due to splinting to relieve the pain.

2. *Progression of simple pneumothorax or open pneumothorax to tension pneumothorax:* You must reassess these patients frequently. The pulse oximeter is very helpful here.

3. *Taking too long on-scene with patients who have penetrating chest injuries:* Patients who have penetrating chest trauma and shock are at the top of the list of load-and-go patients. Nothing should delay transport.

4. *Underestimating the severity of injury in patients who have blunt chest trauma:* Multiple rib fractures with or without flail chest can cause hypoxia from mechanical ventilatory problems as well as pulmonary contusion. The patient (especially older patients) must be closely monitored for hypoxia and respiratory failure. The pulse oximeter is very helpful here.

SUMMARY

Chest injuries are common and often life-threatening in the multiple-trauma patient. If you follow the BTLS assessment priorities, you will identify the injuries while performing the BTLS Primary Survey. These are often load-and-go patients. The primary goals in treating the patient with chest trauma are the following:

1. Ensuring an airway while protecting the C-spine
2. Administering high-flow oxygen
3. Early transport to the appropriate hospital
4. Monitoring the heart if you have monitoring equipment

The thoracic injuries discussed are life-threatening, but treatable by prompt intervention and transport to the appropriate hospital. It is mandatory that the injuries presented are recognized in the field and treated appropriately to salvage these patients.

BIBLIOGRAPHY

1. American College of Surgeons Committee on Trauma. *Advanced Trauma Life Support,* pp. 147–163. Chicago: American College of Surgeons, 1997.

2. Blair, E., C. Topuzulu, and R. S. Deane. "Major Chest Trauma." *Current Problems in Surgery* (May 1969), pp. 2–69.

3. Eckstein, M., and D. Suyehara. "Needle Thoracostomy in the Prehospital Setting." *Prehospital Emergency Care,* Vol. 2, No. 2 (1998), pp. 132–135.

4. Jones, K. W. "Thoracic Trauma." *Surgical Clinics of North America* (1980), pp. 60–95.

5. Kirsh, M. M., D. M. Behrendt, M. B. Orringer, and others. "The Treatment of Acute Traumatic Rupture of the Aorta: A 10–Year Experience." *Annals of Surgery* (1976), pp. 184–308.

6. Richardson, J.D., L. Adams, and L. M. Flint. "Selective Management of Flail Chest and Pulmonary Contusion." *Annals of Surgery,* Vol. 196, No. 4 (1982), pp. 481–487.

CHAPTER 7

Shock Evaluation and Management

Raymond L. Fowler, M.D., F.A.C.E.P.
Paul E. Pepe, M.D., M.P.H., F.A.C.E.P., F.C.C.M.
Roger J. Lewis, M.D., Ph.D., F.A.C.E.P.

OBJECTIVES

UPON COMPLETION OF THIS CHAPTER, YOU SHOULD BE ABLE TO:

1. List the four components necessary for normal tissue perfusion.
2. Describe symptoms and signs of hemorrhagic shock.
3. Explain the pathophysiology of hemorrhagic shock and compare to the pathophysiology of high-space shock.
4. Describe the three common clinical shock syndromes.
5. Describe the management of the following:
   a. Hemorrhage that can be controlled
   b. Hemorrhage that cannot be controlled
   c. Nonhemorrhagic shock syndromes
6. Discuss the routine priorities in the prehospital management of shock.
7. Discuss the current indications and contraindications for the use of the antishock garment in the treatment of traumatic shock.

The management of shock has been the subject of intensive research during the past few years, and recently changes have been made in the recommendations for prehospital treatment of the patient with hemorrhagic shock. Some excellent studies on the treatment of hemorrhagic shock secondary to penetrating trauma have suggested new thinking in this area, while research in the treatment of the patient with blunt trauma has been less revealing. This chapter will review the present knowledge about the pathophysiology and treatment of shock in the traumatized patient.

BASIC PATHOPHYSIOLOGY

The normal perfusion of body tissues requires four intact components:

1. An intact vascular system to deliver oxygenated blood throughout the body
2. Adequate air exchange in the lungs to allow oxygen to enter the blood
3. An adequate volume of fluid in the vascular system, including blood cells and plasma
4. A functioning pump: the heart

The preservation of these components can be related to the basic rules of emergency care, which are:

1. Maintain the airway.
2. Control oxygenation and ventilation.
3. Control bleeding.
4. Maintain circulation.

The term *shock* describes a condition that occurs when the perfusion of the body's tissues with oxygen, electrolytes, glucose, and fluid becomes inadequate. Several processes cause this drop in perfusion. The loss of red blood cells in hemorrhaging patients results in less oxygen transport to the body tissues. Decreased circulating blood volume leads to lowered glucose, fluid volume, and electrolytes to the cells. The above circulatory disturbances result in the cells of the body becoming "shocked," and grave changes in body tissue begin to occur. Eventually, cell death follows.

Deprived of oxygen, cells begin to use "backup" processes that utilize energy sources less efficiently, producing toxic by-products such as lactic acid. Although these backup (anaerobic) processes may postpone cellular death for a time, the lack of oxygen is compounded by these toxic by-products because they can poison certain cellular functions such as the production of energy by mitochondria. Eventually, accumulating lactic acid in the blood and organs creates a systemic acidosis that further disrupts cellular activity. Respiratory muscle function also weakens, and respiratory failure develops, which worsens hypoxia.

In response to inadequate oxygen delivery, the body responds with increased sympathetic tone and release of circulating catecholamines (epinephrine and norepinephrine). These increase the heart rate and constrict peripheral blood vessels. The midbrain responds to the progressive hypoxia with an increase in the respiratory rate.

As you can see, shock is a condition that begins with an injury, spreads throughout the body as a multisystem insult to major organs, and results in specific symptoms at the bedside as the patient becomes progressively sicker.

Shock is a cellular process with clinical manifestations. The patient with shock may be pale, diaphoretic, and tachycardic. At the cellular level, the patient's cells are starving for oxygen and nutrients. Shock, therefore, is a condition in which poor tissue perfusion can severely and possibly permanently damage the organs of the body causing disability or death. The clinical signs and symptoms of the patient in shock imply that critical processes are threatening every vulnerable cell in the patient's body, particularly those in vital organs.

ASSESSMENT: SIGNS AND SYMPTOMS OF SHOCK

When first considering the concept of shock, you must understand that shock produces signs and symptoms that you can observe during patient assessment. The initial diagnosis of the shock state can be made from the physical assessment findings. Although blood pressure should be monitored frequently to help determine whether organ perfusion is adequate, *remember that assessment tools other than measuring the blood pressure must also be used to recognize shock in the trauma patient.*

Humans vary as to the blood pressure required to maintain *adequate* perfusion. The question of "how low can you go" while maintaining adequate perfusion has not yet been answered. We know that the healthy young patient can often maintain adequate perfusion in the face of hypotension whereas older patients, hypertensive patients, and those with head injury often cannot tolerate hypotension for even short periods. You must rely on physician Medical Direction and your own study of current research on shock.

While this text is about trauma, shock is a clinical condition associated with more medical problems than just trauma. Following is a discussion of shock syndromes, many of which are caused by traumatic conditions. The take-home point, though, is that the shock state is one of low tissue perfusion from many causes in which the body *usually* demonstrates similar signs of its response to this perfusion-deprived condition. (The body may not always demonstrate similar signs; see the discussion of high-space shock that follows.) Therefore, the stabbed and bleeding patient often shows many of the same signs as the burned or dehydrated patient. The classic symptoms and signs associated with hemorrhagic shock include the following:

1. *Weakness:* caused by tissue hypoxia and acidosis
2. *Thirst:* caused by hypovolemia (especially with relatively low fluid amounts in the blood vessels)
3. *Pallor* (pale, white color of the skin): caused by catecholamine-induced vasoconstriction and/or loss of circulating red blood cells
4. *Tachycardia:* caused by catecholamines' effect on the heart
5. *Diaphoresis* (sweating): caused by catecholamines' effect on sweat glands
6. *Tachypnea* (elevated respiratory rate): caused by stress, catecholamines, acidosis, and hypoxia
7. *Decreased urinary output:* caused by hypovolemia, hypoxia, and circulating catecholamines (important to remember in interhospital transfers)
8. *Weakened strength of peripheral pulses:* the thready pulse: caused by vasoconstriction, tachycardia, and loss of blood volume
9. *Hypotension:* caused by hypovolemia, either absolute or relative (see later paragraphs for a discussion of relative hypovolemia)
10. *Altered mental status* (confusion, restlessness, combativeness, unconsciousness): caused by decreased cerebral perfusion, acidosis, and catecholamine stimulation
11. *Cardiac arrest:* caused by critical organ failure secondary to blood or fluid loss, hypoxia, and occasionally arrhythmia caused by catecholamine stimulation

To summarize, many of the symptoms of shock of any etiology, including the classic hemorrhagic shock picture, are caused by the release of catecholamines. When the brain senses that perfusion to the tissues is insufficient, it sends messages down the spinal cord to the sympathetic nervous system and the adrenal glands, causing a release of catecholamines (epinephrine and norepinephrine) into the circulation. The circulating catecholamines cause the tachycardia, anxiousness, diaphoresis, and vasoconstriction. The vasoconstriction in the arterioles shunts blood away from the skin and intestines to the heart, lungs, and brain. Close monitoring early in the shock syndrome may detect an initial rise in the blood pressure due to this shunting. There will almost always be an initial narrowing of the pulse pressure because vasoconstriction raises the diastolic pressure more than the systolic. The shunting of blood from the skin causes the pallor of shock.

Decreased perfusion causes weakness and thirst initially, and then later, a decreased level of consciousness (confusion, restlessness, or combativeness) and worsening pallor. As shock continues, the prolonged tissue hypoxia leads to worsening acidosis. This acidosis can cause a loss of response to catecholamines, worsening the drop in blood pressure. This is often the point at which the patient in "compensated" shock suddenly "crashes." Eventually, the hypoxia and acidosis cause cardiac dysfunction, including cardiac arrest, and ultimately death.

Although the individual response to post-traumatic hemorrhage may vary, many patients will have the following classic patterns of "early" and "late" shock:

Early shock (loss of approximately 15 to 25% of the blood volume): enough to stimulate slight to moderate tachycardia, pallor, narrowed pulse pressure, thirst, weakness, and possibly delayed capillary refill

Late shock (loss of approximately 30 to 45% of the blood volume): enough to cause *hypotension* as well as the other symptoms of hypovolemic shock listed earlier

Note that during the Initial Assessment, early shock presents as a fast pulse with pallor and diaphoresis while late shock may present as weak pulse or loss of the peripheral pulse.

Prolonged capillary refill was previously thought to be useful for detecting early shock. Low blood volume and catecholamine-induced vasoconstriction cause decreased perfusion of the capillary bed in the skin. Capillary refill is tested by pressing on the palm of the hand or, in a child, squeezing the whole foot. The test is suspicious for shock if the blanched area remains pale for longer than 2 seconds. Scientific evaluation of this test has shown it to have a high correlation with late shock but of little value for detecting early shock. The test was associated with both frequent false positive as well as false negative results. Measurement of capillary refill is useful for small children in whom it is difficult to get an accurate blood pressure, but it is of little use for detecting early shock in adults.

EVALUATION OF TACHYCARDIA

One of the first signs of illness, and arguably one of the most common, is that of tachycardia. You will frequently be confronted with the patient with an elevated pulse rate and must make some sort of distinction as to the cause. First, remember that you must *always* attempt to explain why a patient has tachycardia. An elevated pulse rate is never normal. Humans can transiently raise their pulses in the setting of anxiety, but such elevation quickly returns to normal or fluctuates in rate depending on the waxing and waning of the anxiety state. *A persistently elevated pulse rate while at rest is always an indication of something medically wrong with the patient, including the possibility of occult hemorrhage.*

Second, remember that an elevated pulse rate is one of the first signs of shock. Any adult trauma patient with a *sustained* pulse rate above 100 must be suspected as having occult hemorrhage until proven otherwise. However, during the brief Initial Assessment, a pulse rate greater than 120 should be a red flag for possible shock.

THE SHOCK SYNDROMES

While the most common shock states seen in trauma patients are associated with hemorrhage and the accompanying hypovolemia, there are actually three major classifications of shock. These three shock states can be categorized according to their causes as follows:

1. *Low-volume shock* (absolute hypovolemia): caused by hemorrhage or other major body fluid loss
2. *High-space shock* (relative hypovolemia): caused by spinal injury, vasovagal syncope, sepsis, and certain drug overdoses
3. *Mechanical (obstructive) shock:* caused by pericardial tamponade, tension pneumothorax, or myocardial contusion

There are notable differences in the appearance of patients with these conditions, and it is critical that you be aware of the signs and symptoms that accompany each one.

LOW-VOLUME SHOCK (ABSOLUTE HYPOVOLEMIA)

Loss of blood from injury is called *post-traumatic hemorrhage* and, in addition to head injury, hemorrhagic shock is the number one cause of *preventable* death from injury.

The amount of volume that the blood vessels *can* hold is many liters more than that which actually flows through the vasculature. The sympathetic nervous system keeps the vessels constricted, reducing their volume and maintaining blood pressure high enough to perfuse vital organs. If blood volume is lost, "sensors" in the major vessels signal the adrenal gland and the nerves of the sympathetic nervous system to secrete catecholamines, which cause vasoconstriction and thus further shrink the vascular space and maintain perfusion pressure to the brain and heart. If the blood loss is minor, the sympathetic system can shrink the space enough to maintain blood pressure. If the loss is severe, the vascular space cannot be shrunk down enough to maintain blood pressure, and hypotension occurs.

Normally, the blood vessels are elastic and are distended by the volume that is in them. This produces a radial artery pulse that is full and wide. Blood loss allows the artery to shrink in width, becoming more threadlike in size; hence the term "thready" pulse in shock.

HIGH-SPACE SHOCK (RELATIVE HYPOVOLEMIA)

As mentioned earlier, the volume that the blood vessels *can* hold is many liters more than the normal blood volume. Again, it is the steady-state action of the sympathetic nervous system that keeps the vascular bed mildly constricted in order to maintain perfusion to the heart and brain. Anything that disturbs the sympathetic nervous system to result in the loss of this normal vasoconstriction can cause the vascular space to become much "too large" for the usual amount of blood. If the blood vessels dilate, the 5 liters or so of blood flowing through the normal adult's vascular space may not be sufficient to maintain blood pressure and vital tissue perfusion. The condition causing the vascular space to be too large for a normal amount of blood has been called *high-space shock* or *relative hypovolemia*. Although several types of high-space shock exist (e.g., sepsis syndrome and drug overdoses), neurogenic shock, commonly called *spinal shock,* will be addressed here.

Neurogenic shock occurs most typically after an injury to the spinal cord. Although circulating catecholamines (already present) may preserve the blood pressure for a short time, the disruption of the sympathetic nervous system outflow from the spinal cord results in loss of the normal vascular tone and in the inability of the body to compensate for any accompanying hemorrhage. The clinical presentation of neurogenic shock differs from hemorrhagic shock in that there is no catecholamine release, thus no pallor, tachycardia, or sweating. The patient will have a decreased blood pressure but the heart rate will be normal or slow, the skin warm, dry, and pink. The patient may also have accompanying paralysis and/or sensory deficit corresponding to the spinal cord injury. You may also see a lack of chest wall movement and only simple diaphragmatic movement when the patient is asked to take a deep breath. The important point is that this form of shock does not have the typical picture of hemorrhagic shock, *even when associated with severe bleeding.* The neurologic assessment is therefore very important, and you should not rely on typical shock symptoms and signs to suspect internal bleeding or accompanying hemorrhage-associated shock. A neurogenic shock patient may "look better" than his or her actual condition.

Certain overdoses (including drinking alcohol) can also result in vasodilatation and relative hypovolemia. Very often injuries result after such intoxication, and their effect on typical clinical signs and symptoms (like neurogenic shock) should be considered. You may find that intoxication is an accompanying problem in many injury victims. Other examples of overdoses that produce relative hypovolemia include nitroglycerin and calcium channel blockers.

MECHANICAL (OBSTRUCTIVE) SHOCK

In the normal adult's resting state, the heart pumps *out* about 5 liters of blood per minute. This means, of course, that the heart also must take *in* about 5 liters of blood per minute. Therefore, any traumatic condition that slows or prevents the venous return of blood can cause shock by lowering cardiac output and thus oxygen delivery to the tissues. Likewise, anything that obstructs the flow of blood to or through the heart can cause shock. The following are traumatic conditions that can cause mechanical shock:

Tension pneumothorax is so named because of the high air tension (pressure) that develops in the pleural space (between the lung and chest wall). This very high positive pressure is transmitted back to the right heart and prevents the venous return of blood. Shifting of mediastinal structures may also lower venous return. See Figure 7-1 and turn to Chapter 6 for a complete description of the signs, symptoms, and treatment of tension pneumothorax.

Cardiac or pericardial tamponade occurs when blood fills the space around the heart, squeezing the heart and preventing the heart from filling or pumping well (see Figure 7-2). The net result is that the heart cannot fill properly and cardiac output falls. Pericardial tamponade may occur in more than 75% of cases of penetrating cardiac injury. *On-scene interventions should be avoided if the diagnosis is suspected because any time wasted on the scene could result in death of the patient.* Definitive surgical care in the nearest appropriate facility for pericardial decompression may be the only lifesaving measure available. See Chapter 6 for a more complete discussion.

Myocardial contusion can result in diminished cardiac output because the heart loses pumping ability due to direct injury. Myocardial contusion often cannot be differentiated from cardiac tamponade in the field. Therefore, rapid transport, supportive care, and cardiac monitoring are the mainstays of therapy.

A word of caution is important here. Patients with shock from mechanical causes can be very near death. *Delay on the scene may prevent salvage of the patient.* Urban studies suggest that, in applicable cases, the time from development of a tamponade to circulatory arrest may be as little as 5 to 10 minutes. Survival following traumatic circulatory arrest, even in the best of trauma systems, is rarely achieved if surgery is not performed within 5 to 10 minutes.

MANAGEMENT OF POST-TRAUMATIC SHOCK STATES

CONTROL BLEEDING: Red blood cells are necessary to carry oxygen. Control of bleeding must be obtained either by direct pressure or rapid transport to surgery.

GIVE OXYGEN: Cyanosis is an extremely late sign of hypoxemia and may not occur at all if there has been extensive blood loss. Give high-flow oxygen to all patients at risk for shock.

TRANSPORT: Patients in shock are in the load-and-go category. Transport as soon as you finish the Primary Survey (Initial Survey and Rapid Trauma Survey). Almost all critical interventions should be done in the ambulance (see Chapter 2).

TREATMENT OF POST-TRAUMATIC HEMORRHAGE

Prehospital management of the patient in shock is controversial at this time. There is no question of the need for control of hemorrhage, supplemental oxygen, and early transport, but the indications for most other therapies are still being debated. Since the early days of modern shock treatment (about the middle of this century), intravenous crystalloid solutions (and sometimes colloid) have been tested and/or utilized to reverse the effects of hypovolemia. In addition, it has been previously proposed that intra-abdominal and pelvic bleeding may possibly be diminished by use of the pneumatic antishock garment (military antishock trousers, PASG, MAST). Now, recent research suggests a modified approach. Patients in hypovolemic shock due to hemorrhage may be generally thought of as falling into one of the following two categories: those with

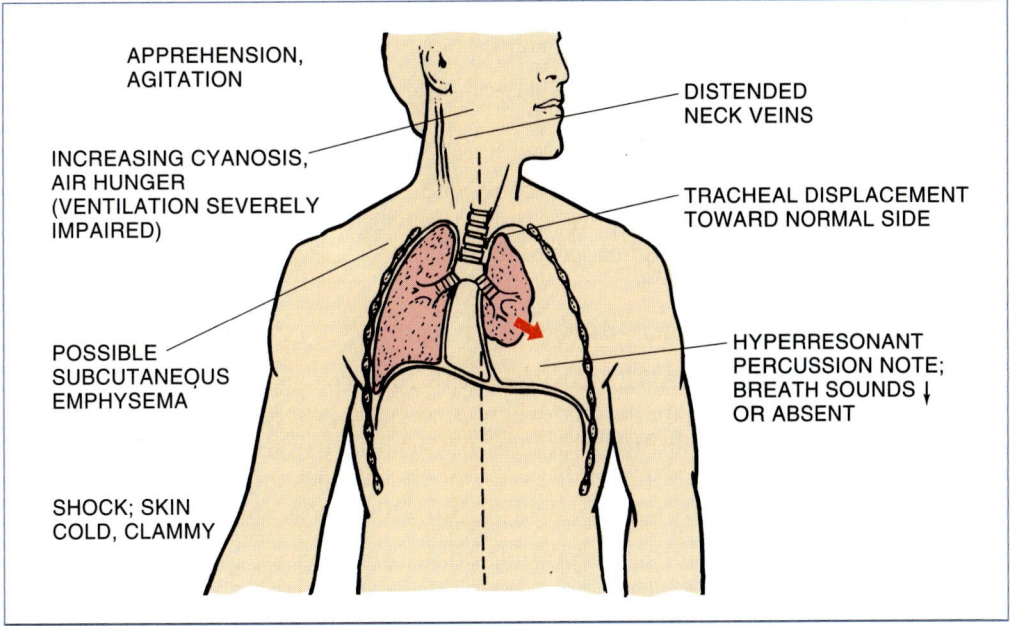

FIGURE 7-1   Physical findings of tension pneumothorax.

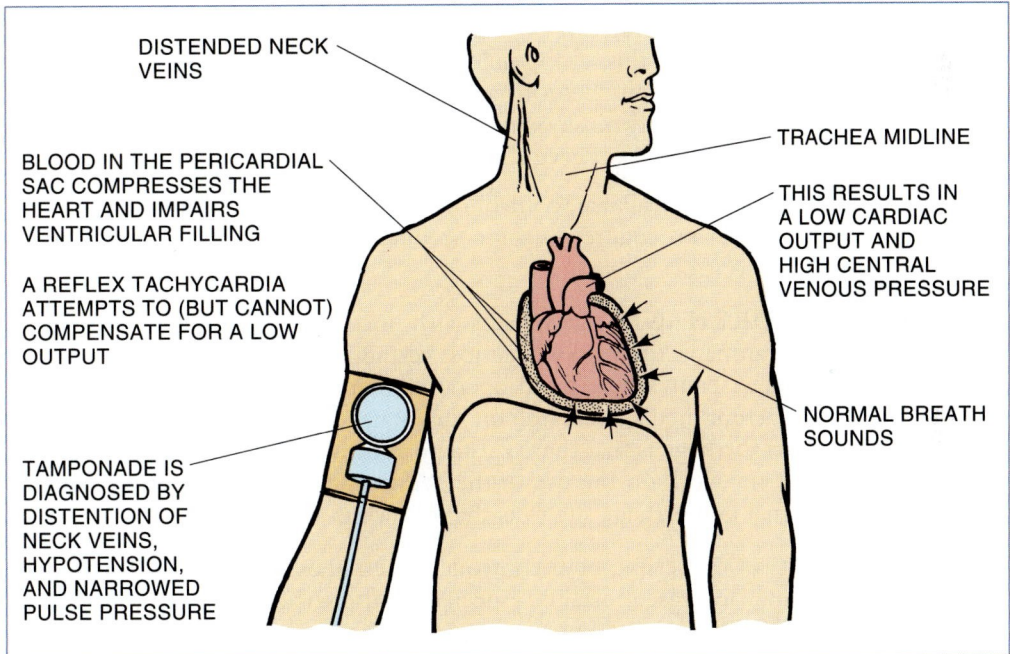

FIGURE 7-2   Pathophysiology and physical findings of cardiac tamponade.

bleeding that you can control (e.g., extremity injury) and those with bleeding that you cannot control (e.g., internal injury). We will consider each type of bleeding and discuss current concepts of therapy for each type.

HEMORRHAGE THAT CAN BE CONTROLLED

A patient with this type of injury is fairly easy to manage. Stop the bleeding by direct pressure. Only in the most extreme circumstances should a tourniquet be applied. A reasonable guide is that you should apply a tourniquet only to the extremity that you are prepared to sacrifice to save a life.

If the patient has clinical evidence of shock that persists after direct control of the bleeding, you should take the following steps:

1. Put the patient's body in a horizontal or slightly head-down position.
2. Administer high-flow oxygen.
3. Transport immediately and rapidly.
4. Apply the PASG, if local protocols recommend, until IV fluid therapy is available.
5. Monitor the heart, and apply pulse oximetry if available.
6. Perform Ongoing Exam and observe closely.

HEMORRHAGE THAT CANNOT BE CONTROLLED

EXTERNAL HEMORRHAGE: A patient with this type of injury must be rapidly transported to an appropriate facility where necessary procedures to gain surgical hemostasis can be performed. Although most physicians advocate fluid resuscitation to treat hemorrhagic shock, you must also remember that elevating blood pressure can increase uncontrolled hemorrhage. To manage this patient, you should:

1. Apply as much direct pressure as possible on the bleeding site (e.g., femoral artery, facial hemorrhage).
2. Put the patient's body in a horizontal or slightly head-down position.
3. Apply tourniquets to a bleeding extremity only as a desperate attempt to stop severe bleeding that cannot be otherwise controlled (discussed earlier).
4. Administer high-flow oxygen.
5. Transport immediately and rapidly.
6. Do not utilize the PASG in this setting unless it can be used to tamponade otherwise uncontrollable lower extremity hemorrhage.
7. Monitor the heart, and apply pulse oximetry if available.
8. Perform Ongoing Exam and observe closely.

Note: If assistance is not available, control of hemorrhage, even if minimal, should remain the priority. Other procedures become secondary if they interrupt attempts to maintain hemorrhage control.

INTERNAL HEMORRHAGE: The patient with uncontrolled internal hemorrhage is the classic critical trauma victim who will almost certainly die unless you rapidly transport to an appropriate facility where rapid operative hemostasis can be obtained. The results of the most current medical research on the management of patients with exsanguinating internal hemorrhage is that there exists no substitute for gaining surgical control of bleeding. Recent work on the use of the PASG and IV fluids in shock patients with presumed internal hemorrhage suggests the following:

1. Use of the PASG in the setting of uncontrolled internal exsanguination due to penetrating injury may increase mortality, especially in the setting of intrathoracic hemorrhage. The PASG raises blood pressure, and raising blood pressure in the setting of bleeding vessels within the thorax, abdomen, and pelvis probably increases internal bleeding, raising the chance of death due to exsanguination.
2. Any delay in providing rapid transport of such patients should not occur unless *absolutely* unavoidable, as in the case of a patient requiring prolonged extrication.
3. Moribund trauma patients (ones in very deep shock with blood pressures under 50 mmHg systolic) usually die, but PASG may be indicated to maintain some degree of circulation. Treatment of this extreme amount of hemorrhage may override the concerns for increased hemorrhage secondary to the use of this intervention. However, this approach is still controversial. Local Medical Direction should guide such therapy.

The recommendations, therefore, for a patient with probable exsanguinating internal hemorrhage *secondary to penetrating injuries* are the following:

1. Transport immediately and rapidly.
2. Put the patient's body in a horizontal or slightly head-down position.

3. Administer high-flow oxygen.
4. Do not utilize the PASG in this setting except as indicated by local Medical Direction.
5. Monitor the heart, and apply pulse oximetry if available.
6. Perform Ongoing Exam and observe closely.

Current published research has not yet adequately addressed the treatment of the patient with presumed internal hemorrhage in the setting of blunt injuries (MVCs, falls, etc.). This creates a dilemma because many patients with blunt injuries can lose a significant amount of blood and fluid from the intravascular space into the sites of large-bone fractures (hematoma and edema). This loss can be enough to cause shock, and yet the blood loss is usually self-limited. This situation should be treated with oxygen and rapid transport.

TREATMENT OF NONHEMORRHAGIC SHOCK SYNDROMES—(MECHANICAL AND HIGH-SPACE)

Treatments for the other shock syndromes, namely, mechanical and high-space (relative hypovolemia) are somewhat different. All patients require high-flow oxygen, rapid transport, shock positioning.

MECHANICAL SHOCK

The patient with mechanical shock must first be accurately assessed to determine the cause of the problem. The patient with tension pneumothorax needs transport to the nearest appropriate hospital for decompression of the elevated pleural pressure.

The patient with suspected pericardial tamponade must be rapidly transported to an appropriate facility, because the time of onset of tamponade to the time of cardiac arrest can be a matter of minutes.

In two separate studies, one prospective and one retrospective, there was an increase in mortality of patients with tamponade when the PASG was applied in the prehospital setting. This may be due to the increase in field time taken to apply the PASG. By increasing peripheral resistance, the PASG also may decrease cardiac output, which may be another cause of increased mortality in such patients with an already low cardiac output. Therefore, the PASG is contraindicated in this setting.

Myocardial contusion rarely causes shock. Recent reports indicate that most contusions cause no clinical findings. However, severe contusion may cause acute heart failure, manifested by distended neck veins, tachycardia, or arrhythmias. These are the same signs seen with pericardial tamponade. These patients require rapid transport for proper care. Give high-flow oxygen and perform cardiac monitoring on the patient with suspected myocardial contusion.

HIGH-SPACE SHOCK

High-space shock, in theory, resembles controlled hemorrhage, in that there is relative hypovolemia with an "intact" vasculature (no leak). Therefore, initial management includes possible short-term use of the PASG. In the absence of a head injury, the patient's level of consciousness is a reasonable end point to follow. Be aware of possible internal injuries, and keep in mind that raising the blood pressure may increase internal bleeding in that situation.

CURRENT USES FOR THE PNEUMATIC ANTISHOCK GARMENT (PASG OR MAST)

The PASG is an inflatable compressive device that encircles the abdomen and legs. The PASG exerts its effect by compression of the arteries of the abdomen and legs, and this increases the peripheral vascular resistance (PVR). As the PVR is a component of blood pressure, it (blood pressure) typically rises with the application and inflation of the PASG. However, as the PVR rises, cardiac output (CO) may fall. Therefore, you must be cautious about elevating the PVR in settings of low blood pressure because of the possibility of lowering the cardiac output. Furthermore, if uncontrolled bleeding is occurring within the patient, raising the blood pressure may increase bleeding.

Until recently, it was commonplace to utilize the PASG for any patient with post-traumatic hypotension. Unfortunately, these well-intentioned recommendations came in the absence of real clinical proof of the effectiveness of the PASG.

In the last few years, controlled clinical trials have been conducted to determine if PASG will improve vital signs, survival to hospital admission, and survival to discharge. From these studies have come the following indications and contraindications for the use of the PASG in trauma patients.

Indications for Use of the Antishock Trousers in Trauma Patients:

1. Shock secondary to hemorrhage that can be controlled
2. Neurogenic shock without evidence of other internal injuries
3. Isolated fractures of legs without evidence of other internal injuries (blow up to only air-splint pressures)
4. Systolic blood pressure less than 50 mmHg (controversial)

Contraindications for Use of Antishock Trousers:

1. *Absolute:*
   a. Pulmonary edema
   b. Bleeding that cannot be controlled, such as penetrating chest or abdominal trauma
2. *Conditional:* Pregnancy—may use leg compartments

Local Medical Direction should guide the use of the PASG.

SUMMARY

The patient with shock is often not diagnosed early enough. Shock may not be obvious until the patient is near death. The importance of careful assessment and reassessment cannot be overemphasized. You must understand the risk of any shock state to the patient. Further, you need to study and memorize the shock syndromes, especially in regard to the rapid provision of the proper treatment for such conditions as internal hemorrhage, pericardial tamponade, and tension pneumothorax. Finally, you should be aware of the controversy on the use of IV fluid resuscitation and the PASG for cases of *uncontrolled* hemorrhage. Rely on your local Medical Direction to keep you current on the standard of care in these areas.

BIBLIOGRAPHY

1. Bickell, W. H., P. E. Pepe, M. L. Bailey, and others. "Randomized Trial of Pneumatic Antishock Garments in the Prehospital Management of Penetrating Abdominal Injury." *Annals of Emergency Medicine,* Vol. 16 (June 1987), pp. 653–658.
2. Bickell, W. H., M. J. Wall, P. E. Pepe, and others. "Immediate Versus Delayed Fluid Resuscitation for Hypotensive Patients with Penetrating Torso Injury." *New England Journal of Medicine,* Vol. 331 (October 1994), pp. 1105–1109.
3. Chestnut, R. M., L. F. Marshall, M. R. Klauber, and others. "The Role of Secondary Brain Injury in Determining Outcome from Severe Head Injury." *Journal of Trauma,* Vol. 34 (1993), pp. 216–222.
4. Domeier, R. M., R. E. O'Conner, and others. "Use of the Pneumatic Anti-Shock Garment (PASG)." *Prehospital Emergency Care,* Vol. 1, No. 1 (1997), pp. 32–44.

5. Kowalenko, T., S. Stern, S. Dronen, and X. Wang. "Improved Outcome with Hypotensive Resuscitation of Uncontrolled Hemorrhagic Shock in a Swine Mode." *Journal of Trauma,* Vol. 33 (1992), pp. 349–353.

6. Mattox, K. L., W. H. Bickell, P. E. Pepe, and others. "Prospective Mast Study in 911 patients." *Journal of Trauma,* Vol. 29 (1989), pp. 1104–1112.

7. Pigula, F. A., S. L. Wald, S. R. Shackford, and others. "The Effect of Hypotension and Hypoxia on Children with Severe Head Injuries." *Journal of Pediatric Surgery,* Vol. 28 (1993), pp. 310–316.

8. Schriger, D. L., and L. J. Baraff. "Capillary Refill—Is It a Useful Predictor of Hypovolemic States?" *Annals of Emergency Medicine,* Vol. 20 (June 1991), pp. 601–605.

9. Vassar, M. J., R. P. Fischer, P. E. O'Brien, and others. "A Multicenter Trial for Resuscitation of Injured Patients with 7.5% Sodium Chloride. The Effect of Added Dextran 70. The Multicenter Group for the Study of Hypertonic Saline in Trauma Patients." *Archives of Surgery,* Vol. 128 (1993), pp. 1003–1011.

CHAPTER 8

Head Trauma

John E. Campbell, M.D., F.A.C.E.P.
Roy L. Alson, Ph.D., M.D., F.A.C.E.P.

(Photo courtesy of Don Resch)

OBJECTIVES

UPON COMPLETION OF THIS CHAPTER, YOU SHOULD BE ABLE TO:

1. Describe the anatomy of the head and brain.
2. Describe the pathophysiology of traumatic brain injury.
3. Explain the difference between primary and secondary brain injury.
4. Describe the mechanisms for the development of secondary brain injury.
5. Describe the assessment of the patient with a head injury.
6. Describe the management of the patient with a head injury.
7. Describe the management of the cerebral herniation syndrome.
8. Identify potential problems in the management of the patient with a head injury.

Head injuries represent a significant problem in the multiple-trauma patient, with 40% having central nervous system (CNS) injuries. This group has a death rate twice as high (35% versus 17%) as that of patients without CNS injuries. Head injuries account for an estimated 25% of all trauma deaths and up to one-half of all motor vehicle fatalities. Head injuries may result in bruising of the brain tissue with swelling and increased intracranial pressure, injury to blood vessels with bleeding and increased intracranial pressure, or penetrating injuries of the skull that directly damage brain tissue. As with other injuries, prompt and organized evaluation and treatment give the patient the greatest chance for complete recovery. To most effectively manage the head-injured patient, you should have a working knowledge of the basic anatomy and physiology of the head and brain. *You must always assume that a serious head injury is accompanied by an injury to the cervical spine and spinal cord.*

ANATOMY OF THE HEAD

The head (excluding the face and facial structures) includes the following (see Figure 8-1):

1. Scalp
2. Skull
3. Fibrous coverings of the brain (meninges: dura, arachnoid, pia)
4. Brain tissue
5. Cerebrospinal fluid
6. Vascular compartments

The scalp is a protective covering for the skull, but it is very vascular and bleeds freely when lacerated. The skull is like a closed box; the only significant opening through which pressure can be released is the foramen magnum at the base where the brain stem becomes the spinal cord. The rigid and unyielding bony skull contributes to several injury mechanisms in head trauma. Because the brain "floats" inside the cerebrospinal fluid and is anchored at its base, there is greater movement at the top of the brain than at the base.

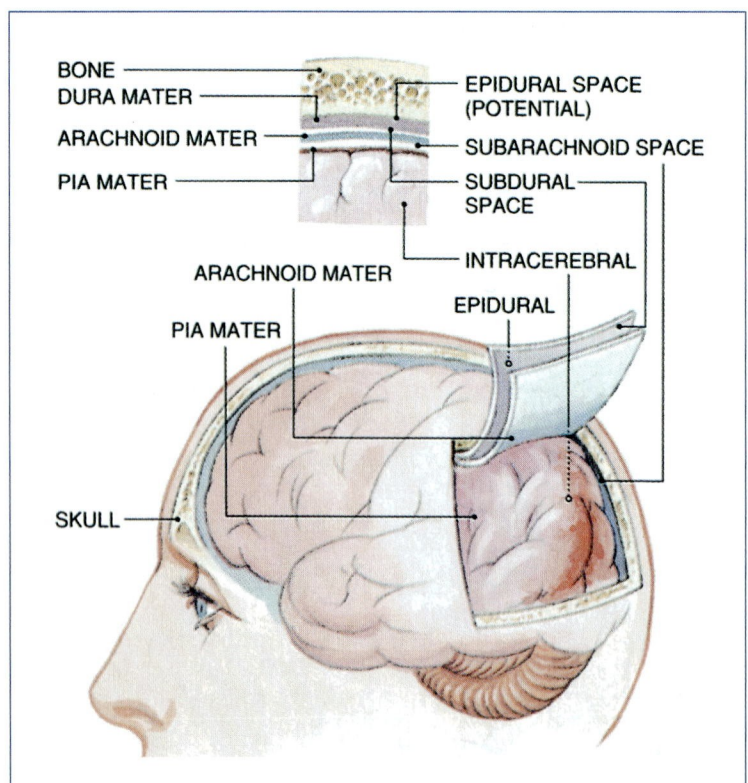

FIGURE 8-1   Anatomy of the head.

On impact, the brain is able to move within the skull and can strike bony prominences within the cranial cavity. This is the "third collision" described in mechanisms of injury in Chapter 1. The temporal bone (temple) is quite thin and easily fractured. The fibrous coverings of the brain include the dura mater ("tough mother"), which covers the entire brain; the thinner pia arachnoid (called simply the arachnoid), which lies underneath the dura and in which are suspended both arteries and veins; and the very thin pia mater ("soft mother"), which lies underneath the arachnoid and is adherent to the surface of the brain. The cerebrospinal fluid is found beneath the arachnoid and pia mater.

The brain fills the entire skull; this fact virtually excludes any adaptation to swelling. This is of great importance in the pathophysiology of head trauma. Following injury, the brain, like all injured tissue, will swell. Because of the fixed space, as the tissue swells and the volume of fluid inside the skull increases, so does the pressure.

Cerebrospinal fluid (e.g., spinal fluid) is a nutrient fluid that bathes the brain and spinal cord. Spinal fluid is continually created within the ventricles of the brain at a rate of 0.33 mL/min. It is reabsorbed by the arachnoid membrane that covers the brain and spinal cord. Anything obstructing the flow of spinal fluid will cause an accumulation of spinal fluid within the brain (hydrocephalus) and an increase in intracerebral pressure.

PATHOPHYSIOLOGY OF HEAD TRAUMA

Brain injury can be divided into two components, primary and secondary. Primary brain injury is the initial damage to the brain tissue that is the direct result of the injury force. Secondary brain injury is the result of hypoxia or decreased perfusion of brain tissue. Management of primary brain injury is best directed at prevention with such measures as better occupant restraint systems in autos, the use of helmets in sports and cycling, firearms education, and so forth. Good prehospital care can help prevent the development of secondary brain injury.

While penetrating wounds to the brain always cause primary injury, most primary injuries occur either as a result of external forces applied against the exterior of the skull or from movement of the brain inside the skull. In deceleration injuries the head usually strikes an object such as the windshield of an automobile, which causes a sudden deceleration of the skull. The brain continues to move forward, impacting first against the skull in the original direction of motion and then rebounding to hit the opposite side of the inner surface of the skull. Thus, injuries may occur to the brain in the area of original impact ("coup") or on the opposite side ("contracoup"). The interior base of the skull is rough, and movement of the brain over this area may cause various degrees of injury to the brain tissue or to blood vessels supporting the brain (see Figure 8-2).

The secondary injuries are caused by the brain's response to the primary injury (swelling with decreased perfusion) or from complications of other injuries (hypoxia or hypotension). The initial response of the injured brain is swelling. Bruising causes vasodilatation with increased blood flow to the injured area and thus an accumulation of blood that takes up space and exerts pressure on surrounding brain tissue. There is no extra space inside the skull, so swelling of the injured area increases intracerebral pressure and decreases blood flow to the brain. The increase in cerebral water (edema) does not occur immediately but develops over hours. Early efforts to maintain perfusion of the brain can be lifesaving.

The brain normally adjusts its own blood flow in response to metabolic needs. The flow of blood is adjusted based on the level of carbon dioxide (CO_2) in the blood. The normal level of CO_2 is 35 to 40 mmHg. An *increase* in the level of CO_2 (hypoventilation) promotes cerebral *vasodilatation* and increased swelling, while *lowering* the level of CO_2 (hyperventilation) causes *vasoconstriction* and cerebral ischemia. In the past, it was thought that hyperventilation (lowering of CO_2) in the head-injured patient would decrease brain swelling and improve cerebral blood flow. More recent research has shown that hyperventilation actually has only a slight effect on brain swelling, but causes a significant decrease in cerebral perfusion from vasoconstriction, which results in cerebral hypoxia. The injured brain does not tolerate hypoxia. *Thus, both hyperventilation*

FIGURE 8-2   The rough inner base of the skull.

and hypoventilation cause cerebral hypoxia and increase mortality. Maintaining good ventilation (not hyperventilation) at a rate of about one breath every 4 to 5 seconds with high-flow oxygen is very important. *Prophylactic hyperventilation for head injury is no longer recommended.*

INTRACRANIAL PRESSURE

Within the skull and fibrous coverings of the brain are the brain tissue, cerebrospinal fluid, and blood. An increase in the volume of any one of these components must be at the expense of the other two because the adult skull (a rigid box) cannot expand. Although there is some give to the volume of cerebrospinal fluid, it accounts for little space and cannot offset rapid brain swelling. Blood supply cannot be compromised, for the brain requires a constant supply of blood (oxygen and glucose) to survive. Thus, since none of the supporting components of the brain can be compromised, brain swelling can be rapidly catastrophic.

The pressure of the brain contents within the skull is termed *intracranial pressure* (ICP). This pressure is usually very low. Intracranial pressure is considered dangerous when it rises to 15 mmHg, and cerebral herniation may occur at pressures above 25 mmHg. The pressure of the blood flowing through the brain is termed the *cerebral perfusion pressure* (CPP). Its value is obtained by subtracting the intracranial (intracerebral) pressure from the mean arterial blood pressure (MAP):

$$CPP = MAP - ICP$$

If the brain swells or if bleeding occurs inside the skull, ICP increases and the perfusion pressure decreases, resulting in cerebral ischemia (hypoxia). If the swelling of the brain is severe enough, the ICP equals the MAP and blood flow to the brain ceases. The body has a protective reflex (Cushing's response or reflex) that attempts to maintain a constant perfusion pressure. When the ICP increases, the systemic blood pressure increases to try to preserve blood flow to the brain. As the situation becomes more critical, the pulse rate drops (bradycardia), and eventually the respiratory rate declines. The pressure within the skull continues in an upward spiral until a critical point at which there is no cerebral perfusion, all vital signs deteriorate, and the patient dies. Because CPP depends on both the arterial pressure and the ICP, hypotension will have a devastating effect if the ICP is high. You must maintain a cerebral perfusion pressure of at least 70 mmHg (see earlier formula), which requires maintaining a systolic blood pressure of at least 110 to 120 mmHg in the patient with a severe head injury. Your only option may be rapid transport to a trauma center where fluids and vasopressors can be given.

CEREBRAL HERNIATION SYNDROME

When the brain swells, particularly after a blow to the head, a sudden rise in ICP may occur. This may force portions of the brain downward, obstructing the flow of cerebrospinal fluid and applying great pressure to the brain stem. This is a life-threatening situation characterized by a decreasing level of consciousness that rapidly progresses to coma, dilation of the pupil and an outward-downward deviation of the eye on the side of the injury, paralysis of the arm and leg on the side opposite the injury, or decerebrate posturing (arms and legs extended). When this is occurring the vital signs frequently reveal increased blood pressure and bradycardia (Cushing's response). The patient may soon cease all movement, stop breathing, and die. This syndrome often follows an acute epidural or subdural hemorrhage. If these signs are developing in a head injury patient, cerebral herniation is imminent and aggressive therapy is needed. As noted earlier, hyperventilation will decrease ICP. In this situation the danger of immediate herniation outweighs the risk of ischemia. *The cerebral herniation syndrome is the only situation in which hyperventilation (you must ventilate every 3 seconds) is still indicated.*

HEAD INJURIES

SCALP WOUNDS

The scalp is very vascular and often bleeds briskly when lacerated. Because many of the small blood vessels are suspended in an inelastic matrix of supporting tissue, the normal protective vasospasm that would limit bleeding is inhibited, which may lead to prolonged bleeding and significant blood loss. This can be very important in children who bleed as freely as adults but do not have the same blood volume. Though an uncommon cause of shock in an adult, a child may develop shock from a briskly bleeding scalp wound. As a general rule, *if you have an adult patient with a scalp injury who is in shock, look for another cause for the shock* (such as internal bleeding). However, do not underestimate the blood loss from a scalp wound. Most bleeding from the scalp can be easily controlled in the field with direct pressure if your exam reveals no unstable fractures under the wound.

SKULL INJURIES

Skull injuries can be linear nondisplaced fractures, depressed fractures, or compound fractures (see Figure 8-3). Suspect an underlying skull fracture in adults with a large contusion or darkened swelling of the scalp. There is very little that can be done for skull fractures in the field except to avoid placing direct pressure upon an obvious depressed or compound skull fracture. The forces that caused the skull fracture may have also caused a brain injury. Treat the brain injury with adequate oxygenation and maintain perfusion. Penetrating objects in the skull should be left in place (*not removed*) and the patient transported immediately. If your patient has a gunshot wound to the head, unless there is a clear entrance and exit wound in a perfectly linear path, assume that the bullet may have ricocheted and is lodged in the neck near the spinal cord.

Suspect child abuse when you find a child with a head injury and no clear explanation of its cause. Pay particular attention to the setting from which you rescued the child and request police or social service assistance if the circumstances suggest child abuse.

BRAIN INJURIES

CONCUSSION: A concussion implies no structural injury to the brain. The injury causes a brief disruption of neural function. There is usually a history of trauma to the head with a variable period of unconsciousness or confusion and then a return to nor-

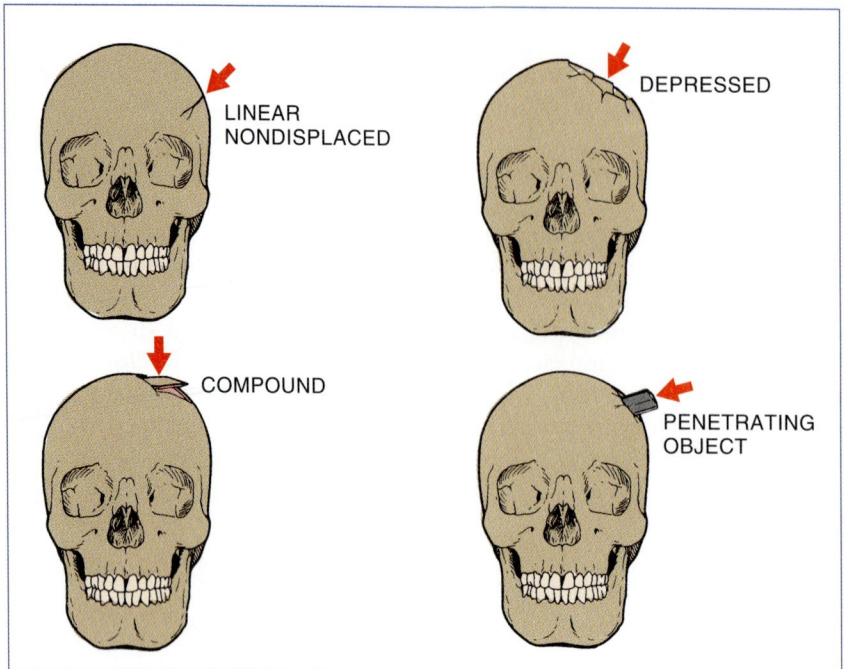

FIGURE 8-3 Types of skull fractures.

mal consciousness. There may be amnesia from the injury. This amnesia usually extends to some point before the injury (retrograde short-term amnesia), so often the patient will not remember the events leading to the injury. Short-term memory is often affected, and the patient may repeat questions over and over as if she hasn't been paying attention to your answers. There may be dizziness, headache, ringing in the ears, and/or nausea.

CEREBRAL CONTUSION: A patient with cerebral contusion (bruised brain tissue) will have a history of prolonged unconsciousness or serious alteration in level of consciousness (e.g., profound confusion, persistent amnesia, abnormal behavior). Brain swelling may be rapid and severe. The patient may have focal neurological signs or appear to have suffered a cerebrovascular accident (stroke). Depending upon the location of the cerebral contusion, the patient may have personality changes such as inappropriately rude behavior.

DIFFUSE AXONAL INJURY: This is the most common type of injury with severe blunt head trauma. The brain is injured so diffusely that there is generalized edema and subarachnoid bleeding. The subarachnoid blood causes irritation that results in fluid "leaking" into the brain and thus more edema. Seizure activity, coma, and vomiting from the irritation is common. These patients often have so much brain swelling that they develop the cerebral herniation syndrome.

ANOXIC BRAIN INJURY: Injuries to the brain from lack of oxygen (e.g., cardiac arrest, airway obstruction, near-drowning) affect the brain in a serious fashion. Following an anoxic episode, perfusion of the cortex is interrupted because of spasm that develops in the small cerebral arteries. After 4 to 6 minutes of anoxia, restoring oxygenation and blood pressure will not restore perfusion of the cortex (no-reflow phenomenon), and there will be continuing anoxic injury to the brain cells. If the brain is without oxygen for a period greater than 4 to 6 minutes, irreversible damage almost always occurs.

Hypothermia seems to protect against this phenomenon, and there have been reported cases of hypothermic patients being resuscitated after almost an hour of anoxia. Current research is directed toward finding medications that either reverse the persistent postanoxic arterial spasm or protect against the anoxic injury to the cells.

INTRACRANIAL HEMORRHAGE: Hemorrhage can occur between the skull and dura (the fibrous covering of the brain), between the dura and the arachnoid, or directly into the brain tissue.

1. *Acute epidural hematoma.* This injury is most often caused by a tear in the middle meningeal artery that runs along the inside of the skull in the temporal region. The arterial injury is often caused by a linear skull fracture in the temporal or parietal region (see Figure 8-4). Because the bleeding is arterial (although it may be venous from one of the dural sinuses), the bleeding and pressure can occur rapidly, and death may occur quickly. Symptoms of an acute epidural hematoma include a history of head trauma with initial loss of consciousness often followed by a period during which the patient is conscious and coherent (the "lucid interval"). After a period of a few minutes to several hours, the patient will develop signs of increasing ICP (vomiting, headache, altered mental status), lapse into unconsciousness, and develop body paralysis on the side opposite of the head injury (see earlier section on Cerebral Herniation Syndrome). There is often a dilated and fixed (no response to bright light) pupil on the side of the head injury. These signs are usually followed rapidly by death. The classic example is the boxer who is knocked unconscious, wakes up, and is allowed to go home, only to be found dead in bed the next morning. If the underlying brain tissue is not injured, surgical removal of the blood and ligation of the ruptured blood vessel often allows full recovery.

2. *Acute subdural hematoma.* This is caused by bleeding between the dura and the arachnoid and is associated with injury to the underlying brain tissue (see Figure 8-5). Because the bleeding is venous, pressure increases more slowly, and the diagnosis often is not apparent until hours or days after the injury. The signs and symptoms include headache, fluctuations in the level of consciousness, and focal neurologic signs (e.g., weakness of one extremity or one side of the body, altered deep tendon reflexes, and slurred speech). Because of underlying brain tissue injury, prognosis is often poor. Mortality is very high (60–90%) in patients who are comatose when found. Always suspect a subdural hematoma in an alcoholic with any degree of altered mental status following a fall. Elderly patients and those taking anticoagulants are also at high risk for this injury.

3. *Intracerebral hemorrhage.* This is bleeding within the brain tissue (see Figure 8-6). Traumatic intracerebral hemorrhage may result from blunt or penetrating injuries of the head. Unfortunately, surgery is often not helpful. The signs and symptoms depend upon the regions involved and the degree of injury. They occur in patterns similar to those that accompany a stroke. Alteration in the level of consciousness is commonly seen.

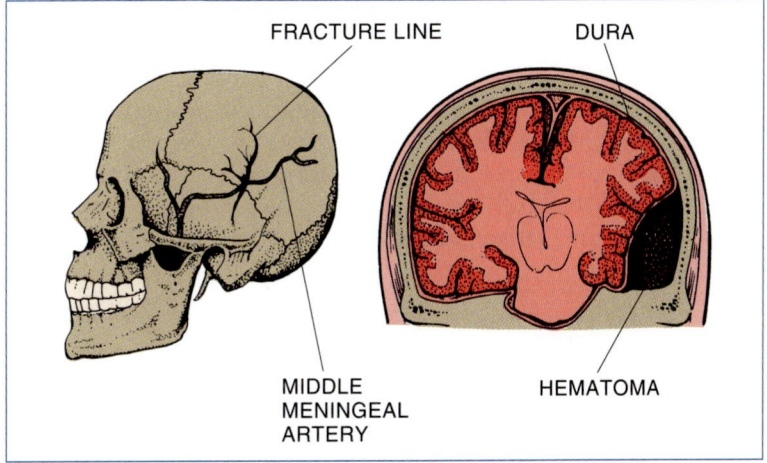

FIGURE 8-4 Acute epidural hematoma. This hemorrhage may follow injury to the extradural arteries. The blood collects between the fibrous dura and the periosteum.

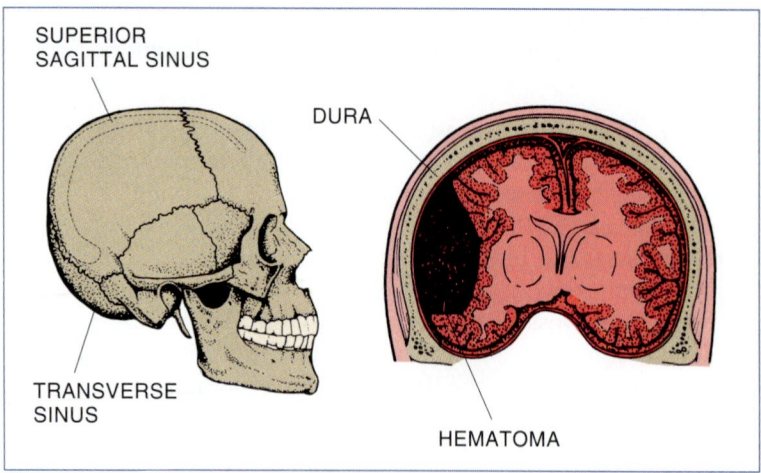

FIGURE 8-5 Acute subdural hematoma. This usually occurs following the rupture of dural veins. Blood collects and often severely compresses the brain.

FIGURE 8-6 Intracerebral hemorrhage.

EVALUATION OF THE HEAD TRAUMA PATIENT

Head-injured patients may be difficult to manage because they are often uncooperative and may be under the influence of alcohol or drugs. As a rescuer, you must pay extraordinary attention to detail and never lose your patience with an uncooperative patient. Remember that every trauma patient is initially evaluated in the same sequence (see Figure 8-7).

SCENE SIZE-UP

The results of the scene size-up will begin to determine if you have a priority patient. Dangerous *generalized mechanisms* (MVC, fall from a height) will require a complete examination (Rapid Trauma Survey) during the BTLS Primary Survey. Dangerous *focused mechanisms* (hit in head with baseball bat) will allow you to "focus" your exam (ABCs, with head and neurologic exams) rather than having to perform a complete exam.

INITIAL ASSESSMENT

The goals of the Initial Assessment are the following:

1. To determine if this is a priority patient
2. To find immediate life-threats

The Initial Assessment in the head trauma patient is to quickly determine if the patient is brain injured and, if so, is the patient's condition a deteriorating one? Obviously, a patient with a history and physical examination that indicates an epidural hematoma

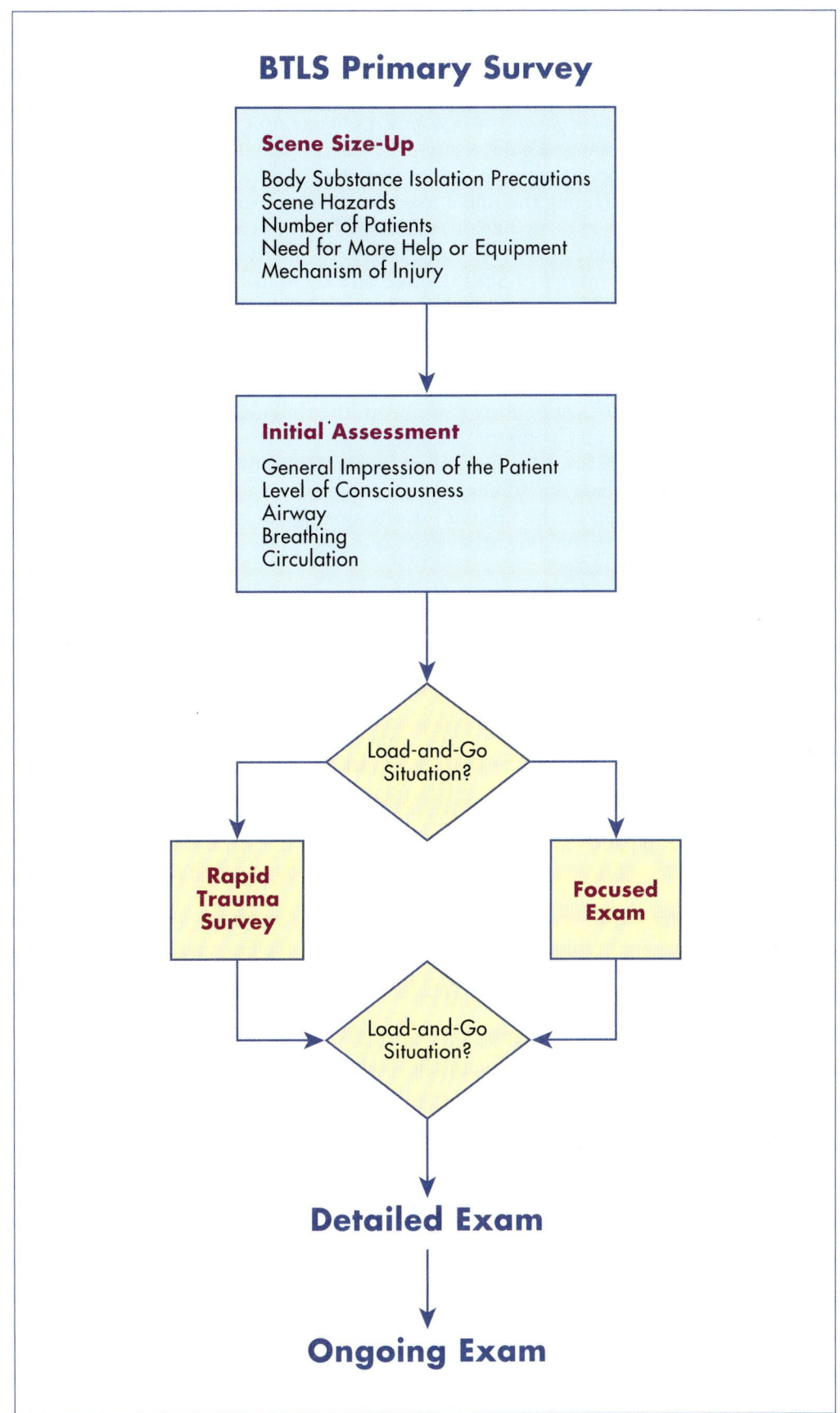

FIGURE 8-7 Steps in the assessment and management of the trauma patient.

should be transported in greater haste than one who is alert and only postconcussion. It is very important that all observations be recorded (but don't interrupt patient care to do this) because later treatment is often dictated by detection of the deterioration of clinical stability.

All patients with head or facial trauma have a C-spine injury until proven otherwise. Stabilization of the C-spine should accompany airway and breathing management. Evaluation for head injury is begun as you obtain your initial level of consciousness by speaking to the patient. During the Initial Assessment your neurological exam is limited to level of consciousness and any obvious paralysis. Level of consciousness is the most sensitive indicator of brain function. Initially, the AVPU method is quite adequate (see Chapter 2). If there is a history of head trauma, or if the initial exam reveals an altered mental status, the Rapid Trauma Survey will include a more complete neurological exam. A change in the level of consciousness is the first indicator of a brain injury or rising ICP.

Control of the airway cannot be overemphasized. The supine, restrained, and unconscious patient is prone to airway obstruction from the tongue, blood, vomit, or other secretions. Vomiting is very common within the first hour following a head injury. Protect the airway of the unconscious patient by placement of an oral or nasal airway. Be prepared for immediate suctioning. Be prepared to turn the patient on his side (maintaining stabilization of the C-spine) in the case of vomiting. Do not allow the head-injured patient to become hypoxic. Even one brief episode of hypoxia can have a significant effect on mortality.

RAPID TRAUMA SURVEY

All patients with an abnormal level of consciousness get a Rapid Trauma Survey (see Chapter 2).

HEAD: Once the initial exam is completed, continue on with the exam guided by the mechanism of injury. Begin with the scalp and quickly, but carefully, examine for obvious injuries such as lacerations or depressed or open skull fractures. The size of a laceration is often misjudged because of the difficulty in assessment through hair matted with blood. Feel the scalp gently for obvious unstable areas of the skull. If none are present, you may safely apply a pressure dressing or hold direct pressure upon a bandage to stop scalp bleeding.

A basilar skull fracture may be indicated by any of the following: bleeding from the ear or from the nose, clear fluid running from the nose, swelling and/or discoloration behind the ear (Battle's sign), and/or swelling and discoloration around both eyes (raccoon eyes) (see Figures 8-8a and 8-8b).

PUPILS: The pupils (see Figure 8-9) are controlled in part by the third cranial nerve. This nerve takes a long course through the skull and is easily compressed by brain swelling and thus may be affected by increasing ICP. Following a head injury, if both pupils are dilated and do not react to light, the patient probably has a brain-stem injury and the prognosis is grim. If the pupils are dilated but still react to light, the injury is often still reversible, so every effort should be made to quickly transport the patient to a facility capable of treating a head injury. A unilaterally dilated pupil that remains reactive to light may be the earliest sign of increasing ICP. The development of a unilaterally dilated pupil ("blown pupil") while you are observing the patient is an extreme emergency and mandates rapid transport. Other causes of dilated pupils that may or may not react to light include hypothermia, lightning strike, anoxia, optic nerve injury, drug effect (e.g., atropine), or direct trauma to the eye. *Fixed and dilated pupils signify head injury only in patients with a decreased level of consciousness.* If the patient has a normal level of consciousness, the dilated pupil is not from head injury.

Fluttering eyelids are often seen with hysteria. Slow lid closure (like a curtain falling) is rarely seen with hysteria. Testing for a blink response (corneal reflex) by touching the cornea, or by applying overly noxious stimuli to a patient to test for response to pain, are techniques that are unreliable and do *not* contribute to prehospital care.

FIGURE 8-8A Battle's sign—evidence of a posterior basilar skull fracture. *(Photo courtesy of David Effron, M.D., FACEP)*

FIGURE 8-8B Raccoon eyes—evidence of an anterior basilar skull fracture. *(Photo courtesy of David Effron, M.D., FACEP)*

EXTREMITIES: Note sensation and motor function in the extremities. Can the patient feel you touch his hands and feet? Can he wiggle his fingers and toes? If the patient is unconscious, note his response to pain. If he withdraws or localizes to the pinching of his fingers and toes, he has grossly intact sensation and motor function. This usually indicates that there is normal or only minimally impaired cortical function.

FIGURE 8-9 Pupils of the eyes.

DILATED

CONSTRICTED

UNEQUAL

Figure 8-10 Decorticate and decerebrate posturing.

Both decorticate posturing or rigidity (arms flexed, legs extended) and decerebrate posturing or rigidity (arms and legs extended) are ominous signs of deep cerebral hemispheric or upper brain-stem injury (see Figure 8-10). *Flaccid paralysis usually denotes spinal cord injury.*

To be consistent with the Revised Trauma Score and other field triage scoring systems (see Appendix F), you should be familiar with the Glasgow Coma Score (GCS), which is simple, easy to use, and has good prognostic value for eventual outcome (see Table 8-1). **In the head trauma patient, a Glasgow Coma Score of 8 or less is considered evidence of a severe brain injury.**

VITAL SIGNS (should be obtained by team member while you are performing the exam): Vital signs are extremely important in following the course of a patient with head trauma. Most importantly, they can indicate changes in ICP (see Table 8-2). You should observe and record vital signs at the end of the BTLS Primary Survey, during the Detailed Exam, and each time you perform the Ongoing Exam.

1. *Respirations:* Increasing intracranial pressure causes the respiratory rate to increase, decrease, and/or to become irregular. Unusual respiratory patterns may reflect the level of brain/brain-stem injury. Just before death the patient may develop a rapid, noisy respiratory pattern called *central neurogenic hyperventilation*. Because respiration is affected by so many factors (e.g., fear, hysteria, chest injuries, spinal cord injuries, diabetes), it is not as useful an indicator as are the other vital signs in monitoring the course of head injury.

Table 8-1 **Glasgow Coma Score.**

Eye Opening	Points	Verbal Response	Points	Motor Response	Points
Spontaneous	4	Oriented	5	Obeys commands	6
To voice	3	Confused	4	Localizes pain	5
To pain	2	Inappropriate words	3	Withdraws	4
None	1	Incomprehensible sounds	2	Abnormal flexion	3*
		Silent	1	Abnormal extension	2**
				No movement	1

*Decorticate posturing to pain
**Decerebrate posturing to pain

Table 8-2   Comparison of Vital Signs in Shock and Head Injury.

	SHOCK	HEAD INJURY WITH INCREASED INTRACRANIAL PRESSURE
Level of consciousness	Decreased	Decreased
Respiration	Increased	Varies but frequently decreased
Pulse	Increased	Decreased
Blood pressure	Decreased	Increased
Pulse pressure	Narrows	Widens

2. *Pulse:* Increasing ICP causes the pulse rate to decrease.
3. *Blood pressure:* Increasing ICP causes increased blood pressure. This hypertension is usually associated with a widening of the pulse pressure. Other causes of hypertension include fear and pain. Hypotension associated with head injury is usually caused by hemorrhagic or neurogenic shock and should be treated as if caused by hemorrhage. The brain-injured patient does not tolerate hypotension. A single instance of hypotension (BP ≤ 90 mmHg systolic) in an adult may increase the mortality rate by 150% (mortality rate even worse in children).

HISTORY (Begin obtaining the history before *and* during the exam.): It is essential to obtain as thorough a history about the event as possible. The circumstances of the head injury may be extremely important for patient management and may be of prognostic importance to the ultimate outcome. Pay particular attention to reports of near-drowning, electrocution, lightning strike, drug abuse, smoke inhalation, hypothermia, and seizures. Always inquire about the patient's behavior from the time of the head injury until the time of your arrival.

DETAILED EXAM

Head trauma patients with altered mental status are load-and-go. The Detailed Exam (see Chapter 2) will be done during transport (or not at all if a short transport).

ONGOING EXAM

Each time you perform the Ongoing Exam, record the level of consciousness, the pupil size and reaction to light, the Glasgow Coma Score, and the development (or improvement) of focal weakness or paralysis. This, along with the vital signs, provides enough information to monitor the condition of the head-injured patient. Decisions on the management of the head trauma patient are based on the changes in all the parameters of the physical and neurologic examination. You are establishing the baseline from which later judgments must be made; record your observations.

MANAGEMENT OF THE HEAD TRAUMA PATIENT

Your job is to prevent secondary injury. It is extremely important to make a rapid assessment and then transport the patient to a facility capable of managing head trauma. The important points of management in the prehospital phase are listed below:

1. Secure the airway and provide good oxygenation. The injured brain does not tolerate hypoxia, so good oxygenation is mandatory. If possible, monitor the oxygen saturation with a pulse oximeter. Maintain good ventilation (not hyperventilation) with high-flow oxygen at a rate of about one breath every 5 seconds. Because head-injured patients are prone to vomiting, be prepared to log-roll the immobilized patient and to suction the oropharynx.

2. Stabilize the patient on a spineboard. The neck should be immobilized in a rigid collar and a padded head immobilization device.
3. Record baseline observations. Record vital signs (describe rate and pattern of breathing), the level of consciousness, the pupils (size and reaction to light), the Glasgow Coma Score, and the development (or improvement) of focal weakness or paralysis. If the patient develops hypotension, suspect hemorrhage or spinal injury.
4. Monitor the observations listed above continuously. Record them every 5 minutes.

PITFALLS AND POTENTIAL PROBLEMS

1. *Cervical spine injury:* Always anticipate a C-spine injury in the head-injured patient.

2. *Hypoxia:* Patients with serious head injuries can't tolerate hypoxia or hypotension. Give high-flow oxygen and monitor oxygenation with a pulse oximeter.

3. *Shock:* Any unexplained shock in a patient with head injury is hypovolemic until proven otherwise. Treat hypotension.

4. *Seizures:* Head trauma, particularly intracranial hemorrhage, may cause seizures. The seizing patient becomes hypoxic and hyperthermic, so persistent seizure activity may worsen his condition. It is not uncommon for seizures to be related to poor airway control, so remember that oxygenation and ventilation are of extreme importance.

5. *Vomiting:* Patients with head trauma frequently vomit. You must remain alert to prevent aspiration. Keep mechanical suction available and be prepared to log-roll the patient onto his side (maintaining immobilization of the C-spine).

6. *Rapidly deteriorating condition:* A patient who shows rapid deterioration of vital signs or rapid progression of brain injury (e.g., unresponsive, dilated pupil; decorticate or decerebrate posturing; or a decrease in the Glasgow Coma Score of ≥2 after correction of hypoxia and hypotension) should be transported rapidly to a trauma center. This is the only situation in which hyperventilation is still indicated. Hyperventilation, while known to cause ischemia, may decrease brain swelling temporarily. Although a desperate measure, this might buy enough time to get the patient to surgery that might be lifesaving. Radio ahead so that a neurosurgeon can be available and the operating room prepared by the time you arrive at the hospital.

7. *Nontraumatic causes of altered mental status:* Remember that hypoglycemia, hypoxia, cardiac dysrhythmias, and drugs can also cause altered mental status. If possible, check the blood glucose level on all patients with altered mental status.

SUMMARY

Head injury is a serious complication of trauma. In order to give your patient the best chance of recovery, you should be familiar with the important anatomy of the head and central nervous system and understand how trauma to the various areas presents clinically. The most important steps in the management of the head-injured patient are rapid assessment, good airway management, prevention of hypotension, rapid transport to a trauma center, and frequent Ongoing Exams. In no other area of trauma care is the recording of repeated assessments so important to future management decisions.

BIBLIOGRAPHY

1. Chestnut, R. M., L. F. Marshall, M. R. Klauber, and others. "The Role of Secondary Brain Injury in Determining Outcome from Severe Head Injury." *Journal of Trauma*, Vol. 34 (1993), pp. 216–222.

2. LaHaye, P.A., G. F. Gade, and D. P. Becker. "Injury to the Cranium." In *Trauma,* eds. K. L. Mattox, E. E. Moore, and D. V. Feliciano, pp. 237–249. Norwalk, CT: Appleton & Lange, 1988.

3. Rimel, R.W., J. A. Jane, and R. F. Edlich. "An Injury Severity Scale for Comprehensive Management of Central Nervous System Trauma." *Annals of Emergency Medicine* (December 1979), pp. 64–67.

4. The Brain Trauma Foundation. *Guidelines for the Management of Severe Head Injury.* Oakwork, IL: American Association of Neurological Surgeons, 1995.

CHAPTER 9

Spinal Trauma

James J. Augustine, M.D., F.A.C.E.P.

(Photo courtesy of Bob Page, NREMT-P)

OBJECTIVES

UPON COMPLETION OF THIS CHAPTER, YOU SHOULD BE ABLE TO:

1. Explain the normal anatomy and physiology of the spinal column and spinal cord.
2. Describe mechanisms of injury that indicate spinal column immobilization may be required.
3. Describe the process of spinal immobilization from extrication through transportation, including airway maintenance.
4. Describe history and assessment criteria that identify patients who do not need spinal immobilization.
5. Give examples of special situations for which spinal immobilization techniques may need to be altered.
6. Using the clinical evaluation, differentiate neurogenic shock from hemorrhagic shock.

Spinal cord injury is a devastating and life-threatening result of modern trauma. If a patient with a spinal cord injury survives, it will cost an average of $1.5 million to support him for a lifetime. The management of trauma patients requires continuous vigilance for spinal injuries. However, the use of spinal immobilization is also associated with complications. EMS providers must skillfully assess the mechanism of injury and the patient to provide safe and appropriate immobilization to trauma patients. In this chapter we review the process of evaluating the mechanism of injury, providing a structured assessment, and packaging, treating, and transporting patients with known or potential spinal cord injuries.

THE NORMAL SPINAL COLUMN AND CORD

SPINAL COLUMN

It is important to differentiate the spinal column from the spinal cord. The spinal column is a bony tube composed of 33 vertebrae (see Figure 9-1). It supports the body in an upright position, allows the use of our extremities, and protects the delicate spinal cord. The column's 33 vertebrae are aligned in an S-shaped curve and are identified by their location: 7 cervical (the C-spine), 12 thoracic (the T-spine), 5 lumbar (the L-spine), and the remainder fused together as the posterior portion of the pelvis (sacrum and coccyx). The vertebrae are then numbered in each section from the head down to the pelvis. The third cervical vertebra from the head is designated C-3, the sixth is called C-6, and so forth. The thoracic vertebrae are T1 through T12, and each attaches to 1 of the 12 pairs of ribs. The lumbar vertebrae are numbered L1 through L5, with L5 being the last vertebra above the pelvis.

The vertebrae are each separated by a fibrous disc that acts as a shock absorber. The alignment is maintained by strong ligaments between the vertebrae and by muscles that run along the length of the bony column from head to pelvis (these are the muscles strained when one lifts improperly). The S-curve is most prominent at the C5–C6 and T12–L1 levels in adults, making these areas the most susceptible to injury.

SPINAL CORD

The spinal cord is an electrical conduit, an extension of the brain stem that continues down to the level of the first lumbar vertebra. The cord is 10 to 13 mm in diameter and

FIGURE 9-1   Anatomy of the spinal column.

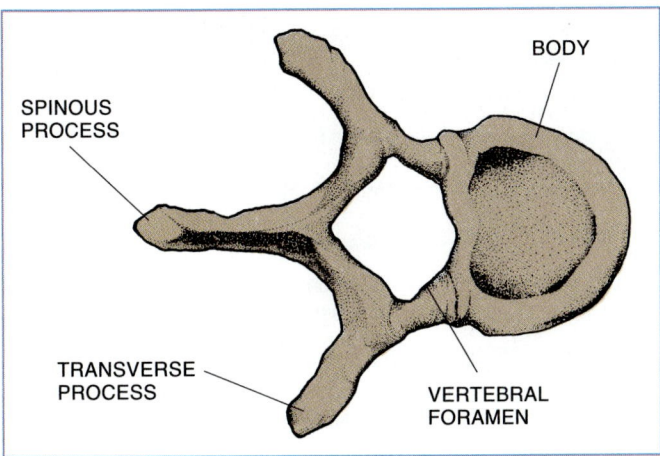

FIGURE 9-2 Vertebra viewed from above. The spinal cord passes through the vertebral foramen.

is suspended in the middle of the vertebral foremen (see Figure 9-2). The cord is soft and flexible, like a cotton rope, and is surrounded and bathed by cerebrospinal fluid along its entire length. The fluid and the flexibility provide some protection to the cord from injury. The cord is composed of specific bundles of nerve tracts, much as a rope is composed of individual strands of fiber that are arranged in a predictable manner. The spinal cord passes down the vertebral canal and gives off pairs of nerve roots that exit at each vertebral level (see Figure 9-3). The roots lie next to the intervertebral discs and the lateral part of the vertebrae, making the nerve roots susceptible to injury when trauma occurs in these areas (see Figure 9-4). The nerve roots carry sensory signals from the

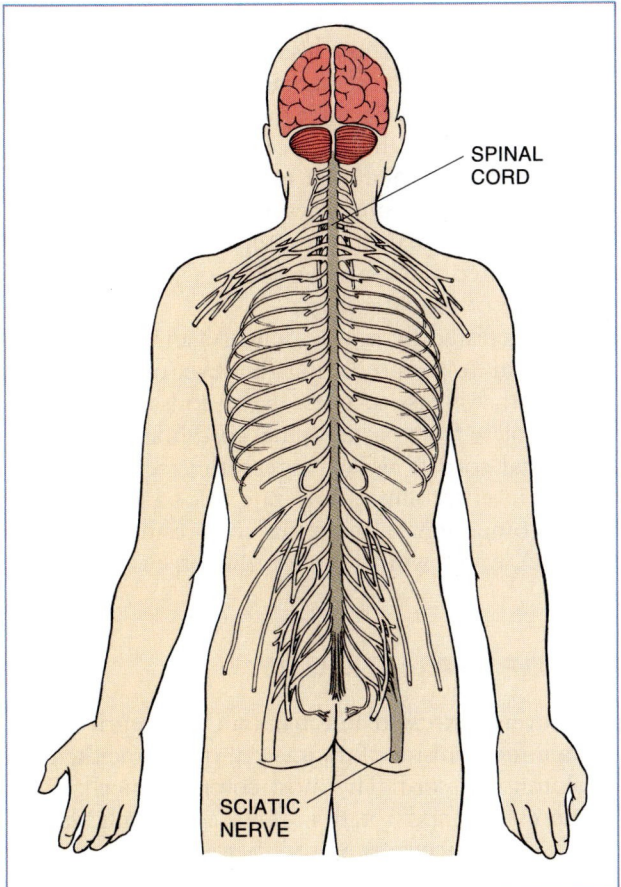

FIGURE 9-3 Spinal cord. The spinal cord is a continuation of the central nervous system outside the skull.

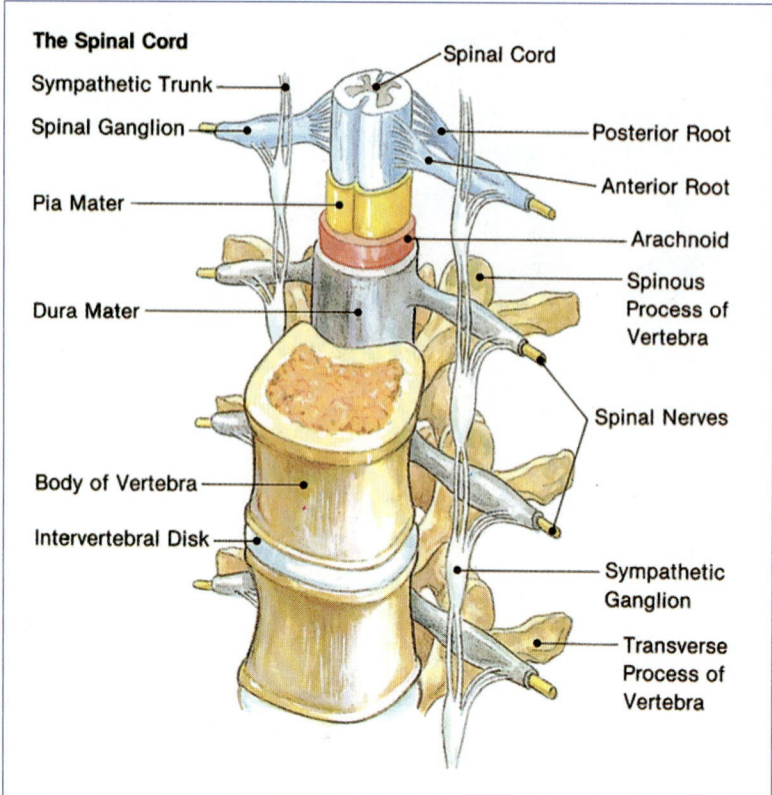

The Spinal Cord

Sympathetic Trunk

Spinal Ganglion

Pia Mater

Dura Mater

Body of Vertebra

Intervertebral Disk

Spinal Cord

Posterior Root

Anterior Root

Arachnoid

Spinous Process of Vertebra

Spinal Nerves

Sympathetic Ganglion

Transverse Process of Vertebra

FIGURE 9-4   Relationship of spinal cord to vertebra. Note how the nerve roots exit between the vertebrae.

body to the spinal cord and then to the brain. The roots also carry signals from the brain to specific muscles, causing them to move. These signals pass back and forth rapidly, and some are strong enough to cause actions on their own, called *reflexes*. This reflex system is demonstrated by a strong tap below the knee causing the lower leg to jerk. If you accidentally put your finger on a hot burner, your reflex system causes your hand to move even before your brain receives the warning message. Strong signals also can overwhelm the spinal cord's ability to keep signals moving separately to the brain, which is why a trauma patient with a fractured hip may complain of knee pain or a patient with a ruptured spleen may complain of shoulder pain.

The integrity of spinal cord function is tested by motor, sensory, and reflex functions. The level of sensory loss is most accurate for predicting the level of spinal cord injury. Muscle strength is another function that is easy to assess in the conscious patient. Reflexes are helpful for distinguishing complete from partial spinal cord injuries, but are best left for hospital assessment. The spinal cord is also an integrating center for the autonomic nervous system, which assists in controlling heart rate, blood vessel tone, and blood flow to the skin. Injury to this component of the spinal cord results in neurogenic shock (commonly called *spinal shock*), which will be discussed later.

MECHANISMS OF BLUNT SPINAL INJURY

A normal healthy spinal column can be severely stressed and maintain its integrity without damage to the spinal cord. But certain mechanisms of trauma can overcome the protective defenses, injuring the spinal column and cord. The most common mechanisms are hyperextension, hyperflexion, compression, and rotation. Less commonly, lateral stress or distraction will injure the cord. These mechanisms and their subsequent blunt injuries are illustrated in Table 9-1.

Table 9-1   **Mechanisms of Blunt Spinal Injury.**

DESCRIPTION	DIAGRAM	EXAMPLES
Hyperextension Excessive posterior movement of head or neck		Face into windshield in MVC Elderly person falling to the floor Football tackler Dive into shallow water
Hyperflexion Excessive anterior movement of head onto chest		Rider thrown off of horse or motorcycle Dive into shallow water
Compression Weight of head or pelvis driven into stationary neck or torso		Dive into shallow water Fall of greater than 10 to 20 feet onto head or legs
Rotation Excessive rotation of the torsoor head and neck, moving one side of the spinal column against the other		Rollover MVC Motorcycle accident
Lateral Stress Direct lateral force on spinal column, typically shearing one level of cord from another		"T-bone" MVC Fall
Distraction Excessive stretching of column and cord		Hanging Child inappropriately wearing shoulder belt around neck Snowmobile or motorcycle under rope or wire

SPINAL COLUMN INJURY

The head is a relatively large ball perched on top of the neck. Sudden movement of the head or trunk will produce flexion, extension, or lateral stresses that may damage the bony or connective tissue components of the spinal column. Injury to the spinal column is like injury to any other bone in the body. It requires a significant amount of force, unless there is a preexisting weakness or defect in the bone. For that reason, the elderly and those with severe arthritis are at higher risk for spinal injuries. Like other bone injuries, pain is the most common symptom, but it may be unnoticed by the patient. This is especially true if the patient has other painful injuries. At the site of a bone injury, local muscle spasm may occur. Injury to individual nerve roots can result from bony spinal column injury, with resulting localized pain, paralysis, or sensory loss. Therefore, signs that may indicate spinal injury include back pain, tenderness along the spinal column, pain with movement of the back, obvious deformity or wounds of the back, paralysis, weakness, or paresthesias (tingling or burning feeling to the skin).

Fortunately, spinal column injury can occur without injuring the spinal cord. Statistically, only 14% of all *column* injuries have evidence of spinal *cord* damage. In the cervical spine region it is much more common to have cord injury, with almost 40% of column injuries having cord damage. Only 63% of spinal *cord* injuries have evidence of spinal *column* damage. This means that almost half of the patients with some degree of paralysis will have no obvious bone or ligament injury to the spinal column (even by x-ray). The unconscious trauma patient carries a high risk (15–20%) of spinal column injury. The injuries are frequently in more than one place, and therefore the unconscious trauma patient should be immediately and consistently immobilized.

SPINAL CORD INJURY

Spinal cord injury is devastating. It is most common in patients aged 16 to 35, typically those who are active and productive. There are 15,000 to 20,000 spinal cord injuries in the United States each year—56% involve MVCs (including pedestrians), 19% falls, 12% penetrating wounds, 7% recreational activities, and the remaining 6% are from all other causes. Under age 16, falls are the most common cause of spinal injury. Under age 8, the relatively large size of the head makes the upper end of the cervical cord the most common site of injury, which can be extremely devastating.

Spinal cord injury results in a defective signal conducting function, presenting as a loss of motor function and reflexes, loss or change in sensation, and/or neurogenic shock. The delicate structure of the spinal cord's nerve tracts make it very sensitive to any form of trauma. What is termed *primary damage* occurs at the time of the trauma itself. Primary damage results from the cord being cut, torn, or crushed or by its blood supply being cut off. This damage is usually irreversible despite the best trauma care. *Secondary damage* occurs from hypotension, generalized hypoxia, injury to blood vessels, swelling, or compression of the cord from surrounding hemorrhage. Emergency efforts are directed at preventing secondary damage through attention to the ABCs and careful packaging of the patient.

NEUROGENIC SHOCK

Injury to the cervical or thoracic spinal cord can produce high-space shock (see Chapter 7). Neurogenic shock results from the malfunction of the autonomic nervous system in regulating blood vessel tone and cardiac output. Classically, this means a patient is hypotensive, with normal skin color and temperature and an inappropriately slow heart rate. In the healthy patient, blood pressure is maintained by the controlled release of catecholamines (epinephrine and norepinephrine) from the adrenal glands. Catecholamines cause constriction of the blood vessels, increase the heart rate and the strength of heart contraction, and stimulate sweat glands. Sensors in the aortic and carotid arteries monitor the blood pressure. The brain and spinal cord signal the adrenal glands to release catecholamines to keep the blood pressure in the normal range. In pure *hemorrhagic shock,* these sensors detect the hypovolemic state and compensate by constricting the blood vessels and speeding the heart rate. The high levels of catecholamines cause pale skin, tachycardia, and sweating. The mechanism of shock from spinal cord injury is just the opposite. There is no significant blood loss, but there is no signal going to the adrenals (the spinal cord cable is out), so no catecholamines are released. The blood vessels dilate, the blood pools, and the blood pressure cannot be maintained. The brain cannot correct this because it cannot get the message to the adrenal glands. The patient with neurogenic shock cannot show the signs of pale skin, fast heart beat, and sweating because the cord injury prevents release of catecholamines. Since neurogenic shock is caused by blood vessel dilation, it may respond to antishock trousers that work by circumferential compression of the blood vessels in the lower part of the body. This use is discouraged unless you are *sure* that there is no internal bleeding (review Chapter 7). Intra-abdominal injury and bleeding can be difficult to determine because the patient with neurogenic shock usually has no sensation in the abdomen. The multiple-trauma patient may have both neurogenic shock and hemorrhagic shock. Neurogenic shock is a diagnosis of exclusion, after all other potential causes of shock have been ruled out. In the prehospital setting, neurogenic shock is treated in the same way as hemorrhagic shock (see Chapter 7).

PATIENT ASSESSMENT

All trauma patients are evaluated in the same manner using the assessment priority plan, of which evaluation of spinal cord function is a part. Clues to spinal cord injury are given in Table 9-2. Parts of the neurological exam are performed during the BTLS Primary Survey. The remainder of the neurological exam is performed during the Detailed Exam. This is frequently done after the patient is loaded into the ambulance. The patient that requires extrication is a special situation. Before beginning extrication you should check sensory and motor function in the hands and feet, and document these

Table 9-2   **Clues to Spinal Cord Injury on Patient Assessment.**

The following are indicators that the spine may have been injured. These patients *may* need to be immobilized (see Figure 9-9).

MECHANISM OF INJURY:

- Blunt trauma above the clavicles
- Diving accident
- Motor vehicle or bicycle accident
- Fall
- Stabbing or impalement anywhere near the spinal column
- Shooting or blast injury to the torso
- Any violent injury with forces that could act on the spinal column or cord

WHEN THE PATIENT COMPLAINS OF:

- Neck or back pain
- Numbness or tingling
- Loss of movement or weakness

WHEN ON EXAM YOU FIND:

- Pain on movement or palpation of the spinal column
- Obvious deformity of back or spinal column
- Guarding against movement of back
- Loss of sensation
- Weak or flaccid muscles
- Loss of control of bladder or bowels
- Erection of the penis (priapism)
- Neurogenic shock

findings later in the written report. Not only does this pre-extrication neurological exam alert you to any spinal injury; it also provides documentation on whether there was loss of function before extrication was begun. Sadly, there are a few reports of patients who have claimed that their spinal injuries were caused by their rescuers. You will not have time to perform the pre-extrication neurological exam on the patient who requires rapid extrication.

The neurological exam is described in more detail in Chapters 2 and 8, but we will review the exam of the peripheral nervous system here. This exam is kept brief and simple. If the conscious patient can move his fingers and toes, the motor nerves are intact. Anything less than normal sensation (tingling or decreased sensation) is suspicious for cord injury. The unconscious patient may withdraw if you pinch his fingers and toes. If so, you have demonstrated intact motor and sensory nerves and thus an intact cord. This does not mean you don't have to immobilize the patient. All unconscious trauma patients should be immobilized. Flaccid paralysis, even in the unconscious head injury patient, usually means spinal cord injury. Document these important findings.

PATIENT MANAGEMENT

Based on the mechanism of injury, it is appropriate to place the head and neck in a neutral position as you first evaluate the patient. The spine is treated as a long bone, with its top being the head and its bottom being the pelvis. The spine is then maintained in stabilization until the patient is securely strapped to the long backboard. The purpose of spinal immobilization is to to minimize spinal movement to avoid aggravating any spinal cord or column injury. Preparation for managing spinal column or cord injury can begin when you are dispatched to the scene of a motor vehicle collision, fall, explosion, head injury, or neck injury.

The critically unstable patient may require rapid extrication from a vehicle or a structure. This form of extrication is used for patients whose Primary Survey indicates a critical degree of ongoing danger. Indications for rapid emergency extrication are the following:

1. Scene size-up identifies a condition that may immediately endanger the patient or rescuers:
   a. Fire or immediate danger of fire
   b. Danger of explosion
   c. Danger of drowning
   d. Structure in danger of collapse
   e. Continuing toxic exposure

2. Initial exam of the patient identifies a condition that requires immediate intervention that cannot be done in the entrapped area:
   a. Airway obstruction that cannot be relieved by modified jaw thrust or finger sweep
   b. Cardiac or respiratory arrest
   c. Chest or airway injuries requiring ventilation or assisted ventilation
   d. Deep shock or bleeding that cannot be controlled

Rapid extrication requires multiple rescuers who remove the patient along the long axis of the body, using their hands to maintain cervical immobilization and to minimize spinal movement (see Chapter 10). When the rapid extrication technique is used, the written report should be carefully reviewed to insure appropriate documentation of the technique and its indication.

The most easily applied and readily available method of cervical immobilization is with your hands or knees. The rescuer's hands should be placed to stabilize the neck in relation to the long axis of the spinal column (see Figure 9-5). "Pulling traction" is not a prehospital option, and the term *traction* is not an appropriate description for the immobilization of the spine. Traction will usually result in further instability of any

FIGURE 9-5   Stabilize in a neutral position.

spinal column injury. The correct approach is stabilization, without pulling on the neck. When immobilizing the body on a backboard, the neutral in-line position allows the most room for the spinal cord, so that is the optimal position.

If an appropriately sized cervical spinal immobilization collar is available, you can place it on the patient as airway assessment is being done. These one- or two-piece collars are not definitive devices for cervical spine control, but should be used only as a reminder that cervical immobilization is necessary and to prevent gross neck movement. The rescuer's hands can be removed only when the head and spinal column have been definitively immobilized on a spinal board with an attached immobilization device. For the conscious patient, positioning the head and neck in the position of patient comfort is a good guideline. Patient management then proceeds with Initial Assessment and interventions.

C-spine immobilization is completed only when the head and body are secured to a long backboard. Inadequate strapping will torque the neck against the body if the patient moves, rolls, is dropped, or is rotated. Once the patient is secured to the board, a rescuer must be present and capable of rolling the board if the patient begins to vomit or loses his airway. Placing and strapping a patient on the board effectively eliminates the patient's ability to protect the airway, and therefore the rescuer is responsible. This rule continues in effect in the emergency department, where an emergency staff person must assume responsibility for airway protection. Definitive immobilization occurs when the body is strapped securely to the board with cushions, blanket, or towel rolls maintaining the head, C-spine, torso, and pelvis in-line. In the past, sandbags have been used for head immobilization and perform well when the patient is kept supine. However, if the board is tilted or the patient and the board are rotated (to prevent aspiration when the patient vomits), the weight of the sandbags may cause an extreme amount of head movement (see Figure 9-6). Therefore sandbags are an extremely poor option for prehospital immobilization. Lighter-weight bulky objects, such as towel rolls, blanket rolls, or head cushions, are better tools for this job. When applied properly, these devices allow removal of the front portion of the cervical collar and observation of the neck, as in the patient with open neck wounds. Commercial cervical immobilization devices may be left in place on the spineboard.

There are some patients (frightened children and patients with altered mental status) who will struggle so violently that they defeat your attempts to eliminate spinal movement. There may be no good solution to this. The Reeves sleeve (see Figure 9-8a) may be the best device to immobilize the combative adult patient.

Recent studies have suggested that a true neutral position for an adult is obtained with the use of 1 to 2 inches of occipital padding on a long backboard. This slightly elevates the head and tends to make the patient more comfortable. This is accomplished with the head pad on a cervical immobilization device or the padding that is used with many backboard devices. Some padding is a necessity in elderly patients whose necks have a natural flexed posture.

PROPER IMMOBILIZATION

PROPER IMMOBILIZATION. LIGHTWEIGHT CUSHIONS BESIDE HEAD.

IMPROPER IMMOBILZATION WITH SANDBAGS. GROSS HEAD MOVEMENT WHEN BOARD IS ROLLED.

FIGURE 9-6
Proper immobilization.

In certain situations, once the patient is packaged onto the backboard, the board and patient may have to be rolled up onto his or her side (see Figure 9-7a through c). Women who are more than 20 weeks pregnant should always be transported with the backboard tilted 20 to 30 degrees to the patient's left side to keep the uterus off the inferior vena cava. Patients with airway problems are better transported on their side. This is especially critical when there is uncontrolled bleeding into the airway or if there is massive face or neck trauma. In these situations gravity helps drain fluids out of the airway and may prevent aspiration if the patient vomits. Because of the danger of vomiting and aspiration, unconscious patients should be transported rolled to the side.

LOG-ROLL

This technique is used for moving a patient onto a backboard. It is commonly used because it is easy to perform with a minimum number of rescuers. As yet no movement technique has been devised that maintains complete spinal immobilization while mov-

FIGURE 9-7A   Pregnant patient immobilized and board tilted to the left.

FIGURE 9-7B Patient in vacuum backboard turned on side. Notice that the body is maintained in a straight line.

FIGURE 9-7C Immobilized patient turned on side. This may be necessary for the patient who is vomiting. The patient must be secured well enough so that the spine remains straight.

ing a patient onto a backboard. Properly performed, the log-roll technique will minimize movement of the spinal column as well as any other technique.

The log-roll technique moves the spinal column as a single unit with the head and pelvis. It can be performed on patients lying prone or supine. Using three or more rescuers, controlled by the rescuer at the patient's head, the patient (with her arms by her side) is rolled onto the uninjured side, a board is slid underneath, and the patient is rolled face up onto the board. The log-roll technique is then completed when the patient's chest, pelvis, and head are secured to the board. Log-roll may be modified for patients with painful arm, leg, and chest wounds who need to be rolled onto their uninjured side. The side to which you turn the patient during the log-roll procedure is not critical and can be changed in situations in which you can only place the backboard on one side of the patient. The log-roll technique is useful for most trauma patients, but for those patients with a fractured pelvis it may aggravate the injury to roll their weight onto the pelvis. If the pelvic fracture appears stable, the log-roll should be carefully performed, turning the patient onto the uninjured side (if it can be identified). Patients with obviously unstable pelvic fractures should not be log-rolled but rather should be lifted carefully onto a board by four or more rescuers. The scoop stretcher could also be used for unstable pelvic fractures.

SPINAL IMMOBILIZATION DEVICES

There is a wide range of devices currently marketed to provide immobilization for injured patients (Figure 9-8a through e). No device has yet been proven to excel over all others, and no device will ever be produced that can immobilize all patients. No device is better than the crew that is using it, so training with the available tools is the most critical factor in providing good patient care.

FIGURE 9-8A Reeves sleeve.

FIGURE 9-8B Miller body splint.

FIGURE 9-8C Pediatric immobilization device.

FIGURE 9-8D   Kendrick immobilization device.

FIGURE 9-8E(1)   Short backboard.

FIGURE 9-8E(2)   Short backboard.

THE COMPLICATIONS OF SPINAL IMMOBILIZATION

There are complications of immobilizing a patient to a board. The patient will be uncomfortable and will often complain of head and low back pain that is directly related to being immobilized on the hard backboard. The head and airway are in a fixed position, which can produce airway compromise and aspiration if the patient vomits. Obese patients and those with congestive heart failure can suffer life-threatening hypoxia. On a rigid board there is uneven skin pressure that can result in pressure sores. Lifting the patient and the board can cause injuries to rescue personnel. Immobilization should be applied appropriately to those who will most likely benefit, and it should be avoided if not necessary.

INDICATIONS FOR SPINAL IMMOBILIZATION

Recent studies have documented the circumstances under which spinal column or cord injury is very unlikely, and therefore you can manage the patient without spinal immobilization. These studies have resulted in a clinical pathway referred to as the Maine Protocol for Spinal Immobilization (see Figure 9-9; written by Peter Goth, M.D.). You must assess the mechanism of injury, interview and examine the patient, then use this

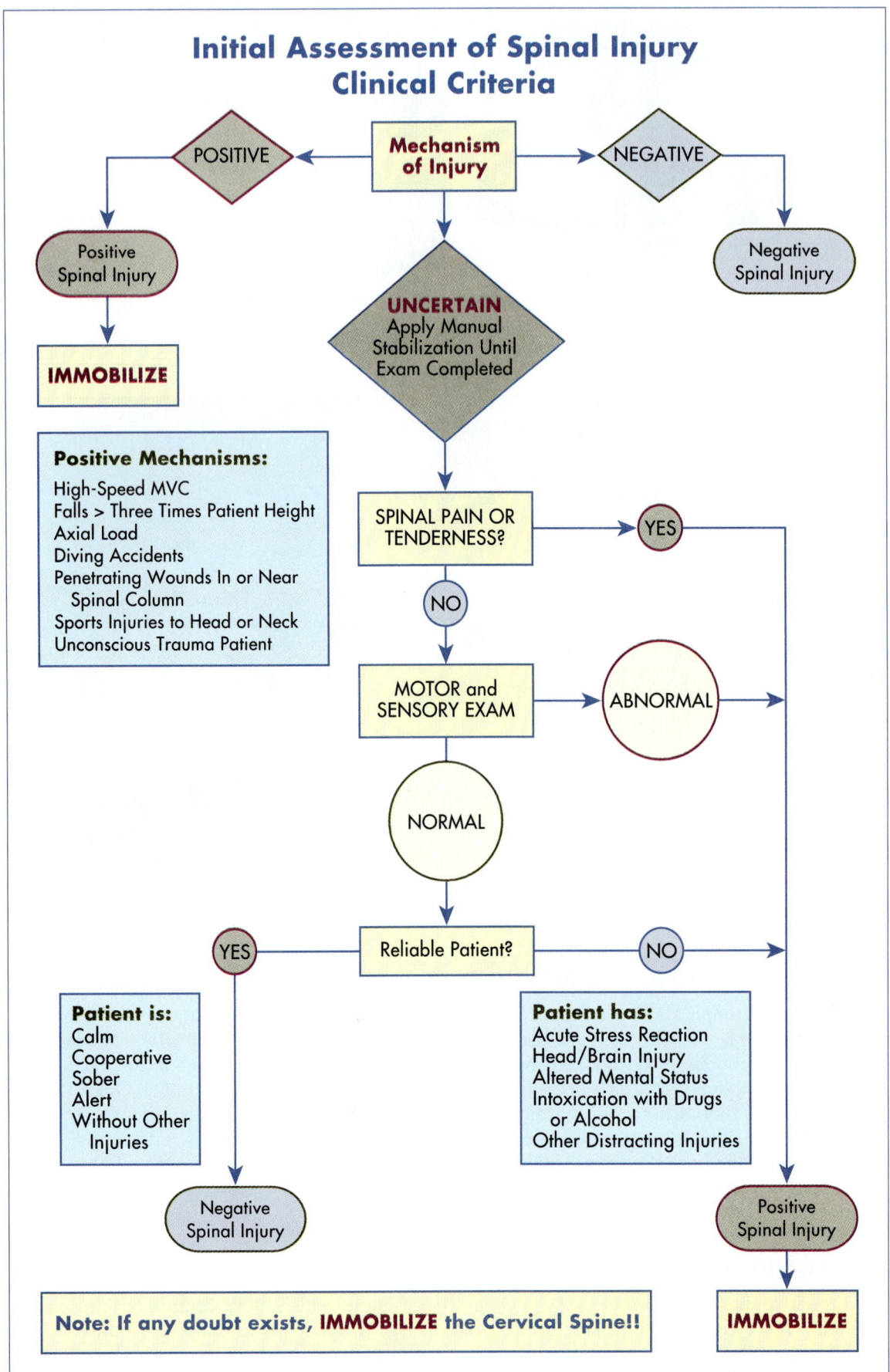

FIGURE 9-9 Decision tree for spinal immobilization. (*Reprinted by permission of Peter Goth, M.D.*)

information to determine which patients need immobilization. From the scene survey, history and assessment come the clues that identify those patients who do not need spinal immobilization.

Under the Maine pathway, the rescuer first assesses the mechanism of injury. Immobilization is not required if there is no mechanism of injury that would damage the spine (foot crushed by a car). If the mechanism is a high-risk event, the patient is immobilized regardless of other clinical findings. These high-risk situations include high-speed MVCs, falls of greater than three times the patient's height, penetrating wounds into or near the spinal column, sports injuries to the head or neck, diving accidents, and any trauma situation in which the patient is still unconscious. If the danger of spinal injury is uncertain (ground-level fall, low-speed "fender bender"), the rescuer will manually stabilize the spine and then assess the patient for signs of spinal injury. The patient must be reliable enough to understand the EMS provider and answer the questions accurately, so children and patients with altered mental status or acute stress reactions are excluded. Then the patient is assessed for evidence of intoxication or distracting injuries that may not allow the patient to clearly feel the pain associated with a spinal injury. The patient is asked if he has pain in the area of the spinal column. If no pain is present in the neck or back, and no other injuries are so painful as to distract the patient from comprehending back or neck pain, the rescuer then carefully examines the spinal column and performs a neurological exam. If there is any tenderness on palpation of the spinal column area or if the patient complains of midline pain when asked to move his back, the patient is immobilized. The patient is also immobilized if there are alterations in the motor or sensory exam.

If the patient has no high-risk mechanism of injury, no alteration of mental status, no distracting injuries, is not intoxicated, has no pain or tenderness along the spine, and has no neurological deficits, the patient may be treated and transported without spinal immobilization. This protocol has proven effective in research studies but, like all protocols, must be approved for local use by Medical Direction and followed up with a quality assurance program.

AIRWAY INTERVENTION

When the rescuer performs spinal immobilization in any manner, the patient loses some of her ability to maintain her own airway. As mentioned earlier, the rescuer must then assume this responsibility until the patient has a controlled airway or has the spinal column cleared in the emergency department and is released from the immobilizing equipment (see Figure 9-10). This is particularly critical in children, who have a greater potential for vomiting and aspiration after a traumatic injury.

Airway manipulations in the trauma patient require careful application. Current research indicates that any airway intervention will cause some movement of the spinal column. In-line manual stabilization is the most effective manner for minimizing this movement. Cervical collars are only a partial assist to prevent movement. Your priority plan should include *manual immobilization,* then the use of the airway control method that you are most skilled at performing. When weighing the risks and benefits of each airway procedure, recall that the risk of dying with an uncontrolled airway is greater than the risk of inducing spinal cord damage using a careful approach to airway intervention.

SPECIAL IMMOBILIZATION SITUATIONS

You must be prepared to stabilize the spinal column of all patients who sustain major trauma. In some patients (see below), traditional techniques must be modified to provide safe and effective spinal immobilization:

1. Patients in closed spaces
2. Patients in water
3. Patients in a prone or standing position

FIGURE 9-10 You are responsible for the patient's airway once the patient is immobilized.

4. Pediatric patients
5. Elderly patients
6. Patients in protective helmets
7. Very large or obese patients
8. Patients with disfiguring or penetrating neck wounds

Closed-space rescues are performed in a manner appropriate for the clinical condition of the patient. The only general rules that can be applied to these rescues are to prevent gross C-spine movement and to move patients in-line with the long axis of the body (see Figure 9-11). Safety of the rescuer is of prime importance in all closed-space rescues. Asphyxia, poison gas, or cave-ins are dangers of closed-space rescue. Never enter a closed space until you are properly trained, equipped (air pack, safety line, etc.), and sure of scene safety.

You can perform water rescues by moving the patient in-line, preventing gross cervical movement. When the rescuers are in a stable position for immobilizing the patient, the backboard is floated under the patient, and the patient is then secured and removed from the water (see Figure 9-12). Safety of both rescuers and patients is of paramount importance.

Prone and standing patients are immobilized in a manner that minimizes spinal column movement, ending with the patient in the conventional supine position. Prone patients are log-rolled onto a long board with careful coordination of head and chest rescuers. Seated patients may be immobilized using short backboards or their commercial adaptations. Used appropriately, these provide initial stabilization of the cervical and thoracic spine and then facilitate the movement of the patient onto a long backboard. Standing patients may be placed against the long board while upright and then, while supporting the head and torso, the board is gently lowered to the supine position and the patient strapped in place.

1. SPLINT HEAD AND NECK WITH ARMS.

2. ROLL PATIENT OVER INTO SUPINE POSITION.

3. ENSURE AIRWAY AND BREATHING
   • PATIENT NOT BREATHING: BEGIN RESCUE BREATHING (WITH A MASK IF POSSIBLE) AND RESCUE FROM WATER AS SOON AS POSSIBLE.
   • PATIENT BREATHING: SLIDE BACKBOARD UNDER PATIENT.

4. APPLY A RIGID EXTRICATION COLLAR.

5. TIE DOWN TORSO, THEN HEAD AND NECK WITH STRAPS OR CRAVATS. FLOAT BOARD TO EDGE OF WATER.

6. REMOVE PATIENT FROM WATER (WITH AS MUCH ASSISTANCE AS NEEDED).

NOTE: THE TECHNIQUE FOR REMOVING PATIENTS FROM WATER ASSURING INTEGRITY OF THE SPINE IS CRITICAL. INTERVIEWS OF PARAPLEGICS WHOSE PARALYSIS RESULTED FROM WATER-RELATED ACCIDENTS INDICATE THAT MANY WERE ABLE TO TREAD WATER AFTER THE INJURY AND PRIOR TO BEING IMPROPERLY REMOVED FROM THE WATER.

FIGURE 9-12 Extricating suspected diving accident patient.

FIGURE 9-13   Most children require padding under back
and shoulders to keep the cervical spine in a neutral position.
(Courtesy of Bob Page, NREMT-P)

It is best to provide initial immobilization of the pediatric patient with the your hands, and then use cushions or towel rolls to help secure the child on an appropriate board or device. Some pediatric trauma specialists suggest padding beneath the *back and shoulders* on the board in a child under the age of 3 (see Figure 9-13). These children normally have a relatively large head that flexes the neck when placed on a straight board. Padding under the back and shoulders will prevent this flexion and also make the child more comfortable. With the exception of load-and-go situations, children who have sustained trauma while restrained in a child safety seat may be packaged in the safety seat for transport to the hospital (See Pediatric BTLS textbook). Using towel or blanket rolls, cloth tape, and a little reassurance, you can secure the child in the safety seat and then belt the seat into the ambulance (see Figure 9-14). This technique minimizes movement of the child and provides a secure method for child transport in the ambulance. Some autos come with built-in child-restraint seats that cannot be removed. Children in such seats will have to be extricated onto a spine board or another pediatric immobilization device. For the child who is frightened and struggling there may be no good way to obtain immobilization. Careful reassurance, the presence of a comforting

FIGURE 9-14   Infant immobilized in car seat. *(Courtesy of David Effron, M.D., FACEP)*

family member, and gentle management will help prevent more complications and further struggling.

Elderly patients require flexibility in packaging techniques. Many elderly patients have arthritic changes of the spine and very thin skin. Such patients will be very uncomfortable when placed on a backboard. Some arthritic spines are so rigid that the patient cannot be laid straight on the board, and some elderly patients have rigid flexion of the neck that will result in a large gap between the head and the board. You can make use of towels, blankets, and pillows to pad the elderly patient and prevent movement and discomfort on the backboard (see Figure 9-15). This is a situation in which the vacuum backboard (which conforms to the shape of the patient) works very well.

Athletes and cyclists wearing helmets are another special set of patients. Large helmets used in these sports must be removed at some point to permit complete assessment and care. Helmets used in different sports present different management problems for rescuers. Football and ice hockey helmets are custom fitted to the individual. Unless special circumstances exist, such as respiratory distress coupled with an inability to access the airway, the helmet should not be removed in the prehospital setting. Athletic helmet design will generally allow easy airway access once the face guard is removed. The face guard can easily be removed with a screwdriver or cut off using rescue scissors (see Figure 9-16). The athlete wearing shoulder pads has his neck in a neutral position when on the backboard with the helmet in place. If the helmet is removed, padding must be inserted under the head to keep the neck from extending (see Figure 9-17a and b). After arrival at the emergency facility the C-spine can be x-rayed with the helmet in place. Once the spine is evaluated, the helmet can be removed by stabilizing the head and neck, removing the cheek pads, releasing the air inflation system, and then sliding the helmet off in the usual manner.

In contrast, motorcycle helmets often must be removed in the prehospital setting. The removal technique is modified to accommodate the different design. Motorcycle helmets are often designed with a continuous solid face guard that limits airway access. These helmets are not custom designed and frequently are poorly fitted to the patient. Their large size will usually produce significant neck flexion if left in place when the patient is placed on a backboard (see Figure 9-18). Motorcycle accidents are usually associated with much more violent forces than are athletic injuries. The motorcycle helmet will make it difficult to stabilize the neck in a neutral position, may obstruct access to the airway, and may hide injuries to the head or neck; it should be removed in the prehospital setting using the techniques described in Chapter 10.

Very large or obese patients may not fit appropriately in standard equipment. You must be flexible, even using sheets of plywood and head cushions or towel rolls to stabilize. In cold-weather climates, patients in bulky warm clothing will need to be snugly secured to prevent excessive movement.

Patients with penetrating or disfiguring wounds of the neck or lower face must be continually observed. Cervical collars will prevent continued examination of the wound site and may compromise the airway in wounds with expanding hematomas or subcuta-

FIGURE 9-15 Elderly patients often require padding under the shoulders and head to stabilize the spine.

FIGURE 9-16   The face guard of football helmets can be removed with rescue scissors or a screwdriver.

FIGURE 9-17   (a) Patients with shoulder pads and helmets are usually best immobilized with the helmet in place. The spine is maintained in a neutral position with a minimum of movement. (b) Patients with shoulder pads must have padding under the head to maintain a neutral position if the helmet is removed.

FIGURE 9-18   Full-face helmets obstruct access to the patient's airway. Notice that the helmet flexes the neck in a patient who is not wearing shoulder pads. *(Courtesy of Bob Page, NREMT-P)*

neous air. If the mandible is fractured, the collar may again cause airway compromise. Therefore, for patients with these injuries, it may be wise to avoid collars, using manual stabilization and then head cushion devices or blanket rolls for cervical immobilization.

Trauma patients with paralysis or neurogenic shock have lost vascular control and thus cannot control blood flow to the skin. They may lose heat rapidly so it is important for you to prevent hypothermia.

SUMMARY

Spinal cord injury is a devastating consequence of modern-day trauma. Unstable or incomplete damage to the spinal column or cord is not predictable, and therefore trauma patients who are unconscious or have any dangerous mechanism of injury affecting the head, neck, or trunk should have their spines immobilized. Those trauma patients with uncertain mechanisms may not require immobilization if they meet the physical exam criteria. Special trauma cases may require special immobilization techniques. Once the patient is immobilized, he loses some ability to control his airway so you must be prepared at all times to intervene should the patient vomit or have evidence of airway compromise.

BIBLIOGRAPHY

1. Aprahamian, L. "Experimental Cervical Spine Injury Model: Evaluation of Airway Management and Splinting Techniques." *Annals of Emergency Medicine,* Vol. 13 (1994), p. 584.

2. Goth, P. C. *Spine Injury, Clinical Criteria for Assessment and Management,* pp. 1–36. Augusta, ME: Medical Care Development, 1994

3. Henry, G. L., and N. Little. *Neurologic Emergencies.* New York: McGraw-Hill, 1985.

4. Illinois State Medical Association. *Guidelines for Helmet Fitting and Removal in Athletes.* Chicago: The Association, 1990.

5. Jacobs, L. M. "Prospective Analysis of Acute Cervical Spine Injury." *Annals of Emergency Medicine,* Vol. 15 (1986), p. 44.

6. Johnson, R. M. "Clinical Orthoses, A Guide to Their Selection and Use." *Clinical Orthopedics,* Vol. 154 (1981), p. 34.

7. Majernick, T. G. "Cervical Spine Movement During Orotracheal Intubation." *Annals of Emergency Medicine,* Vol. 15 (1986), p. 417.

8. Podolsky, S. "Efficacy of Cervical Spine Immobilization Methods." *Journal of Trauma,* Vol. 23 (1983), p. 461.

9. Seaman, P. J. "Log-Roll Technique." *Emergency,* Vol. 24 (1992), p. 18.

CHAPTER 10

Spine Management Skills

Donna Hastings, EMT-P

OBJECTIVES

UPON COMPLETION OF THIS CHAPTER, YOU SHOULD BE ABLE TO:

1. Explain when to use spinal immobilization.
2. Perform spinal immobilization with a short backboard.
3. Perform log-rolling of a patient onto a long backboard.
4. Properly secure a patient to a long backboard.
5. Immobilize a patient from a standing position.
6. Immobilize the head and neck when a neutral position cannot be safely attained.
7. Perform emergency rapid extrication.
8. Explain when helmets should and should not be removed from injured patients.
9. Properly remove a motorcycle helmet.
10. Demonstrate proper stabilization of the neck in patients who are wearing shoulder pads and helmets.

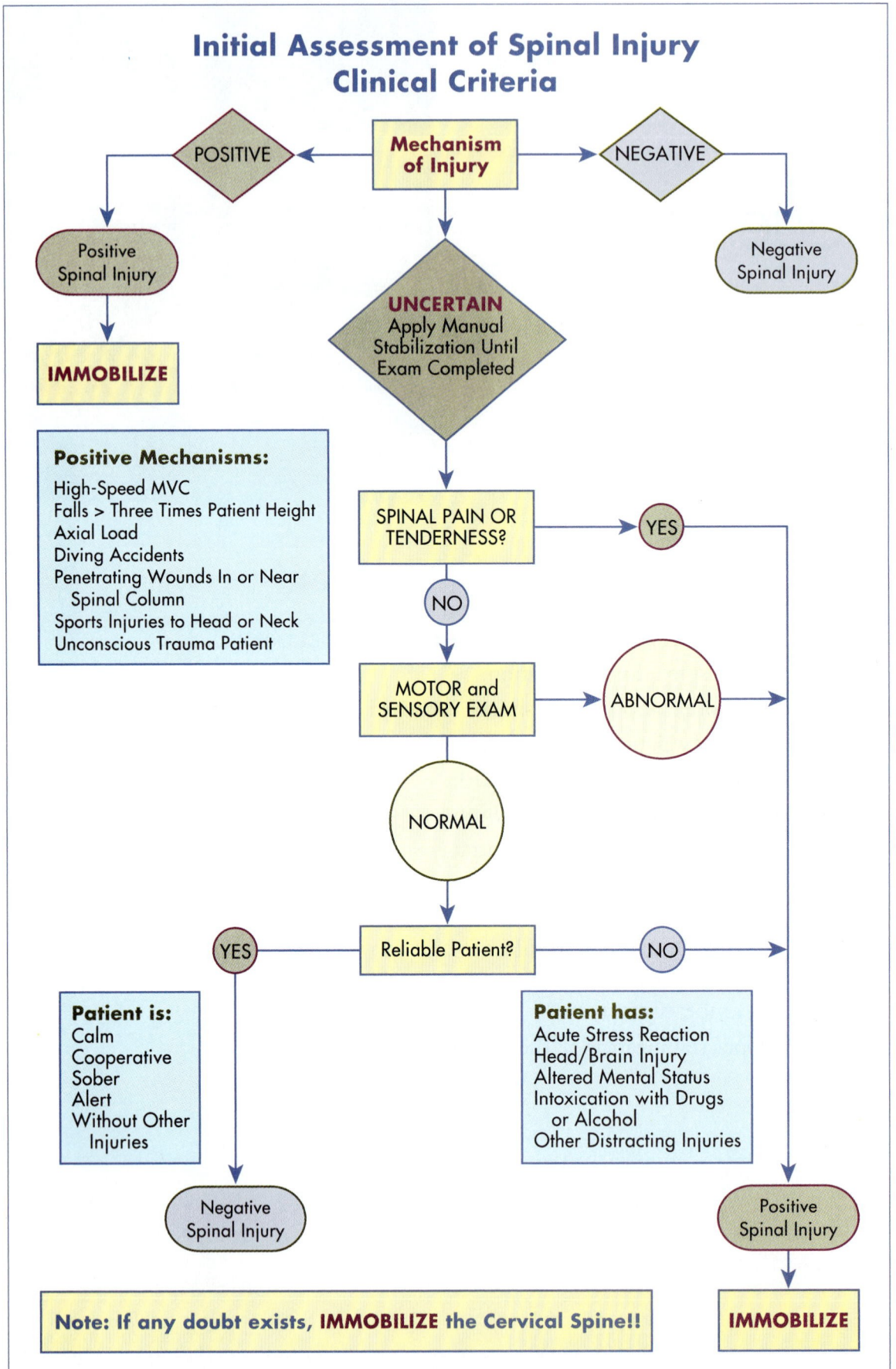

FIGURE 10-1   Decision tree for spinal immobilization. *(Reprinted by permission of Peter Goth, M.D.)*

PATIENTS REQUIRING SPINAL IMMOBILIZATION

The goal of spinal immobilization is to limit movement of the spine and thus prevent further harm. When in doubt, immobilize the patient. Patients requiring immobilization must have it done before they are moved at all. In the case of an automobile collision, you must immobilize the patients before removing them from the wreckage. More movement is involved in extrication than at any other time, so you must immobilize the neck and spine before beginning extrication. *Remember:* Traction can cause permanent paralysis. You are stabilizing the spine, not pulling on it. Except in situations requiring rapid emergency extrication, always try to document sensation and motor function in the extremities before you move the patient.

SPINAL IMMOBILIZATION USING THE SHORT BACKBOARD

The short backboard is used for patients who are in a position (such as in a motor vehicle) that does not permit use of the long backboard. There are several different devices of this type: some of them have different strapping mechanisms from the one explained here. You must first practice with a piece of equipment before employing it in an emergency.

TECHNIQUE

(These steps are illustrated in Figures 10-2 through 10-14.)

1. Remember that the priorities of evaluation and management are done before the immobilization devices go on.
2. One rescuer must, if possible, station himself behind the patient, place his hands on either side of the patient's head, and immobilize the neck in a neutral position. This step is part of the ABCs of evaluation. It is done at the same time that you begin evaluation of the airway.
3. When you have the patient stable enough to begin splinting, you must apply a semirigid extrication collar. If you have enough people, this can be done while someone else is doing the ABCs of evaluation and management. If you have limited help, apply the collar after finishing the Rapid Trauma Survey, but before transferring the patient to the backboard.
4. Position the short backboard behind the patient. The first rescuer continues to immobilize the neck while the short backboard is being maneuvered into place. The patient may have to be moved forward to get the backboard into place; great care must be taken so that moves are coordinated to support the neck and back.
5. Secure the patient to the board: there are usually three straps for this. Place the short strap under the armpits and across the upper chest as an anchor. Bring each long strap over a leg, down between both legs, back around the outside of the same leg, across the chest, and then attach them to the opposite upper strap that was brought across the shoulders.
6. Tighten the straps until the patient is held securely.
7. Secure the patient's head to the board by wide tape or elastic wraps around the forehead. Apply padding under the neck and head as needed to maintain a neutral position.
8. Transfer the patient to a long backboard. Turn the patient so that her back is to the opening through which she is to be removed. Someone must support her legs so that the upper legs remain at a 90-degree angle to her torso. Position the long backboard through the opening until it is under the patient. Lower the patient back onto the long backboard and slide the patient and the short backboard up into position on the long backboard. Loosen the straps on the short board and allow the patient's legs to extend out flat and then retighten the straps. Now secure her to the long backboard with straps, and secure her head with a padded immobilization device. When she is secured in this way, it is possible to turn the whole board up on its side if the patient has to vomit. The patient should remain securely immobilized.

FIGURE 10-2   Stabilize the neck and perform the primary survey.

FIGURE 10-3   Apply a semirigid extrication collar.

FIGURE 10-4   Position the short backboard behind the patient. Coordinate all movement so that the spine is kept immobile.

FIGURE 10-5 Apply straps and tighten securely.

FIGURE 10-6 Turn the patient carefully; then lower onto the long backboard.

FIGURE 10-7 Slide the patient and the short backboard up into position on the long backboard. Loosen the straps and allow the legs to extend out flat; then retighten the straps. Secure the patient and the short backboard to the long backboard. Apply padded immobilization device to secure the patient's head and neck.

FIGURE 10-8 Kendrick extrication device. Stabilize the neck and perform the Primary Survey.

FIGURE 10-9 Apply a semirigid extrication collar.

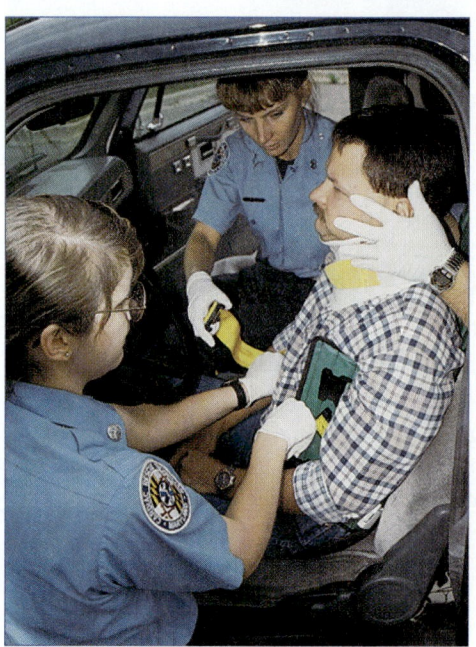

FIGURE 10-10 Position the device behind the patient. Coordinate all movements so that the spine is kept immobile. Position the chest panels up well into the armpits.

FIGURE 10-11   Tighten the chest straps.

FIGURE 10-12   Loop each leg strap around the ipsilateral (same side) leg and back to the buckle on the same side. Fasten snugly.

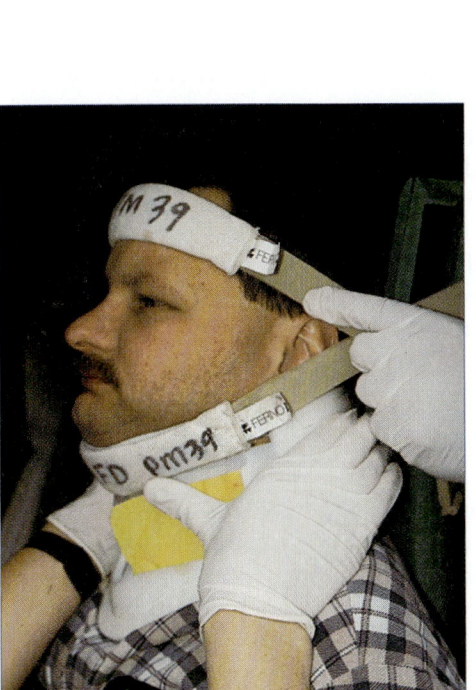

FIGURE 10-13   Apply firm padding as needed between the head and the headpiece to keep the head in a neutral position. Bring the head flaps around to the side of the head and secure firmly with straps, tape, or elastic wrap.

FIGURE 10-14 Turn the patient and the device as a unit; then lower onto a long backboard. Slide the patient and the device up into position on the board. Loosen the leg straps and allow the legs to extend out flat; then retighten the straps. Secure the patient and the device to the backboard.

POINTS TO REMEMBER

1. When you are placing the straps around the legs on a male, do not catch the genitals in the straps.
2. Do not use the short backboard as a "handle" to move the patient. Move both patient and board as a unit.
3. When you are applying the horizontal strap (long backboard) around a woman, place the upper strap above her breasts and under her arms, not across the breasts.
4. When you are applying the lower horizontal strap on a pregnant woman, place it across the pelvis and not across the uterus.
5. You may need to modify how you attach the straps, depending on injuries.
6. Secure the patient well enough so that no motion of the spine will occur if the board is turned on its side. Do not tighten straps so tight that they interfere with breathing.

RAPID EXTRICATION

Patients left inside vehicles following a collision are usually stabilized on a short backboard (or extrication device) and then transferred onto a long backboard. Although this is the best way to extricate anyone with a possible spinal injury, there are certain situations in which a more rapid method must be used. *Note:* BTLS International offers a one-day course (BTLS Access) on basic extrication from automobiles. Call 1-800-495-2857 for information.

SITUATIONS REQUIRING EMERGENCY RAPID EXTRICATION

This procedure is used only in situations in which the patient's life is in immediate danger. Whenever you use this procedure, it should be noted in the written report, and you should be prepared to defend your actions at a review by your Medical Director. You should perform rapid extrication if your BTLS Primary Survey of the patient identifies a condition that requires *immediate* intervention that cannot be done in the vehicle.

EXAMPLES

1. Airway obstruction that you cannot relieve by jaw thrust or finger sweep
2. Cardiac or respiratory arrest
3. Chest or airway injuries requiring ventilation or assisted ventilation
4. Deep shock or bleeding that you cannot control

TECHNIQUE

(These steps are illustrated in Figures 10-15 through 10-22.)

1. One rescuer must, if possible, station himself behind the patient, place his hands on either side of the patient's head, and stabilize the neck in a neutral position. This step is part of the ABCs. It is done at the same time that you begin evaluation of the airway.
2. Do a Rapid Survey; then quickly apply a cervical collar. You should have the collar with you when you begin.
3. If your BTLS Primary Survey of the patient reveals one of the situations above, go to the emergency rapid extrication technique. This requires at least four and preferably five or six persons to perform well.
4. Immediately slide the long backboard onto the seat and, if possible, at least slightly under the patient's buttocks.
5. A second rescuer stands close beside the open door of the vehicle and takes over control of the cervical spine.
6. Rescuer 1 or another rescuer is positioned on the other side of the front seat ready to rotate the patient's legs around.
7. Another rescuer is also positioned at the open door by the patient. By holding the upper torso, he works together with the rescuer holding the legs to turn the patient carefully.
8. The patient is turned so that his back is toward the backboard. His legs are lifted and his back is lowered to the backboard. The neck and back are not allowed to bend during this maneuver.
9. Using teamwork, the patient is carefully slid to the full length of the backboard and his legs are carefully straightened.
10. The patient is then moved immediately away from the vehicle (to the ambulance if available), and resuscitation is begun. He is secured to the backboard as soon as possible.

FIGURE 10-15   Stabilize the neck and perform the Primary Survey.

FIGURE 10-16   Apply a semirigid extrication collar.

FIGURE 10-17   Slide the long backboard onto the seat and slightly under the patient.

FIGURE 10-18   A second rescuer stands close beside the open door of the vehicle and takes over control of the cervical spine.

FIGURE 10-19 Carefully supporting the neck, torso, and legs, the rescuers turn the patient.

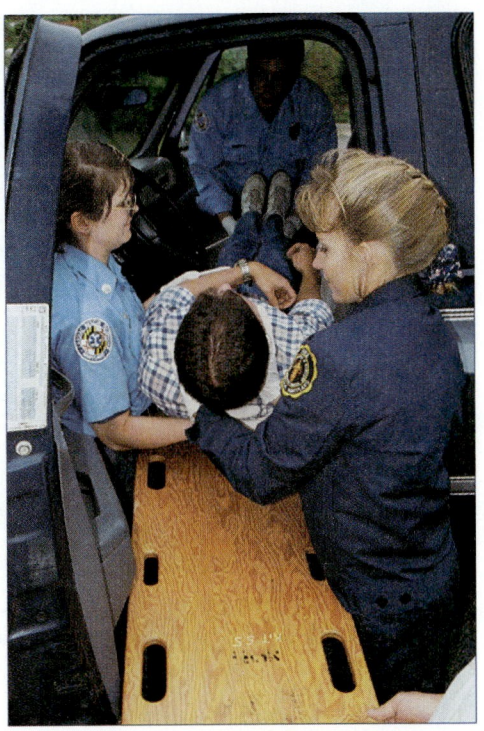

FIGURE 10-20 The legs are lifted and the back is lowered to the backboard.

FIGURE 10-21 Carefully slide the patient to the full length of the backboard.

FIGURE 10-22 The patient is immediately moved away from the vehicle and into the ambulance, if available. Secure the patient to the backboard as soon as possible.

You should also perform rapid extrication when your scene size-up identifies a condition that may *immediately* endanger the patient or you (see Figure 10-23). In some of these situations you may not have time to use any technique other than pulling the patient to safety. This is an example of "desperate situations may demand desperate measures." You must not sacrifice your life in a dangerous situation; use good judgment.

EXAMPLES

1. Fire or immediate danger of fire
2. Danger of explosion
3. Rapidly rising water
4. Structure in danger of collapse
5. Continuing toxic exposure

FIGURE 10-23 Example of a situation in which you may have to perform rapid extrication. *(Courtesy of Bonnie Meneely, R.N.)*

SPINAL IMMOBILIZATION USING THE LONG BACKBOARD

LOG-ROLLING THE SUPINE PATIENT

(These steps are illustrated in Figures 10-24 through 10-32.)

1. Rescuer 1 maintains the spine immobilized in a neutral position. Do not apply traction. Grasp the patient's shoulders at the neck and gently position the patient's head between the rescuer's forearms. A semirigid extrication collar is applied. Even with the collar in place, Rescuer 1 maintains the head and neck in a neutral position until the log-rolling maneuver is completed.
2. The patient is placed with her legs extended in the normal manner and her arms (palms inward) extended by her sides. The patient will be rolled up on one arm with that arm providing proper spacing and acting as a splint for the body.
3. The long backboard is positioned next to the body. If one arm is injured, place the backboard on the injured side so that the patient will roll upon the uninjured arm.
4. Rescuers 2 and 3 kneel at the patient's side opposite the board.
5. Rescuer 2 is positioned at the midchest area and Rescuer 3 is by the upper legs.
6. With his knees, Rescuer 2 holds the patient's near arm in place. He then reaches across the patient and grasps the shoulder and the hip, holding the patient's far arm in place. Usually, it is possible to grasp the patient's clothing to help with the roll.
7. With one hand, Rescuer 3 reaches across the patient and grasps the hip. With his other hand, he holds the feet together at the lower legs.
8. When everyone is ready, Rescuer 1 gives the order to log-roll the patient.
9. Rescuer 1 carefully keeps the head and neck in a neutral position (anteroposterior as well as laterally) during the roll.
10. Rescuers 2 and 3 roll the patient up on her side toward them. The patient's arms are kept locked to her side to maintain a splinting effect. The head, shoulders, and pelvis are kept in line during the log-roll.
11. When the patient is upon her side, Rescuer 2 (or Rescuer 4, if available) quickly examines the back for injuries.
12. The backboard is now positioned next to the patient and held at a 30- to 45-degree angle by Rescuer 4. If there are only three rescuers, the board is pulled into place by Rescuer 2 or 3. The board is left flat in this case.
13. When everybody is ready, rescuer 1 gives the order to log-roll the patient onto the backboard. This is accomplished by keeping head, shoulders, and pelvis in-line.

FIGURE 10-24   Rescuer 1 maintains the neck immobilized in a neutral position.

FIGURE 10-25 The long backboard is positioned beside the patient.

FIGURE 10-26 Rescuer 2 and Rescuer 3 assume their positions at the patient's side opposite the board.

FIGURE 10-27 The patient is carefully rolled upon her side.

FIGURE 10-28 Quickly examine the back for injuries.

FIGURE 10-29 If another person is available, he positions the backboard next to the patient at a 30- to 45-degree angle.

FIGURE 10-30   If no other help is available, Rescuer 2 or 3 positions the backboard and leaves it flat.

FIGURE 10-31   At Rescuer 1's order, the patient is rolled onto the backboard. All movements are coordinated so that the spine is kept straight at all times.

FIGURE 10-32   Log-roll completed.

FIGURE 10-33 New vacuum mattress products hold promise for the packaging of suspected spinal injuries.

LOG-ROLLING THE PRONE PATIENT WITH AIRWAY CONSIDERATIONS

The status of the airway is critical for decisions on the order in which the log-rolling procedure is done. There are three clinical situations that dictate how you should proceed.

1. The patient who is not breathing or who is in severe respiratory difficulty must be log-rolled immediately to manage the airway. Unless the backboard is already positioned, you must log-roll the patient, manage the airway, and then transfer the patient to the backboard (in a second log-rolling step) when ready to transport.
2. The patient with profuse bleeding of the mouth or nose must not be turned to the supine position. Profuse upper airway bleeding in a supine patient is a guarantee of aspiration. This patient will have to be carefully immobilized and transported prone or on his side, allowing gravity to help keep the airway clear (see Chapter 4, Figure 4-8). The vacuum backboard would be very useful here (see Figure 10-33).
3. The patient with an adequate airway and respiration should be log-rolled directly onto a backboard.

LOG-ROLLING THE SUPINE PATIENT WHO HAS AN ADEQUATE AIRWAY

(See Figure 10-34.)

1. Rescuer 1 immobilizes the neck in a neutral position. When placing the hands on the head and neck, the rescuer's thumbs always point toward the patient's face. This prevents having the rescuer's arms crossed when the patient is log-rolled. A semirigid extrication collar is applied.
2. A BTLS Rapid Trauma Survey is done (including the back), and the patient is placed with his legs extended in the normal manner and his arms (palms inward) extended by his sides. The patient will be rolled up on one arm, with that arm acting as a splint for the body.
3. The long backboard is positioned next to the body. The backboard is placed on the side of first rescuer's lower hand (if the first rescuer's lower hand is on the patient's right side, the backboard is placed on the patient's right side). If the arm next to the backboard is injured, carefully raise the arm above the patient's head so he does not roll on the injured arm.
4. Rescuers 2 and 3 kneel at the patient's side opposite the board.
5. Rescuer 2 is positioned at the midchest area, and Rescuer 3 is by the upper legs.

FIGURE 10-34 When immobilizing the neck of the prone (or supine) patient, your thumbs always point toward the face (not the occiput). This prevents having your arms crossed when the patient is rolled over.

6. Rescuer 2 grasps the shoulder and the hip. Usually, it is possible to grasp the patient's clothing to help with the roll.
7. Rescuer 3 grasps the hip (holding the near arm in place) and the lower legs (holding them together).
8. When everyone is ready, Rescuer 1 gives the order to log-roll the patient.
9. Rescuer 1 carefully keeps the head and neck in a neutral position (anteroposterior as well as laterally) during the roll.
10. Rescuers 2 and 3 roll the patient up on his side away from them. The patient's arms are kept locked to his side to maintain a splinting effect. The head, shoulders, and pelvis are kept in line during the roll.
11. The backboard is now positioned next to the patient and held at a 30- to 45-degree angle by Rescuer 4. If there are only three rescuers, the board is pulled into place by Rescuer 2 or 3. The board is left flat in this case.
12. When everyone is ready, Rescuer 1 gives the order to roll the patient onto the backboard. This is accomplished by keeping the head, shoulders, and pelvis in-line.

When log-rolling the patient with chest or abdominal injuries, try to roll onto the uninjured side. The roll should be executed quickly enough to not compromise lung expansion. When log-rolling a patient with injures to the lower extremities, position Rescuer 2 at the feet of the patient to provide in-line support to the injured leg(s) during the log-roll. Again try to roll onto the uninjured side. The side to which you turn the patient during the log-roll procedure is not critical and can be changed in situations where you can only place the backboard on one side of the patient. The log-roll technique is useful for most trauma patients, but for those patients with a fractured pelvis it may aggravate the injury to roll their weight onto the pelvis. If the pelvic fracture appears stable, the log-roll should be carefully performed, turning the patient onto the uninjured side (if it can be identified). Patients with obviously unstable pelvic fractures should not be log-rolled but rather should be lifted carefully onto a board using four or more rescuers. The scoop stretcher is a supplemental device that may help move the patient onto the backboard when specific injuries complicate log-rolling.

SECURING THE PATIENT TO THE BACKBOARD

There are several different methods of securing the patient using straps. Two examples of commercial devices for full body immobilization are the Reeves sleeve and the Miller body splint. The Reeves sleeve is a heavy-duty sleeve into which a standard backboard will slide into. Attached to this sleeve are the following:

1. A head immobilization device
2. Heavy vinyl-coated nylon panels that go over the chest and abdomen and are secured with seat belt-type straps and quick-release connectors
3. Two full-length leg panels to secure the lower extremities
4. Straps to hold the arms in place

5. Six handles for carrying the patient
6. Metal rings (2,500-lb strength) for lifting the patient by rope

When the patient is in this device, he remains immobilized when lifted horizontally, vertically, or even carried on his side (like a suitcase). This device is excellent for the confused, combative patient who must be restrained for his safety (see Figure 10-35).

The Miller body splint is a combination backboard, head immobilizer, and body immobilizer. Like the Reeves sleeve, it does an excellent job of full-body immobilization with a minimum of time and effort.

There are several different commercial strapping systems available. As with all equipment, you should become familiar with your strapping system before using it in an emergency situation.

APPLYING AND SECURING A LONG BACKBOARD TO A STANDING PATIENT

METHOD 1

1. Rescuer 1 stands behind the patient and immobilizes the head and neck in a neutral position. Rescuer 2 applies a semirigid extrication collar while Rescuer 1 maintains immobilization in a neutral position.
2. Resucer 2 places a long backboard on the ground behind the patient.
3. Other rescuers stabilize the shoulders and trunk and allow the patient to carefully sit down on the backboard.
4. The patient is carefully lowered back onto the backboard, maintaining stabilization of the head, neck, and trunk.
5. The patient is centered on the backboard and secured.

METHOD 2

1. Rescuer 1 stands in front of the patient and immobilizes the head and neck in a neutral position. Rescuer 2 applies a semirigid cervical collar while Rescuer 1 continues to maintain immobilization in a neutral position.
2. Rescuer 2 places a long backboard against the patient's back.
3. Rescuer 3 secures the patient to the board using nylon straps. These must include an anchor strap high on the chest as well as ones that cross over the shoulders and the pelvis and legs to prevent movement when the board is tilted down.

FIGURE 10-35 Patient immobilized in a Reeves sleeve. Combative patients can have their arms enclosed within the panels and straps.

4. Rescuer 3 places padding behind the patient's head to maintain a neutral position, and applies and secures a blanket roll or commercial head immobilizer using elastic wraps or wide tape.
5. Rescuers 2 and 3 carefully tilt the board back onto a stretcher and secure the legs.

IMMOBILIZING THE HEAD AND NECK WHEN A NEUTRAL POSITION CANNOT BE ATTAINED SAFELY

If the head or neck is held in an angulated position and the patient complains of pain on any attempt to straighten it, you should immobilize it in the position found. The same is true of the unconscious patient whose neck is held to one side and does not easily straighten with a gentle attempt. You cannot use a cervical collar or commercial head immobilizer in this situation. You must use pads or a blanket roll and careful taping to immobilize the head and neck in the position found.

HELMET MANAGEMENT

IMPORTANT POINTS ABOUT HELMET REMOVAL

1. Patients wearing both helmets and shoulder pads can usually have their spines maintained in a more neutral position by leaving the helmet in place and padding and taping the helmet to the backboard.
2. Patients wearing helmets but no shoulder pads can usually have their spines maintained in a more neutral position by removing the helmet.
3. Face masks on helmets can be removed with screwdrivers or rescue scissors.
4. Full-face motorcycle-type helmets must be removed to evaluate and manage the airway.

REMOVING A MOTORCYCLE HELMET FROM A PATIENT WITH A POSSIBLE CERVICAL SPINE INJURY

(See Figure 10-36.)

1. Position yourself above or behind the patient, place your hands on each side of the helmet, and immobilize the head and neck by holding the helmet and the patient's neck.
2. Your partner positions himself to the side of the patient and removes the chin strap. Chin straps can usually be removed easily without cutting them.
3. Your partner then assumes the stabilization by placing one hand under the neck and the occiput and the other hand on the anterior neck with the thumb pressing on one angle of the mandible and the index and middle fingers pressing on the other angle of the mandible.
4. You now remove the helmet by pulling out laterally on each side to clear the ears and then up to remove. Tilt full-face helmets back to clear the nose (tilt the helmet, not the head).
5. If the patient is wearing glasses, remove them through the visual opening before removing the full-face helmet. Your partner maintains steady immobilization of the neck during this procedure.
6. After removal of the helmet, you again assume immobilization of the neck by grasping the head on either side with your fingers holding one angle of the jaw and the occiput.
7. Your partner now applies a suitable C-collar.

3

Rescuer 2 places one hand on the mandible at an angle—thumb on one side, index and other fingers on the other side. With his other hand, he holds the occipital region. This maneuver transfers the stabilization responsibility to Rescuer 2.

6

After the helmet has been removed, Rescuer 1 places his hands on either side of the head with his palms over the ears to maintain stabilization.

Summary:

The helmet must be maneuvered over the nose and ears while the head and neck are held rigid.

(a) Stabilization is applied from above.
(b) Stabilization is transferred below with pressure on the jaw and occiput.
(c) The helmet is removed.
(d) Stabilization is reestablished from above.

2

Rescuer 2 cuts or loosens the strap at the D-rings while maintaining stabilization.

5

Throughout the removal process, Rescuer 2 maintains in-line stabilization from below in order to prevent head tilt.

7

Stabilization is maintained from above until a cervical collar and a spine board are in place.

1

Rescuer 1 applies stabilization by placing his hands on each side of the helmet with his fingers on the patient's mandible. This position prevents slippage if the strap is loose.

4

Rescuer 1 removes helmet.

Keep in mind the following three factors:

(a) The helmet is egg-shaped and therefore must be expanded laterally to clear the ears.
(b) If the helmet provides full facial coverage, glasses must be removed first.
(c) If the helmet provides full facial coverage, the nose will impede removal. To clear the nose, the helmet must be tilted backward and raised over the nose.

FIGURE 10-36 Helmet removal from injured patient.

ALTERNATE PROCEDURE FOR REMOVING A HELMET

(See Figure 10-37.)

This has the advantage of one person maintaining immobilization of the neck through-out the whole procedure. This procedure does not work well with full-face helmets.

1. Position yourself above or behind the patient and place your hands on each side of the neck at the base of the skull. Immobilize the neck in a neutral position. If nec-essary, you may use your thumbs to perform a modified jaw thrust while doing this.
2. Your partner positions himself over to the side of the patient and removes the chin strap.
3. Your partner now removes the helmet by pulling out laterally on each side to clear the ears and then up to remove. You maintain immobilization of the neck during the procedure.
4. Your partner now applies a suitable C-collar.

1

Rescuer 1 positions himself above or behind the patient and places his hands on each side of the neck at the base of the skull. He maintains steady immobiliza-tion with the neck in a neutral position. He may use his thumbs to perform a modified jaw thrust while doing this.

2

Rescuer 2 positions himself over to the side of the patient and removes or cuts the chin strap.

3

Rescuer 2 now removes the helmet by pulling out laterally on each side to clear the ears and then up to remove. Full-face helmets will have to be tilted back to clear the nose (tilt the helmet, *not* the head). If the patient is wearing glasses, Rescuer 2 should remove them through the visual opening before removing the full-face hel-met. Rescuer 1 maintains steady immobi-lization during this procedure.

4

Rescuer 2 now applies a rigid extrication collar. Rescuer 1 maintains immobilization until the patient is transferred to a back-board and a padded immobilization device is applied.

FIGURE 10-37 Alternate method for removal of helmet.

CHAPTER 11

Abdominal Trauma

Gail V. Anderson Jr., M.D., M.B.A.,
   F.A.C.E.P.
Arthur H. Yancey II, M.D., M.P.H.,
   F.A.C.E.P.

OBJECTIVES

UPON COMPLETION OF THIS CHAPTER, YOU SHOULD BE ABLE TO:

1. Identify the basic anatomy of the abdomen and explain how abdominal and chest injuries may be related.

2. Relate how injuries apparent on the exterior of the abdomen can damage underlying structures.

3. Differentiate between blunt and penetrating injuries and identify complications associated with each.

4. Describe possible intra-abdominal injuries based on findings of history, physical examination, and mechanism of injury.

5. Describe the treatment required for the patient with protruding viscera.

Injury to the abdomen can be a difficult condition to evaluate even in the hospital. In the field it is usually more so. Nevertheless, since *intra-abdominal injury is the second leading cause of preventable traumatic death,* even the possibility of intra-abdominal injury must be recognized, documented, and addressed immediately. Penetrating abdominal injuries obviously need immediate surgical attention; blunt injuries may be more subtle, but potentially are just as deadly. Whether the result of blunt or penetrating trauma, abdominal injury presents two life-threatening dangers: hemorrhage and infection. Hemorrhage has immediate consequences, and thus you must be alert to the danger of early shock in all abdominal injury patients. Infection may be just as deadly, but does not require field intervention because its onset is slower.

The role of prehospital providers in the management of abdominal trauma has been the subject of some controversy. Studies in the mid-1980s demonstrated that appropriate and timely intervention by well-trained paramedics could improve the hemodynamic status of critically injured patients with wounds to the abdomen. More recent studies have suggested that pneumatic antishock garment (PASG) application and vigorous IV fluid resuscitation in the prehospital setting may do more harm than good for patients with penetrating abdominal trauma (see Chapter 8 and the Bibliography for this chapter). The effects in blunt trauma are less well studied.

In the field, you need to remember that rapid patient assessment and rapid transport to the appropriate hospital are keys to management of the patient with abdominal trauma.

ANATOMY

The abdomen is traditionally divided into three regions: the thoracic abdomen, the true abdomen, and the retroperitoneal abdomen. The thoracic portion of the abdomen is located underneath the thin sheet muscle, the diaphragm, and is enclosed by the lower ribs (see Figure 11-1). It contains the liver, gallbladder, spleen, stomach, and transverse colon. Injury to the liver and spleen can result in life-threatening hemorrhage.

The true abdomen contains the small intestines and the bladder (see Figure 11-2). Damage to the intestines can result in infection, peritonitis, and shock. In the female, the uterus, fallopian tubes, and ovaries are considered to be part of the pelvic portion of the true abdomen.

The retroperitoneal abdomen lies behind the thoracic and true portions of the abdomen (see Figure 11-3). This area includes the kidneys, ureters, pancreas, posterior duodenum, ascending and descending colon, abdominal aorta, and the inferior vena cava. Because of its location away from the body surface, injuries here are difficult to evaluate. While hemorrhage in the true abdomen may cause the anterior abdominal wall to become

FIGURE 11-1   Intrathoracic abdomen.

DIAPHRAGM

SPLEEN

LIVER

PANCREAS

KIDNEYS

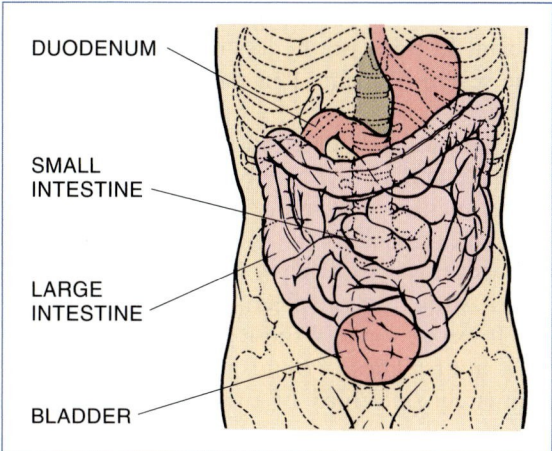

FIGURE 11-2   True abdomen.

distended, hemorrhage severe enough to cause shock may occur in the retroperitoneal space without this dramatic sign. In the pelvic part of the retroperitoneal abdomen are the iliac vessels. These vessels may be damaged by abdominal trauma or pelvic fracture. Injury to them can cause exsanguinating hemorrhage with few early symptoms.

TYPES OF INJURIES

Injuries to the abdomen are usually described as being blunt or penetrating. The penetrating group is subdivided into gunshot and stab wound categories. Blunt trauma is the most common mechanism of abdominal injury. Blunt abdominal injuries have relatively high mortality rates of 10 to 30%, usually because of the frequency of accompanying injuries to the head, chest, or an extremity(s) in as many as 70% of MVC victims. Blunt abdominal injury may be from direct compression of the abdomen, with fracture of solid organs and blowout of hollow organs, or from deceleration, with tearing of organs or their blood vessels. The patient who has suffered blunt trauma may have no pain and little external evidence of injury, which may create a false sense of security in the examiner.

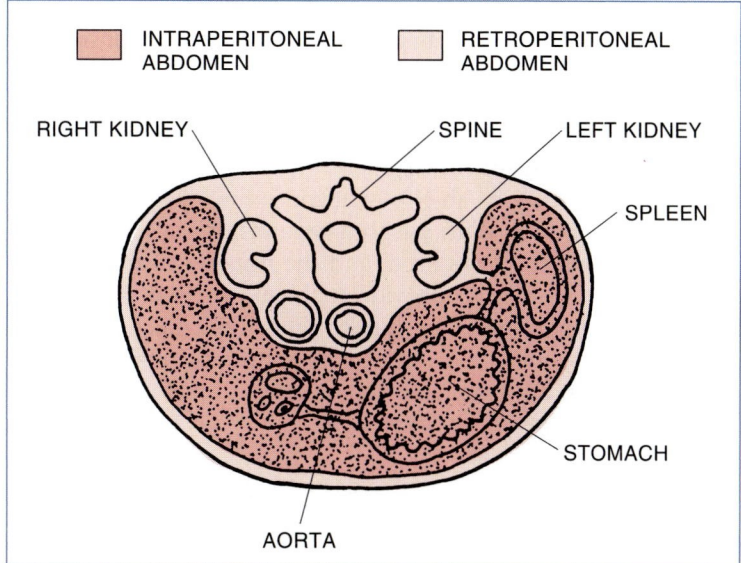

FIGURE 11-3   Retroperitoneal abdomen.

Patients with multiple lower rib fractures are notorious for having severe intra-abdominal injuries without significant abdominal pain. In this case the less noticeable abdominal pain is completely overshadowed by the severe rib pain. This patient may bleed to death because the abdomen is overlooked.

Gunshot wounds to the abdomen, as a rule, will be treated in the operating room. These patients have mortality rates of between 5 and 15%. These rates are much higher than those of stab wounds because of greater incidence of injury to abdominal viscera from the higher energy imparted to the intra-abdominal organs (see Chapter 1).

The mortality rate from abdominal stab wounds is relatively low (1–2%). Unless the knife penetrates a major vessel or organ, such as the liver or spleen, the patient may not initially appear to be in shock at the scene. However, some of these patients can develop life-threatening peritonitis over the next few hours. These wounds need to be carefully evaluated in the hospital because approximately one-third of these patients require surgery.

You should remember that the path of the penetrating object may not be readily apparent from the wound location. A stab to the chest may penetrate the abdomen and vice versa. The course of a bullet may pass through numerous structures in different body locations. It is important to look at the patient's entire posterior surface because penetrating trauma in the gluteal area (iliac crests to the gluteal folds, including the rectum) is associated with up to a 50% incidence of significant intra-abdominal injuries.

In the prehospital phase, with both blunt and penetrating trauma, you must be most concerned about intra-abdominal bleeding with hemorrhagic shock.

EVALUATION AND STABILIZATION

SCENE SIZE-UP

You can glean much important information from the scene by noting the circumstances surrounding the patient's injury. An accurate but rapid assessment of the scene will usually tip you off to the possibility of abdominal trauma. Do circumstances on the scene suggest that the victim has fallen from a height or been hit by a passing vehicle? Has there been an explosion that could have hurled the victim against immobile objects or transmitted blast pressure to organs inside the abdomen? Has the passenger of an automobile crash had the shoulder strap under the arm rather than over the shoulder? Or was the lap belt worn too high over the soft true abdomen instead of correctly across the pelvis? Any of these mechanisms can lead to penetrating or blunt abdominal injury.

If the patient was involved in a motor vehicle crash, as you do your scene survey, quickly observe the damage to the vehicle, such as passenger compartment intrusion, broken windows, bent steering wheel/steering column, and location of occupants. If the patient needs to be extricated, note the location of the safety belts; although they certainly save lives, incorrectly worn safety belts can cause blunt abdominal injuries by compressing the intra-abdominal organs against the spine.

The person who is stabbed or shot may be able to give you some idea as to the size of the instrument or trajectory of the bullet. With gunshot wounds, it is also important to know the caliber, the range from which it was fired, and the number of times it was fired. A bystander or the police may be able to provide such information. When you arrive at the hospital (optimally a trauma center), be sure to report any mechanism that suggests abdominal injury. However, while at the scene, it is important not to spend a great deal of time attempting to obtain a history. The major cause of preventable mortality in abdominal trauma is *delayed diagnosis and treatment*.

EVALUATION

As in treating any other traumatic condition, the patient should first undergo the BTLS Primary Survey. If shock is discovered (Chapter 7) and is not accounted for by injuries elsewhere, intra-abdominal injury must be assumed to be the cause. The essence of the prehospital abdominal examination in the Primary Survey is rapid visual evaluation and palpation. Observe the torso for deformities, contusions, abrasions, and punctures (DCAP), evisceration, and distention. Note any tenderness or tenseness. The chest is only one thin muscle sheet (the diaphragm) away from the abdominal cavity, so injury to both is not uncommon. Be mindful that splenic injury may present with left posterior shoulder pain, and liver injury may present with right posterior shoulder pain. *Distention of the abdomen should be interpreted as a sign of severe hemorrhage as should tenderness or tenseness over the abdominal wall.* Gentle palpation of the iliac crests (pelvic wings) and pubis of the pelvis may reveal the tenderness or the bony crepitus associated with fractures. Pelvic fractures frequently result in hemorrhagic shock. Signs of intra-abdominal injury usually don't appear early, so if signs of intra-abdominal injury are present in the prehospital phase, there is usually significant injury. Shock may be imminent (see Chapter 7). Abdominal tenderness or distention is an indication for immediate transport to the hospital. But remember that tenderness is an unreliable indicator of injury in a patient with an altered mental status and/or spinal injury at or above the level of the abdomen. Little is gained and critical time is lost by auscultation or percussion in the field. Abdominal wounds should never be probed with your finger or with an instrument.

If clothing must be removed to visualize injury, try to preserve important potential legal evidence by cutting around (rather than through) areas that have signs of possible penetration.

STABILIZATION

Interventions should follow the protocol outlined in Chapter 2. They should proceed in the same order in which evaluation occurred: airway (**A**), breathing (**B**), and circulation (**C**). In critically injured patients, evaluation and treatment should occur simultaneously in the foregoing order. This means that even if a patient has only an abdominal injury, supplemental oxygen by mask or nasal cannula should be delivered through a confirmed open airway. Breathing should be verified to be adequate or the patient treated to ensure adequate ventilation. Then, and only then, should the consequences of any abdominal injury be addressed as part of the circulation assessment.

The patient should be readied for rapid transport. If the system in which you practice allows the use of the pneumatic antishock trousers (PASG), these may be placed on the patient but inflated only after consultation with on-line Medical Direction (see Chapter 7). The more critically ill the patient, the more important it is to transport the patient early and apply the PASG en route. Gently cover any organ or viscera protruding from a wound with gauze moistened with saline or water. You can also use a nonadherent material, such as plastic wrap or aluminum foil, to prevent drying of the intestines (see Figure 11-4). If the intestines are allowed to dry, they may become irreversibly damaged. Do not *ever* push any abdominal contents protruding from a wound back into the abdomen. Similarly, if a foreign body (e.g., knife, glass shard) is impaled in the abdomen, do not attempt removal or manipulation. Carefully stabilize the object in place without moving it. Pregnant patients deserve the special considerations addressed in Chapter 17.

PITFALLS

When mechanisms of injury or associated injuries (lower rib fractures, gluteal penetrating wounds) suggest possible intra-abdominal injury, do not be fooled by the patient's lack of abdominal pain or tenderness. Be prepared for shock from occult intra-abdominal bleeding.

A

B

C

D

FIGURE 11-4   Protruding intestines.

SUMMARY

Effective prehospital management of the patient with abdominal trauma entails:

1. Scene size-up for mechanisms and pertinent history from the patient and/or witnesses
2. Rapid patient assessment
3. Rapid transport to the appropriate hospital (optimally a trauma center)
4. Other interventions as needed (usually performed en route)

The enemies of the abdominal trauma patient are bleeding and time from injury to optimal care. If you can minimize on-scene delays, you will help to maximize the patient's chance for survival.

BIBLIOGRAPHY

1. Aprahamian, C., B. M. Thompson, J. B. Towne, and others. "The Effect of a Paramedic System on Mortality of Major Open Intra-Abdominal Vascular Trauma." *Journal of Trauma,* Vol. 23 (1983), pp. 687–690.

2. Bickell, W. H., M. J. Wall, P. E. Pepe, and others. "Immediate Versus Delayed Fluid Resuscitation for Hypotensive Patients with Penetrating Torso Injury." *New England Journal of Medicine,* Vol. 331 (October 1994), pp. 1105–1109.

3. Mattox, K. L., W. H. Bickell, P. E. Pepe, and others. "Prospective MAST Study in 911 Patients." *Journal of Trauma,* Vol. 29 (1989), pp. 1104–1112.

4. Pons, P. T., B. Honigman, C. E. Moore, and others. "Prehospital Advanced Trauma Life Support for Critical Penetrating Wounds to the Thorax and Abdomen." *Journal of Trauma,* Vol. 25 (1985), pp. 828–832.

CHAPTER 12

Extremity Trauma

John E. Campbell, M.D., F.A.C.E.P.

OBJECTIVES

UPON COMPLETION OF THIS CHAPTER, YOU SHOULD BE ABLE TO:

1. Prioritize extremity trauma in the assessment and management of life-threatening injuries.

2. Discuss the major complications and treatment of the following extremity injuries:
   a. Fractures
   b. Dislocations
   c. Amputations
   d. Open wounds
   e. Neurovascular injuries
   f. Sprains and strains
   g. Impaled objects
   h. Compartment syndrome

3. Estimate blood loss from pelvic and extremity fractures.

4. Discuss major mechanisms of injury, associated trauma, potential complications, and management of injury to the following areas:
   a. Pelvis
   b. Femur
   c. Hip
   d. Knee
   e. Tibia/fibula
   f. Clavicle and shoulder
   g. Elbow
   h. Forearm and wrist
   i. Hand or foot

You must never let distorted or wounded extremities occupy your attention when there may be more life-threatening injuries present. These dramatic injuries are easy to identify when you first encounter the patient and may be disabling, but are rarely immediately life-threatening. It is important to remember that the movement of air through the airway, the mechanics of breathing, the maintenance of circulating blood volume, and the appropriate treatment of shock always come before the splinting of any fracture.

Hemorrhagic shock is a potential danger of very few musculoskeletal injuries. Only direct lacerations of arteries or fractures of the pelvis or femur are commonly associated with enough bleeding to cause shock. Injuries to the nerves or vessels that serve the hands and feet are the most common complications of fractures and dislocations. Such injuries cause the loss of function that we lump under the term *neurovascular compromise*. Thus, evaluation of sensation and circulation (PMS: pulse, motor, and sensation) distal to fractures is very important.

INJURIES TO EXTREMITIES

FRACTURES

Fractures may be open (compound) with the broken end of the bone still protruding or having once protruded through the skin (see lead photo in chapter), or they may be closed (simple) with no communication to the outside (see Figure 12-1). Fractured bone ends are extremely sharp and are quite dangerous to all the tissues that surround the bone. Since nerves and arteries frequently travel near the bone, across the flexor side of joints, or very near the skin (hands and feet), they are frequently injured. Such neurovascular injuries may be due to lacerations from bone fragments or from pressure due to swelling or hematomas.

Closed fractures can be just as dangerous as open fractures because injured soft tissues often bleed profusely. It is important to remember that any break in the skin near a fractured bone may be considered to be an opening for contamination.

A closed fracture of one femur can cause the loss of up to a liter of blood; thus two fractured femurs can cause life-threatening hemorrhage (see Figure 12-2). A fractured pelvis can cause extensive bleeding into the abdomen or the retroperitoneal space. The pelvis usually fractures in several places and may have 500 cc of blood loss for each fracture. Pelvic fractures may lacerate the bladder or the large pelvic blood vessels. Either of these structures can cause fatal hemorrhage into the abdomen. Remember, multiple fractures can cause life-threatening hemorrhage without any *external* blood loss.

CLOSED

OPEN

FIGURE 12-1 Basic types of fractures.

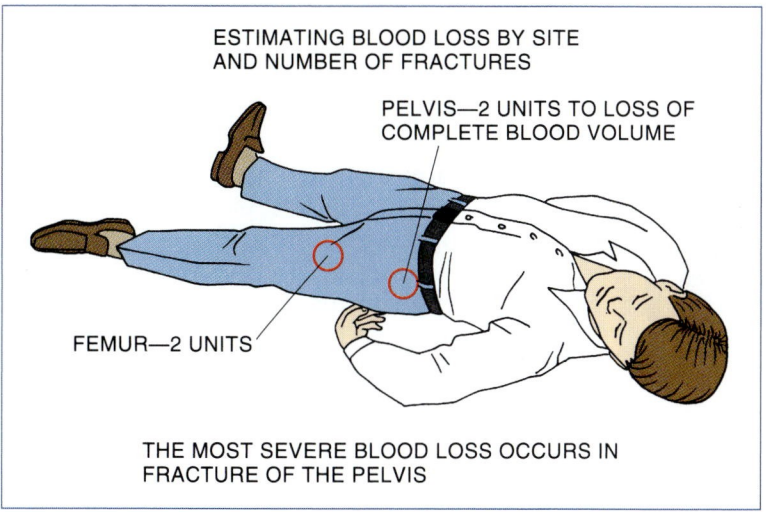

ESTIMATING BLOOD LOSS BY SITE
AND NUMBER OF FRACTURES

PELVIS—2 UNITS TO LOSS OF
COMPLETE BLOOD VOLUME

FEMUR—2 UNITS

THE MOST SEVERE BLOOD LOSS OCCURS IN
FRACTURE OF THE PELVIS

FIGURE 12-2   Internal blood loss from fractures.

Open fractures add the dangers of contamination as well as loss of blood outside the body. If protruding bone ends are pulled back into the skin when the limb is aligned, bacteria-contaminated debris will be pulled into the wound. Infection from such debris may prevent healing of the bone and may even cause death from septic complications.

DISLOCATIONS

Joint dislocations are extremely painful injuries. They are almost always easy to identify because normal anatomy is distorted. Major joint dislocations, though not life-threatening, are often true emergencies because of the neurovascular compromise that can, if not treated quickly, lead to amputation. It is impossible to know whether a fracture exists in combination with a dislocation. It is very important to check for PMS distal to major joint dislocations. Ordinarily, you splint injuries in the position you find them. There are certain exceptions to this rule. It is universally true, however, that one can apply only *gentle* traction to any distorted extremity in an effort to straighten it. In the few instances that you would use traction to straighten, use no more than 10 pounds of force. Most often the best treatment for the patient is padding and splinting the extremity in the most comfortable position and rapidly transporting to a facility that has orthopedic care available.

AMPUTATIONS

These are disabling and sometimes life-threatening injuries. They have the potential for massive hemorrhage, but most often, the bleeding will control itself quite readily with ordinary pressure applied to the stump. The stump should be covered with a damp sterile dressing and an elastic wrap that will apply uniform, reasonable pressure across the entire stump. If bleeding absolutely cannot be controlled with pressure, a tourniquet may be used. In general, a tourniquet is to be avoided whenever possible.

You should make an effort to find the amputated part and bring it with you. This sometimes neglected detail can have serious future implications for the patient, since parts can frequently be used for graft material. Reimplantation is attempted only in very limited situations. For this reason, you should not suggest to the patient that reimplantation will be done. Small amputated parts should be placed in a plastic bag (see Figure 12-3). If ice is available, place the bag in a larger bag or container containing ice and water. Do not use ice alone and *never* use dry ice. Cooling the part slows the chemical processes and will increase the viability from 4 hours to up to 18 hours. It is important to bring amputated parts even if reimplantation appears to be impossible.

AMPUTATED FINGER

FIGURE 12-3 Transportation of amputated part. If ice and time are available, seal part in small container and place this in a larger container of ice and water. Do not use dry ice. Do not place amputated part directly on ice. If no ice is available, place part in plastic bag and seal so that the part will not lose moisture. Do not wrap the part in a moistened dressing.

OPEN WOUNDS

Cover wounds with a sterile dressing and bandage carefully. Gross contamination such as leaves or gravel should be removed from the wound, and smaller pieces of contamination can be irrigated from the wound with a normal saline drip in the same manner that you would irrigate a chemically contaminated eye. Bleeding can almost always be stopped with pressure dressings or pneumatic splints. Tourniquets should almost never be used to stop bleeding from a wound if amputation is not present. If necessary, a blood pressure cuff or pressure on a larger artery proximal to the injury may be appropriate.

NEUROVASCULAR INJURIES

The nerves and major blood vessels generally run beside each other, usually in the flexor area of the major joints. They may be injured together, and loss of circulation and/or sensation can be due to disruption, swelling, or compression by bone fragments or hematomas. Foreign bodies or broken bone ends may well impinge on delicate structures and cause them to malfunction. Always check for PMS before and after any extremity manipulation, application of splint, or traction.

SPRAINS AND STRAINS

These injuries cannot be differentiated from fractures in the field. Treat them as though they are fractures.

IMPALED OBJECTS

Do not remove impaled objects. Apply a very bulky type of padding to hold the object in place and transport the patient with the object in place. The skin is a pivot point in these cases, and any motion outside the body is translated or magnified within the tissues where the end of the object may lacerate or harm sensitive structures. The cheek of the face is the exception to this rule because you can reach inside the mouth to put pressure on the bleeding.

COMPARTMENT SYNDROME

The extremities contain muscle tissue in closed spaces that are surrounded by tough membranes that will not stretch. Trauma (crush injuries, closed or open fracture, or sustained compression) to these areas (forearm and lower leg most commonly) may cause bleeding and swelling within the closed spaces. As the area swells, pressure is transmitted to the blood vessels and nerves. This pressure may compress the blood vessels in such a manner that circulation is impossible. The nerves may also be compromised. These injuries usually develop over a period of hours. Late symptoms are the five Ps: **p**ain, **p**allor, **p**ulselessness, **p**aresthesia, and **p**aralysis. The early symptoms are usually pain and paresthesia. As with shock, you should think of this diagnosis before the later symptoms develop.

ASSESSMENT AND MANAGEMENT

SCENE SIZE-UP AND HISTORY

In extremity trauma, it is especially important to get a history because the apparent mechanism of injury and the condition of the extremity when you first arrive may give you important information on the severity of the injury. If you have enough rescuers, one can obtain the history while you are performing the BTLS Primary Survey. If not, you should not attempt to elicit a detailed verbal history until you have assessed the status of the airway, breathing, and circulation. In the conscious patient, you should obtain most of the history at the end of the Primary Survey.

Foot injuries from long jumps (falls landing on the feet) often have lumbar spine injuries associated with them. Any injury to the knee when the patient is in the sitting position may have associated injuries to the hip. In a like manner, hip injuries may refer pain to the knee, so the knee and the hip are intimately connected and must be evaluated together rather than separately. Falls onto the wrist frequently injure the elbow, and so the wrist and elbow must be evaluated together. The same is true of the ankle and the proximal fibula of the outside of the lower leg.

Any injury that appears to be in the shoulder must be carefully examined because it may easily involve either the neck, chest, or shoulder. Fractures of the pelvis are usually associated with very large amounts of blood loss. Whenever a fracture in the pelvis is identified, shock must be suspected and proper treatment begun.

ASSESSMENT

During the BTLS Primary Survey, you are concerned with obvious fractures to the pelvis and large bones of the extremities. You should also find and control major bleeding from the extremities.

During the Detailed Exam, you should quickly assess the full length of each extremity, looking for deformity, contusions, abrasions, penetrations, burns, tenderness, lacerations, and swelling (DCAP-BTLS). Feel for instability and crepitation (see Chapters 2 and 3). Check the joints for pain and movement. Check and record distal PMS. Pulses may be marked with ballpoint pen to identify the area in which the pulse is best felt (see Figure 12-4). *Crepitation or grating of bone ends is a definite sign of fracture, and once identified, the bone ends should be immediately immobilized to prevent further soft tissue injury.* Checking for crepitation should be done *very gently,* especially when checking the pelvis. Crepitation means bone ends are grating on one another, and this means you are causing further tissue injury.

FIGURE 12-4   (a) Palpation of radial pulse; (b) Location of dorsalis pedis and posterior tibial pulses.

MANAGEMENT OF EXTREMITY INJURIES

Proper management of fractures and dislocations will decrease the incidence of pain, disability, and serious complications. Treatment in the prehospital setting is directed at proper immobilization of the injured part by the use of an appropriate splint.

PURPOSE OF SPLINTING: The objective is to prevent motion in the broken bone ends (see Figure 12-5). The nerves that cause the most pain in a fractured extremity lie in the membrane surrounding the bone. The broken bone ends irritate these nerves, causing a very deep and distressing type of pain. Splinting not only decreases pain, but also eliminates further damage to muscles, nerves, and blood vessels by preventing further motion of the broken bone ends.

WHEN TO SPLINT: There is no simple rule that determines the precise sequence to follow in every trauma patient. In general, the seriously injured patient will be better off if only major (spinal) immobilization is done before transport. The patient who requires a load-and-go approach can be adequately immobilized by careful packaging on the long spineboard. This does not mean that you have no responsibility to identify and protect extremity fractures, but rather implies that it is better to do some splinting in the vehicle en route to the hospital. It is never appropriate to sacrifice time immobilizing a limb to prevent *disability,* when that time may be needed to save the patient's *life.* Conversely, if the patient appears to be stable, extremity fractures should be splinted before moving the patient.

RULES OF SPLINTING

1. You must adequately visualize the injured part. Clothes should be cut off, not pulled off, unless there is only an isolated injury that presents no problem with maintaining immobilization.
2. Check and record distal sensation and circulation before and after splinting. Check movement distal to the fracture if possible (e.g., ask the conscious patient to wiggle his fingers or observe the motion of the unconscious patient when a painful stimulus is applied). Pulses may be marked with a pen to identify where they were last palpated.

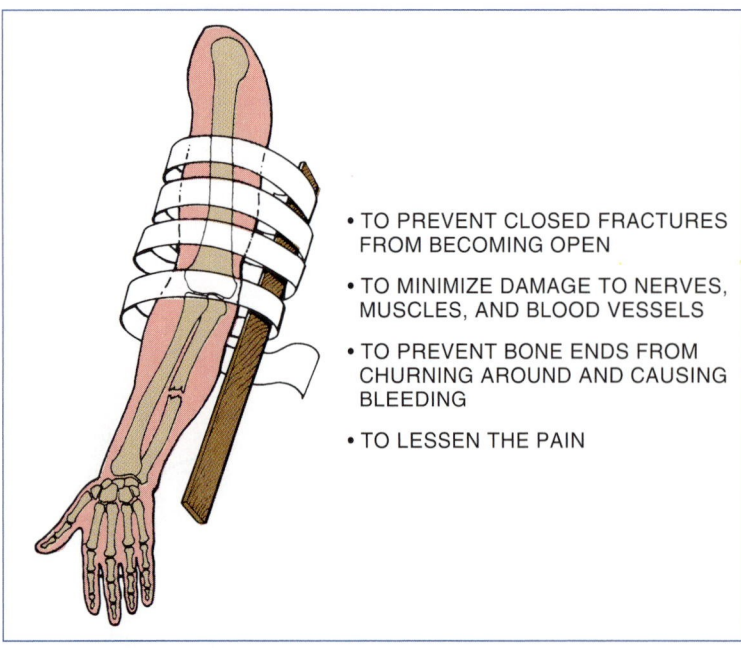

- TO PREVENT CLOSED FRACTURES FROM BECOMING OPEN

- TO MINIMIZE DAMAGE TO NERVES, MUSCLES, AND BLOOD VESSELS

- TO PREVENT BONE ENDS FROM CHURNING AROUND AND CAUSING BLEEDING

- TO LESSEN THE PAIN

FIGURE 12-5   Reasons for splinting.

3. If the extremity is severely angulated and pulses are absent, you should apply gentle traction in an attempt to straighten it (see Figure 12-6). This traction should never exceed 10 pounds of pressure. If resistance is encountered, splint the extremity in the angulated position. When you are attempting to straighten an extremity, it is very important to be honest with yourself with regard to resistance. It takes very little force to lacerate the wall of a vessel or to interrupt the blood supply to a large nerve. If the trauma center is near, always splint in the position found.

4. Open wounds should be covered with a sterile dressing before you apply the splint. Splints should always be applied on the side of the extremity away from open wounds to prevent pressure necrosis.

5. Use the splint that will immobilize one joint above and below the injury.

6. Pad the splint well. This is particularly true if there is any skin defect or if bony prominences might press against a hard splint.

7. Do not attempt to push bone ends back under the skin. If you apply traction and the bone end retracts back into the wound, do not increase the amount of traction. You should not use your hands or any tools to try to pull the bone ends back out, but be sure to notify the receiving physician. Bone ends should be carefully padded by bandages before pneumatic splints are applied to the lower extremities. The healing of bone is improved if the bone ends are kept moist when transport time is prolonged.

8. In a life-threatening situation, extremity injuries may be splinted while the patient is being transported. When the patient is stable, splint all injuries before moving the patient.

9. If in doubt, splint a possible injury.

TYPES OF SPLINTS

RIGID SPLINT: This type of splint can be made from many different materials and includes all the cardboard, hard plastic, metal, or wooden types of splints. The type of splint that is made rigid by evacuating air from a moldable splint (vacuum splint) is also classified as a rigid splint. Rigid splints should be padded well and should always extend one joint above and below the fracture.

1. CONFIRM LOSS OF PULSE

2. GENTLY GRASP EXTREMITY ABOVE AND BELOW BREAK

3. APPLY TRACTION STEADILY AND SMOOTHLY

4. MAINTAIN TRACTION WHILE SPLINT IS APPLIED

5. RECHECK PULSE AND SENSATION

FIGURE 12-6   Straightening angulated fractures to restore pulses.

SOFT SPLINT: This type includes air splints, pillows, and sling and swathe type splints. Air splints are good for fractures of the lower arm and lower leg. The pneumatic anti-shock garment (PASG or MAST) is an excellent air splint (blow up to only air-splint pressures). Air splints have the advantage of compression, which helps to slow bleeding, but they have the disadvantage of increasing pressure as the temperature rises or the altitude increases. They *should not* be put on angulated fractures since they will automatically apply straightening pressure.

Other major disadvantages of air splints include the fact that the extremity pulses cannot be monitored while the splint is in place; the splints also often stick to the skin and are painful to remove.

Inflating the splints requires you to blow the splints up by mouth or by hand or foot pump (never by compressed air) until they give good support and yet *can easily be dented with slight pressure from a fingertip*. When using air splints, you must constantly check the pressure to be sure that the splint is not getting too tight or too loose (they often leak).

Remember that if air splints are applied in a cold environment and the patient is moved into the warm environment of the ambulance, the pressure will increase as the splints warm up. Where air ambulances are available, it must be remembered that the pressure in air splints increases if they are applied on the ground and then subsequently the patient is airlifted to the hospital. Also remember that if pressure is released during the flight, the pressure will be too low when the patient is returned to the ground.

Pillows make good splints for injuries to the ankle or foot. They are also helpful, along with a sling and a swathe, to stabilize a dislocated shoulder.

Slings and swathes are excellent for injuries to the clavicle, shoulder, upper arm, elbow, and sometimes the forearm. They utilize the chest wall as a solid foundation and splint the arm against the chest wall. Some shoulder injuries cannot be brought close to the chest wall without significant force being applied. In these instances, pillows are used to bridge the gap between the chest wall and the upper arm.

TRACTION SPLINT: This device is designed for fractures of the femur. It holds the fracture immobile by the application of a steady pull on the ankle while applying countertraction to the ischium and the groin. This steady traction overcomes the tendency of the very strong thigh muscles to spasm. If traction is not applied, the pain worsens because the bone ends tend to impact or override. Traction also prevents free motion of the ends of the femur, which could lacerate the femoral nerve, artery, or vein. There are many designs and types of splints available to apply traction to the lower extremity, but each must be carefully padded and applied with care to prevent excessive pressure on the soft tissues around the pelvis. It is also necessary to use a great deal of care in applying the ankle hitch so as not to interfere with the circulation of the foot. Many of these devices can be used with a buck's boot as an alternative to the ankle hitch.

MANAGEMENT OF SPECIFIC INJURIES

SPINE: This is covered elsewhere in the book but included here to remind you that if there is any chance of spinal injury, proper immobilization must be done to prevent life-long paralysis or even death from a spinal cord injury (see Figure 12-7). In the most urgent cases, careful packaging of the patient on the long spineboard may be adequate splinting for a number of different extremity injuries. Remember that certain mechanisms of injury, such as a fall from a height in which the patient lands on both feet, may cause lumbar spine fracture because forces are transmitted all the way up the body.

PELVIS: It is practical to include injuries to the pelvis with extremities because they are frequently associated. Pelvic injuries are usually caused by motor vehicle accidents or by severe *trauma such as falls from heights. They are identified by **gentle** pressure being placed on the iliac crests, hips, and pubis during the patient survey.* There is always the potential for serious hemorrhage in pelvic fractures, so shock should be expected and the patient rapidly transported (load-and-go). The patient with a pelvic injury should

PROPER IMMOBILIZATION

PROPER IMMOBILIZATION.
LIGHTWEIGHT CUSHIONS
BESIDE HEAD.

IMPROPER IMMOBILZATION
WITH SANDBAGS. GROSS
HEAD MOVEMENT WHEN
BOARD IS ROLLED.

FIGURE 12-7   Proper immobilization.

always be transported on a spineboard. The vacuum backboard is especially useful here because it is much more comfortable than the hard backboard. Log-rolling a patient with a pelvic fracture can aggravate the injury. Scoop stretchers or adequate manpower is needed to move these patients to the backboard.

FEMUR: The femur usually fractures at the midshaft, although hip fractures are quite common. These fractures may have open wounds associated with them and, if so, they must be presumed to be open fractures. There is a lot of muscle tissue surrounding the femur, and a great deal of bleeding can occur into the tissue of the thigh. Bilateral femur fractures can be associated with a loss of up to 50% of the circulating blood volume. Pneumatic splints such as the PASG are useful in decreasing the internal bleeding around femur fractures.

HIP: Hip fractures are most often in the narrow "neck" of the femur where strong ligaments may occasionally allow this type of fracture to bear weight. The ligaments are very strong, and there is very little movement of the bone ends in the most frequent type of hip fracture.

You must consider hip fractures in any elderly person who has fallen and has pain in the knee, hip, or pelvic region. This type of presentation and pain should be considered a fracture until an x-ray proves otherwise. In this age group, pain is frequently well tolerated and sometimes even ignored or denied. In general, the tissues in the elderly patient are more delicate, and less force is required to disrupt a given structure. Always remember that in the child and in the elderly patient isolated knee pain may well be coming from damage to the hip.

Hip dislocation is a different story. Most hip dislocations are a result of the knees being struck by the dashboard, forcing the relatively loose, relaxed hip out of the posterior side of its cup in the pelvis (see Figure 12-8). Thus, any patient in a severe automobile accident with a knee injury must have the hip examined very carefully. Hip dislocation is an orthopedic emergency and requires reduction as soon as possible to prevent sciatic nerve injury or necrosis of the femoral head due to interrupted blood supply.

FIGURE 12-8 Mechanism of posterior dislocation of the hip, "down and under."

This is a very difficult reduction to perform because the amount of force required is very great and the movement must be quite precise.

The dislocated hip will usually be flexed, and the patient will not be able to tolerate having the leg straightened. The leg will almost invariably be rotated toward the midline. A posterior hip dislocation should be supported in the most comfortable position by the use of pillows and by splinting to the uninjured leg (see Figure 12-9). This patient requires rapid transport.

KNEE: Fractures or dislocation of the knee are quite serious because the arteries are bound down above and below the knee joint and are often bruised or lacerated if the joint is in an abnormal position. There is no way to know whether a fracture exists in an abnormally positioned knee and, in either case, the decision must be based on the circulation and neurological function below the knee in the foot. Some authorities state that about 50% of knee dislocations have associated injuries to the vessels, and many knee

IMMOBLIZE IN POSITION FOUND

MOLD PILLOW AROUND KNEE OR BANDAGE TO WELL-PADDED SPLINT

FIGURE 12-9 Splinting posterior dislocation of the hip.

injuries later require amputation. It is important to restore the circulation below the knee whenever possible.

Prompt reduction of knee dislocation is very important. If there is loss of pulse or sensation, you should apply gentle traction that may be by hand or by a traction splint. You must be careful to apply *no more than 10 pounds* of force, and this force must be applied along the long axis of the leg. If there is resistance to straightening the knee, splint it in the most comfortable position and transport the patient rapidly. This may be considered to be a true orthopedic emergency.

TIBIA/FIBULA: Fractures of the lower leg are often open due to thin skin over the front of the tibia and often have significant internal and/or external blood loss. Internal blood loss can interrupt the circulation to the foot if a compartment syndrome develops. It is rarely possible for patients to bear weight on fractures of the tibia. Fractures of the lower tibia/fibula may be splinted with a rigid splint, an air splint, or a pillow (see Figure 12-10). Pneumatic splints will adequately splint upper tibia fractures. Here again it is important to dress any wound and pad any bone ends that may be put under an air splint or PASG.

CLAVICLE: This is the most frequently fractured bone in the body but rarely causes problems (see Figure 12-11). It is best immobilized with a sling and swathe. Rarely there may be injuries to the subclavian vein and artery or to the nerves of the arm when this area is injured. It is also very important that the ribs and chest be very carefully evaluated whenever an injury to the shoulder or clavicle is discovered.

SHOULDER: Most shoulder injuries are not life-threatening, but they may be associated with severe injuries of the chest or neck. Many shoulder injuries are dislocations or separations of joint spaces and may show up as a defect at the upper outer portion of the shoulder. The upper humerus is fractured with some degree of frequency, however. The radial nerve travels quite close around the humerus and may be injured in humeral fractures. Injury to the radial nerve results in an inability of the patient to lift the hand (wrist drop). Dislocated shoulders are very painful and quite often require a pillow between the arm and body to hold the upper arm in the most comfortable position. Shoulders that are held in abnormal positions should never be forced into a more anatomic alignment (see Figure 12-12).

FIGURE 12-10   Splinting lower leg fractures with air splint or board splint.

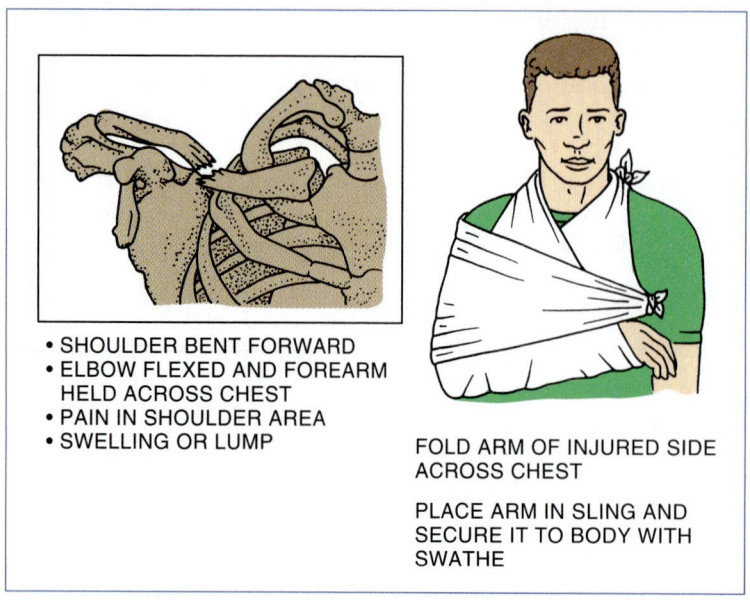

- SHOULDER BENT FORWARD
- ELBOW FLEXED AND FOREARM HELD ACROSS CHEST
- PAIN IN SHOULDER AREA
- SWELLING OR LUMP

FOLD ARM OF INJURED SIDE ACROSS CHEST

PLACE ARM IN SLING AND SECURE IT TO BODY WITH SWATHE

FIGURE 12-11 Fractured clavicle.

FIGURE 12-12 Dislocated shoulder.

ELBOW: It is often difficult to tell whether there is a fracture or dislocation; both can be serious because of the danger of damage to the vessels and nerves that run across the flexor surface of the elbow. Elbow injuries should always be splinted in the most comfortable position and the distal function clearly evaluated (see Figure 12-13). Never attempt to straighten or apply traction to an elbow injury because the tissues are quite delicate and the structure is very complicated.

FOREARM AND WRIST: This a very common fracture, usually as a result of a fall on the outstretched arm. Usually it is best immobilized with a rigid splint or an air splint (see Figure 12-14). If a rigid splint is used, a roll of gauze in the hand will hold the arm in the most comfortable position of function. The forearm is also subject to internal bleeding that can interrupt the blood supply to the fingers and the hand (compartment syndrome).

HAND OR FOOT: Many industrial accidents involving the hand or the foot produce multiple open fractures and avulsions. These injuries are often gruesome in appearance but are seldom associated with life-threatening bleeding. A pillow may be used to support these injuries very effectively (see Figure 12-15). An alternative method of dressing the hand is to insert a roll of gauze in the palm, then arrange the fingers and thumb in

IMMOBILIZE LIMB IN POSITION
IN WHICH IT WAS FOUND

BENT POSITION

STRAIGHT POSITION

FIGURE 12-13 Fractures or dislocations of the elbow.

SECURE FOREARM
IN SPLINT

SECURE ARM
IN SPLINT

FIGURE 12-14 Fractures of the forearm and wrist.

FIGURE 12-15 Pillow splinting an injured foot.

their normal position. The entire hand is then wrapped as though it were a ball inside a very large and bulky dressing. Elevating the isolated hand or foot injury above the level of the heart will almost always reduce bleeding dramatically during transport.

PITFALLS AND IMPORTANT POINTS

1. Be very alert to the mechanism of injury so that you know what fractures to suspect and so that you can predict possible complications.

2. Remember the ABCs.

3. Visualize the injured part.

4. Be prepared for hemorrhagic shock when there is a pelvic or femur fracture.

5. Always record sensation and circulation initially and after any manipulation, particularly splinting.

6. Pad joints and hard spots very carefully. Be sure all splints are padded well.

7. Examine and immobilize one joint above and below any suspected fracture.

8. Splint the patient at an appropriate time. The axial skeleton is splinted after the Primary Survey, but extremities should be splinted en route if a critical situation exists.

9. If in doubt, splint a potential fracture. In major trauma, the axial skeleton is always splinted on a long spineboard.

10. Do not waste the golden hour. Be cautious but be rapid.

SUMMARY

While usually not life-threatening, extremity injuries are often disabling. These injuries may be more obvious than more serious internal injuries, but do not let extremity injuries distract you from following the usual steps of the BTLS Primary Survey. Pelvic and femur fractures can be associated with life-threatening internal bleeding, so patients with these injuries are in the load-and-go category. Proper splinting is important to protect the injured extremity from further injury. Dislocations of elbows, hips, and knees require careful splinting and rapid reduction to prevent severe disability to the affected extremity.

BIBLIOGRAPHY

1. Bledsoe, B. E., R. S. Porter, and B. R. Shade. "Musculoskeletal Injuries." In *Paramedic Emergency Care*, 5th ed., pp. 473–493. Upper Saddle River, NJ: Prentice Hall, 1991.

2. Committee on Trauma, American College of Surgeons. "Musculoskeletal Trauma." In *Advanced Trauma Life Support Program*, pp. 301-320. Chicago: The College, 1997.

3. Grant, H. D., R. H. Murray, and J. D. Bergeron. "The Upper Extremities" and "The Lower Extremities." In *Emergency Care*, 6th ed., pp. 258–323. Upper Saddle River, NJ: Prentice Hall, 1994.

CHAPTER 13

Extremity Trauma Skills

Donna Hastings, EMT-P

OBJECTIVES

UPON COMPLETION OF THIS CHAPTER, YOU SHOULD BE ABLE TO:

1. Explain when to use a traction splint.
2. Describe the complications of using a traction splint.
3. Apply the most common traction splints:
   a. Thomas splint
   b. Hare splint
   c. Sager splint

USE OF TRACTION SPLINTS

Traction splints are designed to immobilize fractures of the femur. They are *not* useful for fractures of the hip, knee, or lower leg. Applying firm traction to a fractured or dislocated knee may tear the blood vessels behind the knee. If there appears to be a pelvic fracture, you cannot use a traction splint because it may cause further damage to the pelvis. Fractures below the midthigh that are not angulated or are severely shortened may just as well be immobilized by air splints or the antishock garment. Traction splints work by applying a padded device to the back of the pelvis (ischium) or to the groin. A hitching device is then applied to the ankle, and countertraction is applied until the limb is straight and well immobilized. Apply the splints to the pelvis and groin very carefully to prevent excessive pressure on the genitalia. Also use care when attaching the hitching device to the foot and ankle so as not to interfere with circulation. To prevent any unnecessary movement, do not apply traction splints until the patient is on a long backboard. If the splint extends beyond the end of the backboard, be very careful when moving the patient and when closing the ambulance door. You must check the circulation in the injured leg, so remove the shoe before attaching the hitching device. In every case at least two people are needed. One must hold steady, *gentle* traction on the foot and leg while the other applies the splint. When dealing with load-and-go situations, do not apply the splint until the patient is in the ambulance (unless the ambulance has not arrived).

APPLYING A THOMAS TRACTION SPLINT (HALF-RING SPLINT)

The Thomas splint was used exclusively prior to the advent of modern traction devices. During World War I its use decreased the mortality rate for battlefield femur fractures from 80 to 40%. At that time it was considered one of the greatest advancements in medical care. It is still used in some countries and in the absence of other options (see Figure 13-1).

1. Support the leg and maintain gentle traction while your partner cuts away the clothing and removes the shoe and sock to check the pulse and sensation at the foot.
2. Position the splint under the injured leg. The ring goes down and the short side goes to the inside of the leg. Slide the ring snugly up under the hip, where it will be pressed against the ischial tuberosity.

FIGURE 13-1   Applying a Thomas traction splint.

3. Position two support straps above the knee and two below the knee.
4. Attach the top ring strap.
5. Apply padding to the foot and ankle.
6. Apply the traction hitch around the foot and ankle (see Figure 13-2).
7. Maintain gentle traction by hand.
8. Attach the traction hitch to the end of the splint.
9. Increase traction by Spanish windlass action using a stick or tongue depressors.
10. Release manual traction and reassess circulation and sensation.
11. Support the end of the splint so that there is no pressure on the heel.

Applying a Hare Traction Splint

This is the modern version of the Thomas splint (see Figure 13-3).

1. Position the patient on the backboard or stretcher.
2. Support the leg and maintain gentle traction, while your partner cuts away the clothing and removes the shoe and sock to check pulse and sensation at the foot.
3. Using the uninjured leg as a guide, pull the splint out to the correct length.
4. Position the splint under the injured leg. The ring goes down and the short side goes to the inside of the leg. Slide the ring up snugly under the hip against the ischial tuberosity.
5. Position two support straps above the knee and two below the knee.
6. Attach the heel rest.
7. Attach the top strap.
8. Apply the padded traction hitch to the ankle and foot.
9. Maintain gentle manual traction.
10. Attach the traction hitch to the windlass by way of the S-hook.
11. Turn the ratchet until the correct tension is applied.
12. Release manual traction and recheck circulation and sensation.
13. Attach support straps around the leg with Velcro straps.
14. To release traction, pull the ratchet knob outward and then slowly turn to loosen.

PADDING   T-STRAP

COLLINS HITCH   SPANISH WINDLASS

PADDING

Figure 13-2   Applying a traction hitch to the ankle.

FIGURE 13-3
Hare traction splint.

APPLYING A SAGER TRACTION SPLINT

This splint is different in several ways. It works by providing countertraction against the pubic ramus and the ischial tuberosity medial to the shaft of the femur; thus it does not go under the leg. The hip does not have to be slightly flexed as with the Hare. The Sager splint is also lighter and more compact than other traction splints. You can also splint both legs with one splint if needed. The current Sager splints are significantly improved over older models and may represent the state of the art in traction splints (see Figure 13-4):

1. Position the patient on a long backboard or stretcher.
2. Support the leg and maintain gentle traction while your partner cuts away the clothing and removes the shoe and sock to check the pulse and sensation at the foot.
3. Using the uninjured leg as a guide, pull the splint out to the correct length.
4. Position the splint to the inside of the injured leg with the padded bar fitted snugly against the pelvis in the groin. The splint can be used on the outside of the leg, using the strap to maintain traction against the pubic ramus. Be very careful not to catch the genitals under the bar (or strap).
5. While maintaining gentle manual traction, attach the padded hitch to the foot and ankle.
6. Extend the splint until the correct tension is obtained.
7. Release manual traction and recheck circulation and sensation.
8. Apply elastic straps above and below the knee.

FIGURE 13-4
Sager traction splint.

CHAPTER 14

Burns

Roy L. Alson, Ph.D., M.D., F.A.C.E.P.
Richard C. Treat, M.D., F.A.C.S.

OBJECTIVES

UPON COMPLETION OF THIS CHAPTER, YOU SHOULD BE ABLE TO:

1. Identify the basic anatomy of the skin including:
   a. Epidermal and dermal layers
   b. Structures found within
2. List the basic functions of the skin.
3. Identify the descriptive categories of burns.
4. Identify complications and describe the management of:
   a. Thermal burns
   b. Chemical burns
   c. Electrical burns
5. List situations and physical signs that may indicate:
   a. Upper airway injury
   b. Inhalation injury
6. List signs and symptoms of carbon monoxide poisoning.
7. Discuss how carbon monoxide causes hypoxia.
8. Describe the treatment for carbon monoxide poisoning.
9. Estimate depth of burn based on skin appearance.
10. Estimate extent of burn using the rule of nines.
11. Identify which patients may require transport to a burn center.

There are over 1 million burn injuries per year in the United States, resulting in more than 5,000 deaths. Many who survive their burns are severely disabled and/or disfigured. Applying the basic principles taught here will help decrease death, disability, and disfigurement from burn injuries. As the rescue and treatment of burn patients can be extremely dangerous, following the rules of scene safety is extremely important. Multiple agents (see below) can cause burn injuries, but in general, pathologic damage to the skin is similar. Specific differences among the types of burns will be discussed in later sections.

TYPES OF BURN INJURIES

1. Flame
2. Electrical
3. Chemical
4. Steam
5. Radiation
6. Scald

ANATOMY AND PATHOLOGY

The largest organ of the body, the skin, is made up of two layers. The outer layer that we can see on the surface is called the *epidermis*. It serves as a barrier between the environment and our body. Underneath the thin epidermis is a thick layer of collagen connective tissue called the *dermis*. This layer contains the important sensory nerves and also the support structures such as the hair follicles, sweat glands, and oil glands (see Figure 14-1). The skin has many important functions, which include acting as a mechanical barrier between the body and the outside world and acting as a protective barrier to seal fluids inside and prevent bacteria and other microorganisms from readily entering the body. The skin is also a vital sensory organ that provides input to the brain on general and specific environmental data and serves a primary role in temperature regulation.

FIGURE 14-1 The skin.

Burn damage to the skin occurs when heat or caustic chemicals come in contact with the skin and damage its chemical and cellular components. In addition to actual tissue injury, the body's inflammatory response to the skin damage may also result in injury or increase the severity of the burn. Burns are characterized as first, second, or third degree, based on the depth of tissue damage and skin response. First-degree burns result in minor tissue damage to the outer epidermal layer only, but do cause an intense and painful inflammatory response. Although no medical treatment is usually required, various medications can be prescribed that significantly speed healing and reduce the painful inflammatory response. Second-degree burns cause damage through the epidermis and into a variable depth of the dermis. These injuries will heal (usually without scarring) because the cell lining at the deep level of the epidermis (which also lines the deeper hair follicles) will multiply and result in the growth of new skin for healing. Antibiotic creams or various specialized types of dressings are routinely used to treat these burns and, therefore, appropriate medical evaluation and care should be provided for patients with these injuries.

Flash burns are virtually always first- or second-degree burns. A flash burn occurs when there is some type of explosion, but no actual fire. The single heat wave traveling out from these explosions results in such short patient–heat contact that only superficial burns occur. Only areas directly exposed to the true heat wave will be injured. *In situations of possible flash explosion risk, you should ALWAYS wear proper protective clothing.* Other injuries (fractures, internal injuries, blast chest injuries, etc.) may well occur as a result of explosion.

Third-degree burns cause damage to all layers of the epidermis and dermis. No more skin cell layers are left, so healing is impossible except in small third-degree burns that usually scar in from the sides. All third-degree burns leave scars. Deeper third-degree burns usually result in skin protein becoming denatured and hard, leaving a firm leatherlike covering that is referred to as eschar. Characteristics of these burns are listed in Table 14-1, and the depth levels are shown in Figure 14-2. Examples of second-degree and third-degree burns are shown in Figures 14-3a and 14-3b.

The inflammatory response to the burn injury results in progressive tissue damage for a day or two following burn injury; this may well result in an increase in burn depth. Any condition that either reduces circulation to this damaged tissue or by itself causes further tissue damage will lead to burn progression with increasing burn depth. Because of the process of burn progression, it is not essential to exactly determine the burn depth in the field. You should, however, be able to clearly discern between superficial and deep burns.

Table 14-1 Characteristics of Various Depths of Burns.

	FIRST DEGREE	**SECOND DEGREE**	**THIRD DEGREE**
Cause	Sun or minor flash	Hot liquids, flashes, or flame	Chemicals, electricity, flame, hot metals
Skin color	Red	Mottled red	Pearly white and/or charred, translucent and parchmentlike
Skin surface	Dry with no blisters	Blisters with weeping	Dry with thrombosed blood vessels
Sensation	Painful	Painful	Anesthetic
Healing	3–6 days	2–4 weeks, depending on depth	Requires skin grafting

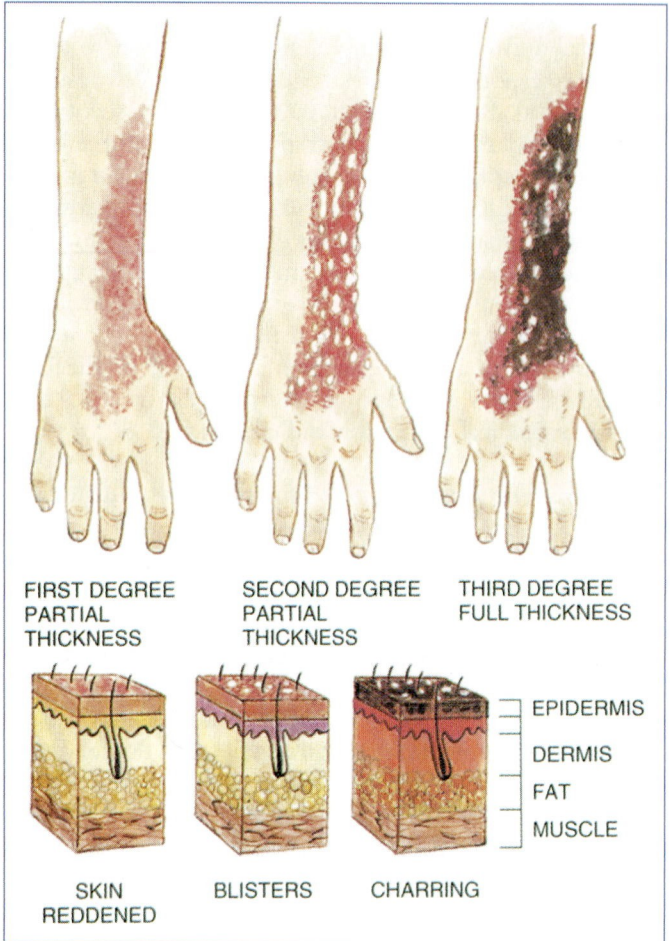

FIGURE 14-2 Degrees of burns.

FIGURE 14-3A Second-degree scald burn. *(Courtesy of Roy Alson, M.D.)*

First-degree and second-degree burns are commonly referred to as partial-thickness burns because there are still some layers of skin cells left that can multiply and result in healing. Third-degree burns are referred to as full-thickness burns because all layers of the skin have been destroyed, and no skin cells are left to allow healing. The magnitude of burn injury depends on the extent and depth of the burn. Initial care that is directed specifically toward the burn should concentrate on limiting any progression of these two factors.

Figure 14-3b Third-degree flame burn. *(Courtesy of Roy Alson, M.D.)*

INITIAL FIELD CARE

Patient Assessment and Management

Evaluation of the burn patient is often complicated by the dramatic nature of the injuries. The responder may be overwhelmed by the extent of the injury. One must remember that even patients with major burns rarely expire in the initial postburn period from the burn injury. They die as a consequence of associated trauma or associated conditions such as airway compromise or smoke inhalation. A careful, systematic approach to patient evaluation will allow the responder to identify and manage critical life-threatening problems and to improve patient outcome.

The steps for assessing a major burn patient are the same as for any other major trauma patient. Begin by performing a scene size-up as outlined in Chapter 1, with an emphasis on your safety. After this is completed, your next priority is to remove the patient from the source of the burn. Removing the burn source is the first step in treating a burn patient, and the most important concept in removing the burn source is the maintenance of safety. This involves both maintaining your safety *and* maintaining patient safety. There are specific and significant dangers in removing the burn source in all types of burn injuries. In the progression of a building fire, there is a point at which flashover occurs. Flashover is the *sudden* explosion into flame of everything in the room with the temperature rising instantaneously to over 3,000 degrees. There is no warning before this happens; thus *removal of patients from burning buildings takes priority over all other treatment*. Remember also that fire produces large quantities of toxic products and smoke. Thus, personnel making entry to carry out rescue should wear breathing apparatus.

Chemicals are not always easy to detect, either on patients or on other objects in the environment. Severe chemical burns to rescuers have occurred because of the inability to note sources of toxic and caustic chemicals. Special training in hazardous materials management is recommended for all rescuers. Electricity is exceptionally dangerous, and handling of high voltage wires is extremely hazardous. Specialized training and knowledge are required to appropriately deal with these situations, and you should not attempt to remove wires unless specifically trained to do so. Even objects commonly felt to be safe, such as wooden sticks, manila rope, and firefighter's gloves, may not be protective and may result in electrocution. If at all possible, the source of electricity should be turned off before any attempt at rescue is made.

People do not actually die rapidly from burn injuries. Even though the burn is highly visible and makes an intense impression at the scene, care of the burn itself has low priority. You should manage burn patients routinely as *trauma* patients and perform a BTLS Primary Survey immediately upon arrival in a safe staging area. The BTLS Primary Survey should follow the standard format described in Chapter 2.

Begin by securing the airway, while simultaneously checking the initial level of consciousness and protecting the C-spine. Assessment of breathing, circulation, and control of major hemorrhage is then carried out. Based upon the findings from the survey of mechanism of injury and the Initial Assessment, a Rapid Trauma Survey is then performed, a baseline set of vital signs is obtained, and if possible, a SAMPLE history obtained. At this point a determination is made on the need for immediate transport and critical interventions. Critical problems in the burn patient that require immediate intervention include airway compromise, altered level of consciousness, or the presence of major injuries in addition to the burn. Clues from the mechanism of injury that point to critical problems include a history of being confined in a closed space with the fire or smoke, electrical burns, falls from a height, or other major blunt force trauma.

The Rapid Trauma Survey of the burn patient is directed towards identification of airway and circulatory compromise. Besides clues from the mechanism of injury, other findings that should alert the responder to potential airway problems are the presence of facial and scalp burns, sooty sputum, and singed nasal hair and eyebrows. Examine the oral cavity and look for soot, swelling, or erythema (redness). Ask the patient to speak. A hoarse voice suggests involvement of deeper airway structures. Auscultate the chest. Wheezing or rales should alert you to the presence of lower airway injury from inhalation. Examine burned areas and check for distal pulses. Circumferential full-thickness burns may lead to neurovascular compromise. While this is rarely a problem on the fire scene, this may become significant during an interfacility transfer. Full-thickness burns of the chest wall, with eschar formation, may compromise chest expansion and ventilation. Escharotomy (by qualified personnel) is necessary. Be sure to alert the receiving facility to the presence of full-thickness circumferential burns.

Once the immediate life-threats have been addressed, you should attend to the burn wound itself. You should try to specifically limit burn wound progression as much as possible. Rapid cooling early in the course of a surface burn injury may help limit progression. Immediately following removal from the source of the burn, the skin is still hot and heat continues to injure the tissues. This will cause an increase in burn depth and seriousness of the injury. Cooling halts this process and, if done appropriately, is beneficial. Cooling should be done with any source of water, but this should be undertaken for a *maximum of one minute* since the burn is only 1 or 2 mm thick. Cooling for longer periods of time is actually detrimental to patients because it will induce hypothermia and subsequent shock.

Following the brief period of cooling, manage the burn by the use of clean, dry sheets and blankets to keep the patient warm and to prevent hypothermia. *It is not necessary to have sterile sheets.* The patient should be covered even when the environment is not cold because damaged skin loses temperature regulation capacity. Patients should never be transported on wet sheets, wet towels, or wet clothing, and *ice is absolutely contraindicated.* Ice will positively worsen the injury because it causes vasoconstriction and thus reduces the blood supply to already damaged tissue. It is better not to cool the burn wound at all rather than cool the burn wound improperly and cause hypothermia or additional tissue damage. Initial management of chemical and electrical burn injuries will be described in the sections on those injuries.

In your assessment of the burn patient, note and record the type of burn mechanism and the particular circumstances such as entrapment, explosion, mechanisms for other possible injuries, smoke exposure, chemical/electrical details, and so forth. An appropriate past medical history should also be documented in writing.

Perform a standard Detailed Exam on stable patients. This survey should specifically include an evaluation of the burn with an estimate of the depth based on appearance and a rough calculation of the burn size. These findings are important in determining the level of medical care that is appropriate for the burn victim. The burn size is best

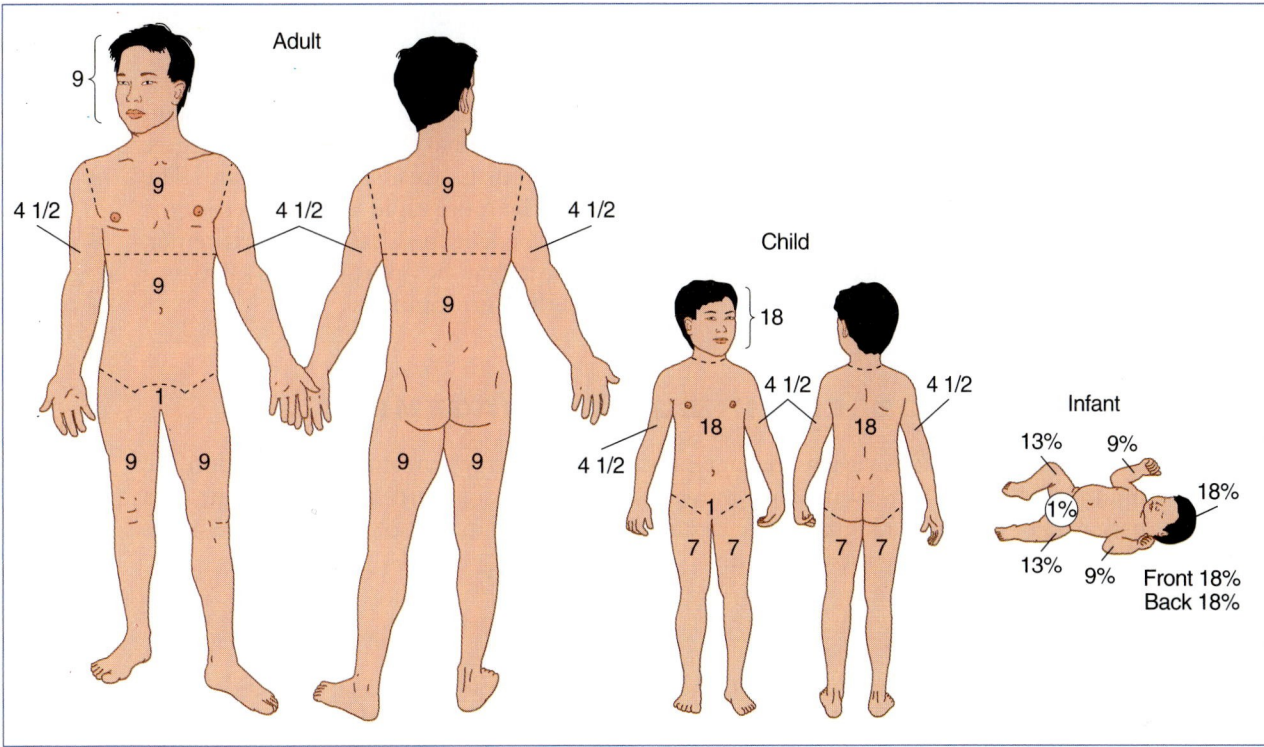

FIGURE 14-4 The rule of nines.

judged by using the rule of nines (see Figure 14-4). The body is divided into areas that are assigned either 9 or 18% of total body sizes, and by roughly drawing in the burned areas, the size can be estimated. There are some differences in body size proportionality in children. For smaller or irregular burns, the size can be estimated using the surface of the patient's hand to represent about 1% of the total body surface area. Even small burns are serious if they involve certain parts of the body (see Figure 14-5).

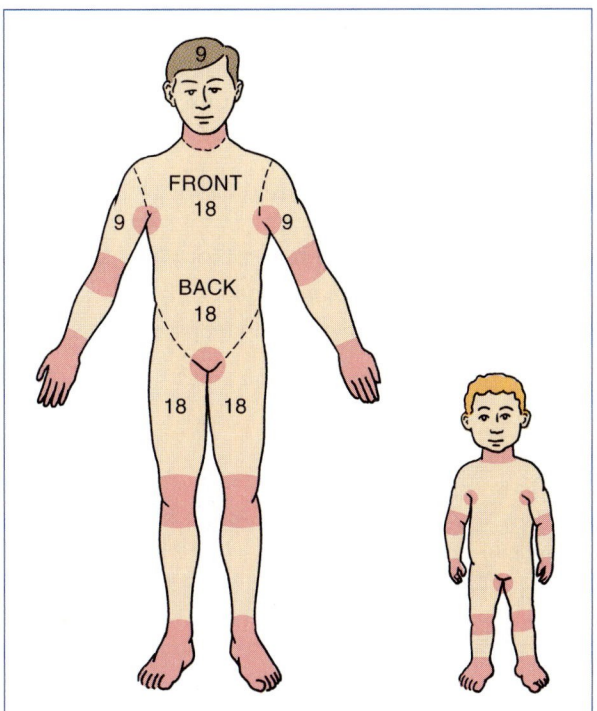

FIGURE 14-5 Areas in which small burns are more serious. Second- or third-degree burns in these areas (shaded portions) should be treated in the hospital.

Next remove the patient's loose clothing and jewelry. Cut around burned clothing that is adherent but do not try to pull the clothing off of the skin.

It is appropriate that burn injuries be seen by a physician. This is important because we now have specialized forms of therapy that offer specific advantages to the treatment of first-degree, second-degree, and third-degree burns. We have all seen second-degree burns become infected and progress to third-degree burns because of poor care. The sooner that specialized burn therapy can be initiated, the more rapid and satisfactory the results will be. Table 14-2 lists conditions that would benefit from care at a burn center. Based upon available local resources and protocols, it may be appropriate to bypass a local facility and transport these patients directly to the burn center.

SPECIAL PROBLEMS IN BURN MANAGEMENT

The following sections review management of specific types of burns, based upon the injury mechanism. Be aware that more than one type of burn can be present in a patient. For example, a high-voltage electrical burn injury may also produce flame burns due to ignition of the patient's clothing.

INHALATION INJURIES

Inhalation injuries accounted for more than half of the 5,000 plus burn-related deaths in the United States in 1995. Inhalation injuries are classified as carbon monoxide poisoning, heat inhalation injuries, or smoke inhalation injuries. Most frequently, inhalation injuries occur when a patient is injured in a confined space or is trapped; however, even victims of fires in open spaces may have inhalation injuries. Flash explosions (no fire) practically never cause inhalation injuries.

Carbon monoxide poisoning and asphyxiation are by far the most common causes of early death associated with burn injury. Carbon monoxide is simply a by-product of combustion and is one of the numerous chemicals in common smoke. It is present in high concentrations in auto exhaust fumes and fumes from some types of home space heaters. Since it is colorless, odorless, and tasteless, its presence is virtually impossible to detect. Carbon monoxide binds to hemoglobin (257 times stronger than oxygen), resulting in the hemoglobin being unable to transport oxygen. Patients quickly become hypoxic even in the presence of very small concentrations of carbon monoxide, and an alteration in their level of consciousness is the most predominant sign of hypoxia (see Table 14-3). A cherry-red skin color or cyanosis is virtually *never* present as a result of carbon monoxide poisoning and, therefore, cannot be used in the assess-

Table 14-2 Injuries That Benefit from Care at a Burn Center.

1. Second- and third-degree burns, 10% body surface area if age <10 or >50
2. Second- and third-degree burns, 20% body surface area, any age
3. Burns of face, hands, feet, genitalia, perineum, and skin overlying major joints
4. Third-degree burns, ≥5% total body surface area
5. Specialized burn types
   a. Electrical, including lightning
   b. Chemical
   c. Inhalation injury
   d. Circumferential chest or extremity injury
6. Presence of significant preexisting medical disorders
7. Presence of significant other injuries

Source: American Burn Association.

Table 14-3 **Symptoms Associated with Increasing Levels of Carboxyhemoglobin Binding.**

CARBOXYHEMOGLOBIN LEVEL (%)	SYMPTOMS
20	Headache common, throbbing in nature; shortness of breath on exertion
30	Headache present; altered central nervous system function with disturbed judgment; irritability, dizziness; decreased vision
40–50	Marked central nervous system alteration with confusion, collapse; also fainting with exertion
60–70	Convulsions; unconsciousness; apnea with prolonged exposure
80	Rapidly fatal

ment of patients for carbon monoxide poisoning. Death usually occurs because of myocardial ischemia and myocardial infarction due to progressive cardiac hypoxia. Treat patients suspected of having carbon monoxide poisoning with high-flow oxygen by mask. If such a patient has lost consciousness, ventilate using 100% oxygen. If a patient is simply removed from the source of the carbon monoxide and allowed to breathe fresh air, it takes up to 7 hours to reduce the carbon monoxide–hemoglobin complex to a safe level. Having a patient breathe 100% oxygen decreases this time to about 90 to 120 minutes, and use of hyperbaric oxygen (100% oxygen at 2.5 atmospheres) will decrease this time to about 30 minutes (see Figure 14-6).

Heat inhalation injuries selectively damage the upper airway, since breathing in flame and hot gases does not result in heat transport down to the lung tissue itself. The water vapor in the air in the tracheal–bronchial tree effectively absorbs this heat. Steam inhalation causes an exception to this rule (since it is already superheated water vapor). As a result of the heat injury, tissue swelling occurs just as it does with surface burns. The vocal cords themselves do not swell because they are dense fibrous bands of connective tissue. The loose mucosa in the supraglottic area (the hypopharynx) is where the swelling occurs, and this can easily progress to complete airway obstruction and death (see Figure 14-7). Airway swelling, like surface burn swelling, usually does not occur until after IV fluids have been running for some time and, therefore, heat airway injury compromise is very uncommon in prehospital burn care.

During secondary transport to a burn center, however, airway swelling can become significant and can cause airway obstruction as volume resuscitation IV fluids are being administered. For this reason, if there is any danger of airway burns, the patient should

FIGURE 14-6 Decay curve for disappearance of carboxyhemoglobin from 50% lethal level to 20% acceptable level in air, 1 atm. O_2 (100% oxygen) and 2.5 atm. O_2 (hyperbaric oxygen—100% at 2.5 atmospheres).

FIGURE 14-7   Heat inhalation can cause complete airway obstruction by swelling of the hypopharynx. Left side—normal anatomy; right side—swelling proximal to cords.

be sedated and intubated before a transfer. Figure 14-8 lists signs that should alert you to the danger of your patient having upper airway burns. Swollen lips indicate the presence of hot gases and burn injury at the airway entry, and hoarseness (indicating altered airflow through the larynx area) is a warning of early airway swelling. Stridor (high-pitched breathing, seal-bark cough) indicates severe airway swelling with more than 85% obstruction and *represents an immediate emergency*. The only appropriate treatment is airway stabilization. Load and go immediately.

Smoke inhalation injuries (see Figure 14-9) are the result of inhaled toxic chemicals that cause structural damage to lung cells. Smoke may contain hundreds of toxic chemicals that damage the delicate alveolar cells. Smoke from plastic and synthetic products is the most damaging. Damage from smoke inhalation usually takes days to develop and is virtually never a problem in initial field management.

CHEMICAL BURNS

There are virtually thousands of different types of chemicals that can cause burn injuries. Chemicals may not only injure the skin, but also may be absorbed into the body and cause internal organ failure (especially liver and kidney damage). Volatile forms of chem-

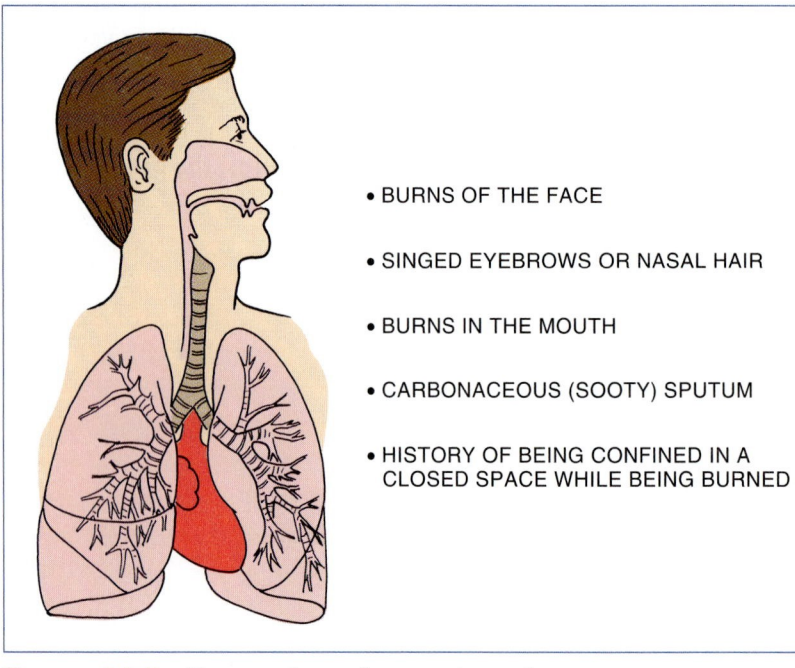

- BURNS OF THE FACE

- SINGED EYEBROWS OR NASAL HAIR

- BURNS IN THE MOUTH

- CARBONACEOUS (SOOTY) SPUTUM

- HISTORY OF BEING CONFINED IN A CLOSED SPACE WHILE BEING BURNED

FIGURE 14-8   Danger signs of upper airway burns.

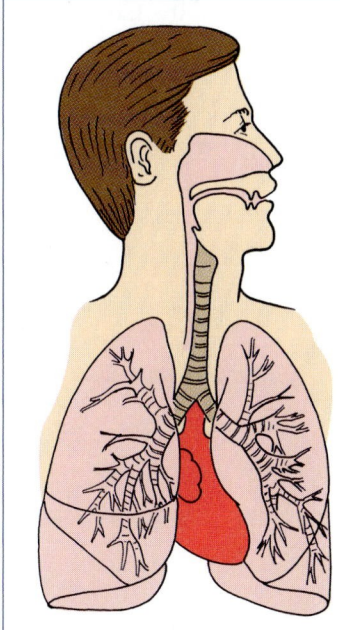

- VICTIMS EXPOSED TO SMOKE IN AN ENCLOSED PLACE
- VICTIMS WHO WERE UNCONSCIOUS WHILE EXPOSED TO SMOKE OR FIRE
- VICTIMS WITH A COUGH AFTER BEING EXPOSED TO SMOKE OR FIRE
- VICTIMS SHORT OF BREATH AFTER BEING EXPOSED TO SMOKE OR FIRE
- VICTIMS WITH CHEST PAIN AFTER BEING EXPOSED TO SMOKE OR FIRE

FIGURE 14-9   Patients in whom you should suspect smoke inhalation injury.

icals may be inhaled and cause lung tissue damage with subsequent severe life-threatening respiratory failure. Chemical injuries are frequently deceiving in that initial skin changes may be minimal even when a severe injury is present. This may cause a secondary problem in that such burns may not be obvious but you can get these chemicals on your own skin unless appropriate precautions are taken. Tissue damage factors include chemical concentration, quantity, manner and duration of skin contact, and the mechanism of action. The pathologic process causing the tissue damage continues until the chemical is either consumed in the damage process or is removed. Attempts at inactivation with specific neutralizing chemicals are dangerous because neutralizing chemicals generate other chemical reactions that may worsen the injury. Therefore, you should aim treatment at chemical removal by following these four steps:

1. Wear protective gloves, eyewear, and so on.
2. Remove all clothing with chemicals on it.
3. Flush most chemicals off the body by irrigating copiously with any source of available water or other irrigant. If dry chemical are on the skin, they should first be thoroughly brushed off before performing copious irrigation.
4. Remove any retained agent adhering to the skin by any appropriate physical means such as wiping or scraping. Follow this by further irrigation.

In all but the most trivial injuries, continue flushing for 15 minutes, unless a critical or unstable situation warrants transport sooner (see Figures 14-10 and 14-11). Irrigation of caustic chemicals in the eye is exceptionally important because irreversible damage will occur in a very short period of time (less than the transport time to get to the hospital). Irrigation of injured eyes may be difficult because of the pain associated with eye opening. However, you must begin irrigation to prevent severe and permanent damage to the corneas (see Figure 14-12). Check for contact lenses and, if present, remove them early during irrigation. Remember that dealing with hazardous materials requires proper training and equipment.

ELECTRICAL BURNS

In cases of electrical burns, damage is caused by electricity entering the body and traveling through the tissues. Extremities usually have more significant tissue damage because

FIGURE 14-10 Chemical burns of the skin.

REMOVE
CONTAMINATED
CLOTHING

FLOOD AREA
WITH WATER

FIGURE 14-11 Acid burn of the ankle being irrigated.
(Courtesy of Roy Alson, M.D.)

their small size results in higher local current density (see Figure 14-13). The factors that determine severity of electrical injury include the following:

1. The type and amount of current
2. Path of the current
3. Duration of contact with the current

The most serious injury that occurs due to electrical contact is immediate cardiac dysrhythmias. *Any patient involved with an electric current injury, regardless of how stable he looks, should have a careful immediate evaluation of his cardiac status and continuous monitoring of cardiac activity.* The most common life-threatening dysrhythmias are premature ventricular contractions, ventricular tachycardia, and ventricular fibrillation. Automated defibrillators are very useful in this situation, since these patients usually have normal healthy hearts and the chances for resuscitation are excellent. For a patient in ventricular fibrillation with only basic life support available, start cardiopulmonary resuscitation (CPR) and transport immediately to a hospital facility. Most of these victims do not have preexisting cardiovascular disease, and their heart muscle tissue is usually not damaged as a result of the electricity. Even under circumstances of prolonged CPR, resuscitation is often possible. Once those efforts at managing cardiac status are complete, provide field care as previously described for thermal burns.

FIGURE 14-12 Chemical burns of the eye.

FIGURE 14-13 Electrical burn of the lower leg and foot.
(Courtesy of Roy Alson, M.D.)

Additional electrical injuries include skin burns at entrance and exit sites because of high temperatures generated by the electric arc (2,500 degrees centigrade) at the skin surface. Additional surface flame burns may be present as a result of the patient's clothing being ignited. Fractures and/or dislocations may be present due to the violent muscle contractions that electrical injuries cause. Internal injuries usually involve muscle damage, nerve damage, and possible intravascular blood coagulation due to electrical current passage. *Internal chest or abdominal organ damage is exceedingly rare.*

At the scene of an electrical injury, your first priority in determining scene safety is to determine if the patient is still in contact with the electrical current. If so, you must remove the patient from contact without becoming a victim yourself (see Figure 14-14). Handling high-voltage electrical wires is extremely hazardous. Special training and special equipment are needed to deal with downed wires; never attempt to move wires with makeshift equipment. Tree limbs, pieces of wood, and even manila rope may conduct high-voltage electricity. Even firefighter's gloves and boots do not protect one in this situation. If possible, leave the handling of downed wires to power company employees or develop a special training program with your local power company to learn how to use the special equipment needed to handle high-voltage lines.

Initially, it is impossible to tell the total extent of the damage in electrical burns; all electrical burn patients should be transported for hospital evaluation.

LIGHTNING INJURY

Lightning kills more Americans each year than any other weather-related phenomenon. Injuries from lightning are very different from other electrical burns in that they involve extremely high voltages (>10,000,000 volts) and currents (>2,000 amps), but the electricity has a very short duration (<100 msec).

Lightning produces a "flashover" phenomenon, in which the current flows around the outside of the victim's body. Consequently, the internal damage due to current flow from contact with generated electricity is not seen with lightning strike. Most of the effects from a lightning strike are the result of the massive dc (direct current) shock that is received. Classic lightning strike burns produce a fern-like pattern across the skin (see Figure 14-15). The victim does not need to be struck directly to sustain an injury. Lightning may strike an adjacent object or nearby ground and still produce an injury to a victim. Often the victim's skin is wet, from either sweat or rain. This water, when heated by the lightning current, is quickly vaporized, producing first-degree and second-degree burns, and may literally explode the clothing off the victim. As these burns are superficial, aggressive fluid resuscitation is not required.

The most serious effect of a lightning strike is cardiorespiratory arrest, with the massive current acting like a defibrillator to briefly stop the heart. Cardiac activity often

FIGURE 14-14   Removal of high-voltage electrical wires. Do not try to remove wires with the safety equipment (or with sticks) unless specially trained. Turn off the electricity at the source or call the power company to remove the wires.

FIGURE 14-15 Classic fern-like burns on the skin of a victim of a lightning strike. *(Courtesy of Roy Alson, M.D.)*

spontaneously resumes within minutes. However, the respiratory drive centers of the brain are also depressed by the current discharge, and these areas take longer to recover and resume the normal respiratory drive. Consequently, the victim remains in respiratory arrest, which is followed by a hypoxic cardiac arrest.

The essential component of the management of the lightning strike victim is restoration of cardiorespiratory function, while protecting the C-spine. Since lightning strikes often occur at sporting events and other outdoor gatherings, strikes often become multiple-casualty events. It must be stressed that in a multiple-casualty lightning strike, the conventional triage approach of a pulseless or nonbreathing patient equaling a dead patient should not be followed. If a patient is awake or breathing after a lightning strike, she will most likely survive without further intervention. Concentrate on those victims who are in respiratory or cardiac arrest, since prompt CPR represents the only chance that these victims have for survival.

Long-term problems have been seen in lightning strike patients, such as the development of cataracts, or neurological and/or psychological difficulties. Perforation of the eardrum is quite common, and rarely long bone or scapular fractures, as seen in the victims of generated high-voltage electrical injuries, may be seen. These fractures are managed as described in Chapter 12.

There are over 200 reported deaths in the United States each year due to lightning strike. This represents only 30% of lightning strike victims, thus it is possible that you will have to care for such a victim. These events often involve multiple victims, with varying degrees of severity. Prompt CPR greatly improves the chances of survival. When confronted with a naked (or partially unclothed) unconscious or confused patient, with perforated eardrums and a fern-like burn pattern on his body, think: lightning strike!

SECONDARY TRANSPORT

Major burns usually do not occur in locations where immediate transport to one of the major burn centers is possible. As a result, transport from a primary hospital to a burn center is commonly necessary. After the initial stabilization (which should require between 1 and 3 hours), immediate movement to a major burn center is best for the patient. During this transport, it is important to be able to continue resuscitation.

Prior to secondary transports, the transferring physician should have completed the following:

1. Stabilization of respiratory and hemodynamic function. This may necessitate intubation, and certainly two large-bore IVs for fluid administration are standard.

2. Assessment and management of associated injuries
3. Review of appropriate lab data (specifically blood gas analysis)
4. Placement of a nasogastric tube in all burns covering more than 20% of the body surface area
5. Assessment of peripheral circulation and appropriate wound management
6. Proper arrangements with the receiving hospital and physician

You should specifically discuss the transport with either the referring or the receiving physician to determine what special functions may need monitoring. It is important for you to maintain careful records indicating patient condition and treatment during the transport. You should also make an in-depth report to the receiving facility.

PEDIATRIC BURNS

Children represent nearly one-half of all patients who seek treatment for burns. Because of their thinner skin, they are more likely to suffer a more severe injury following a burn. Postburn problems, such as hypothermia, are more likely to occur in children because of their larger surface area to body mass ratio. Because of differences in anatomy, the rule of nines needs to be modified, as in small children the head represents a larger portion of the body surface (see Figure 14-4). Another way to estimate the extent of burns in children is to use a Lund and Browder chart.

Burns in children may be the result of intentional abuse and, in fact, 10% of abuse cases involve burns. You should be alert for signs of abuse. These include burns that match shapes of objects, such as curling irons, irons, or cigarette burns. Also suspicious for abuse are multiple stories of how the injury occurred or stories of the burn being caused by activities by the child that are inconsistent with the child's development. Burns to the genitalia, perineum, or in a stocking or glove distribution (see Figure 14-16) should also raise suspicion. If there is a suspicion of abuse, this must be reported to child protective services or law enforcement. Fire and EMS personnel can help reduce burns in children through community education. Programs to teach parents about limiting the temperature on household water heaters to 120 degrees Fahrenheit and programs to teach children about fire safety can make a significant impact on the incidence of pediatric burns in your community. You should also be aware that the elderly may also be victims of abuse by burns (see Chapter 16).

FIGURE 14-16   Full-thickness scald burns on a child caused by abuse.
(Courtesy of Roy Alson, M.D.)

PITFALLS AND IMPORTANT POINTS

1. Maintain appropriate safety when removing patients from the source of a burn injury.

2. Treat burn patients as trauma patients—BTLS Primary Survey, critical interventions, and transport decision, Detailed Exam, and Ongoing Exam.

3. Properly cool the surface thermal injury if early after burn event—don't cause hypothermia.

4. Any type of burn can have some degree of inhalation injury.

5. Early deaths from burns are not due to burn injury but to airway compromise. Perform frequent ongoing assessments of the airway.

6. Chemical injuries, in general, require prolonged and copious irrigation.

7. Immediately check cardiac status of victims of electrical injury.

8. Plan all secondary transports to major burn centers and effectively continue resuscitation during such transports.

9. Do not begin a secondary transport of a patient with a possible airway burn without the patient being intubated before transport.

SUMMARY

Burn injuries are potentially deadly for both you and your patient. You must never forget the rules of scene safety. Half of all burn deaths are from inhalation injuries; do not forget the airway. Give 100% oxygen if there is any chance of inhalation injury. Cool the burn to halt the burning process, but do not cause hypothermia. You must begin irrigating chemical burns in the field, or the burn damage will continue during transport. This is one of the few instances in trauma care when extra time spent in the field may be beneficial to the patient. Electrical burns are commonly associated with cardiac arrest, but rapid evaluation and management are usually lifesaving. High-voltage electricity is extremely dangerous; get trained personnel to turn it off. Do not begin secondary transfer of a burn patient until the patient has been properly stabilized and the airway protected.

BIBLIOGRAPHY

1. Alson, R. "Thermal Burns." *Emedicine: On-line Emergency Medicine Text.* Boston: Boston Medical Publishers, 1998.

2. Committee on Trauma, American College of Surgeons. "Injuries Due to Burns and Cold." *Advanced Trauma Life Support.* Chicago: The College, 1997.

3. Committee on Trauma, American College of Surgeons. *Advanced Burn Life Support.* Chicago: The College, 1988.

4. Criss, E., and others. "Not Just Blowing Smoke." *Emergency Medical Services* (March 1998), pp. 27–39.

5. Wald, D. A. "Burn Management: Systematic Patient Evaluation, Fluid Resuscitation, and Wound Management." *Emergency Medicine Reports,* Vol. 19 (1998), pp. 45–52.

CHAPTER 15

Trauma in Children

Ann Marie Dietrich, M.D., F.A.C.E.P.,
   F.A.A.P.
Jon Groner, M.D.

(Photo courtesy of David Effron, M.D., FACEP)

OBJECTIVES

UPON COMPLETION OF THIS CHAPTER, YOU SHOULD BE ABLE TO:

1. Describe effective techniques for gaining the confidence of children and their parents.
2. Predict pediatric injuries based on common mechanisms of injury.
3. Describe the Primary Survey and Detailed Exam in the pediatric patient.
4. Demonstrate understanding of the need for immediate transport in potentially life-threatening circumstances, regardless of lack of immediate parental consent.
5. Differentiate equipment needs of pediatric patients from those of adults.
6. Describe the various ways to immobilize a child and how this differs from an adult.
7. Discuss the need for involvement of EMS personnel in prevention programs for parents and children.

Note: Because of increasing demand for further training in management of the injured child, BTLS has developed a one-day course (Pediatric BTLS) that covers this subject in greater detail. You may get more information about this course by calling BTLS International at: 1-800-495-2875.

COMMUNICATING WITH THE CHILD AND FAMILY

An injured child is still part of a family unit. Family-centered care is critical for the child, and the one constant factor in their life is their family. Remember that the caregiver of a child will not always be a "parent," but for simplicity we will use the generic term "parents" when referring to the guardian of a child. Following an injury, parents should be involved as much as possible in the care their child receives. The parents should be directed and supported in efforts to provide love and concern to their child. Parents who receive careful instructions and guidance are the best assets in the field. Explain to the parents what you are doing and why you are doing it, and use their trust relationship with the child to enhance your history, physical examination, and care of the patient. Inclusion and respect of the family will improve the performance of all aspects of stabilization of an injured child.

The best way to get the parents' confidence is to demonstrate your competence and compassion in managing the child. Parents are more likely to be cooperative if they see that you are confident, organized, and are using equipment that is designed for children. Show the parents you know how important they are by involving them in the care of their child. Whenever possible, keep parents in physical and verbal contact with the child. They can perform simple tasks such as holding a pressure dressing or holding the child's hand. Parents can explain to the child what is going on or sing their favorite songs.

Show your concern for the child—but don't freeze. One technique is to pretend that the parent is one of your examiners. You can then talk your way through the examination using language that is understandable to both the child and family. You will also be able to better assess mental status. A child who can be consoled or distracted by a person or a toy has a normal mental status (most sensitive indicator of adequate perfusion). On the other hand, a child who cannot be consoled or distracted may have a head injury, be in shock, be experiencing hypoxia, or be in severe pain. Changes in distractibility and consolability are important observations about the level of consciousness of a child. Record and report them just as you would report changes in level of consciousness of an adult.

A child less than 9 months old likes to hear "cooing" sounds, the tinkle and sight of keys, and often feels more comfortable when swaddled. For the child less than age 2, the flashlight is a good distraction. Use appropriate language for the development of the child. Children less than one year of age know many "ah" sounds, like "mama" and "papa." Try to use those. Older children, especially 2-year-old children, are typically negative and often difficult to distract or comfort. Expect all questions to be answered by "no." Therefore, tell the child and the parents what you are going to do and do it. For example, "We are going to hold your head still. Mom, this is important in case he has hurt his neck." Speak simply, slowly, and clearly. Be gentle and firm. The toddler and young child can benefit from a toy or doll being with them. Ask the parent to get one favorite belonging, if easily available, for the ride to the hospital. It will make the trip to and through the hospital easier. If time allows and the patient is stable, you can make an airplane out of two tongue blades or a doll out of a rubber glove (if child is over 3 years old and won't choke on the rubber).

Don't get caught in the trap of asking the child if he wants to take a trip in the ambulance or to be placed in a cervical collar. The child will answer "no" most of the time. Tell the child what you are doing with a smile on your face. Show it does not hurt, perhaps by doing it to a parent or yourself. Size is intimidating. When approaching a child, try to make yourself small by getting on the child's level. In the care of the child, it is appropriate that paramedics spend much field time on their knees. Frightened children, especially around the age of 2 to 4, may try to defend themselves by biting, spitting, or hitting. They are acting out of fear. Stay calm, recognize that the behavior is normal, reassure the child, and use firm, not painful, physical control of the patient as needed. Parents and children do not understand packaging, which makes them more likely to resist it. Explain why packaging is necessary. Most parents will understand if you explain that even though the chances are low that there is anything seriously wrong with the spine, the stakes are high if there is. Make a game of packaging with the child. If the parent refuses to let you package, write it down on your run report and get the parent to sign it.

Many states have consent laws that exist to protect children. Although consent is necessary for children who are stable, and desirable in children who are injured, any critically injured child should NOT have care delayed while attempting to obtain consent. Paramedics have to make a decision on whether it will take too long to find a parent to obtain consent. In a situation in which a child needs emergency care (e.g., a child in a bicycle–auto collision and no parent present), you must treat that child appropriately. Transport before you receive permission, document why you are transporting without permission, and notify Medical Direction of this action. If the parents or legal guardians do not want you to transport or treat, try to persuade them. If you cannot, document your actions on the written report and try to get them to sign it. If you suspect abuse, notify authorities.

Whenever possible, allow parents to accompany their child in the vehicle. It is very frightening for a child and a family to be separated, especially if the injuries are severe. Give the parents specific instructions and position them to provide comfort and support to their child without interfering with the care that must be given.

Before you leave the scene with the child, be sure to ask the parent about other children. Sometimes they are so concerned about one they forget other small children who may be in a high-risk situation, such as alone in the house.

EQUIPMENT

Table 15-1 contains a list of suggested pediatric equipment for the prehospital provider. You would not want to approach a 170-pound man having a heart attack with a 3.5-mm endotracheal tube, nor would you approach a child with adult equipment. Pediatric equipment should be kept in a separate trauma box. Equipment for each size child could be kept in different trauma boxes, so that everything for that size child would be at your fingertips. However, lack of storage space makes multiple boxes impractical for most rescue vehicles and ambulances. In addition, it is impractical to make multiple trips back to the vehicle if the prearrival information was inaccurate. The Broselow tape is a commercial tape measure that, when used to measure the length of a child, gives you the estimated weight of the child, precalculated doses of fluid and medications, and estimated sizes of common equipment needed. You could have equipment and supplies sorted into boxes or bags coded to the color panels on the Broselow tape (a compact bag is commercially available).

Using a length/weight-based drug dose chart or tape (i.e., the Broselow tape) has become an essential component for determining the appropriate equipment and medication doses for a child (see Figure 15-1). These devices allow you to focus on the patient instead of remembering the correct equipment size and drug dose. The Broselow tape is used by placing the end of the tape that says "measure from head" at the top of the child's head. Stretch the tape the length of the child and put your other hand on the tape at the level of the child's heel. The colored section your hand is touching gives you a great deal of information. Estimated weight, precalculated drug dosages, and the proper sizes of endotracheal tubes, suction catheters, nasogastric tubes, and oral airways are all shown on the tape. The Broselow tape estimates weight better than emergency medicine professionals and endotracheal tube size as well as anesthesiologists.

Table 15-1 Prehospital Pediatric Equipment and Supplies.

BLS EQUIPMENT AND SUPPLIES	
ESSENTIAL	**DESIRABLE**
Oropharyngeal airways: infant, child, and adult sizes (sizes 00–5) with tongue blades for insertion	Infant car seat
Self-inflating resuscitation bag, child and adult sizes	Glasgow Coma Score reference
Masks for bag-valve mask device: infant, child, and adult sizes	Small stuffed toy
Nonrebreathing mask: pediatric and adult sizes	Finger-stick blood glucose device
Stethoscope	
Pediatric femur traction splint	
Pediatric backboard with head immobilizer	
Pediatric cervical collars (rigid)	
Blood pressure cuff, infant and child	
Portable suction unit with a regulator	
Suction catheter: tonsil-tip and 6F–14F	
Extremity splints: pediatric sizes	
Bulb syringe	
Obstetric pack	
Thermal blanket	
Broselow tape	

FIGURE 15-1 Broselow tape.

PATIENT ASSESSMENT

COMMON MECHANISMS OF INJURY IN CHILDREN

Children are most commonly injured from falls, MVCs, auto–pedestrian accidents, burns, airway obstruction from a foreign body, and child abuse. Children who fall usually land on their heads because the head is the largest and heaviest part of a small child's body. You should anticipate head injury when a child falls. Auto collisions, especially if lap belt restraints are improperly used, may injure the liver, spleen, or intestines. Any situation in which the injury pattern and mechanism differ may be child abuse. Suspect abuse if the history doesn't match the injury, if there is a delay in seeking health care, or if the story keeps changing.

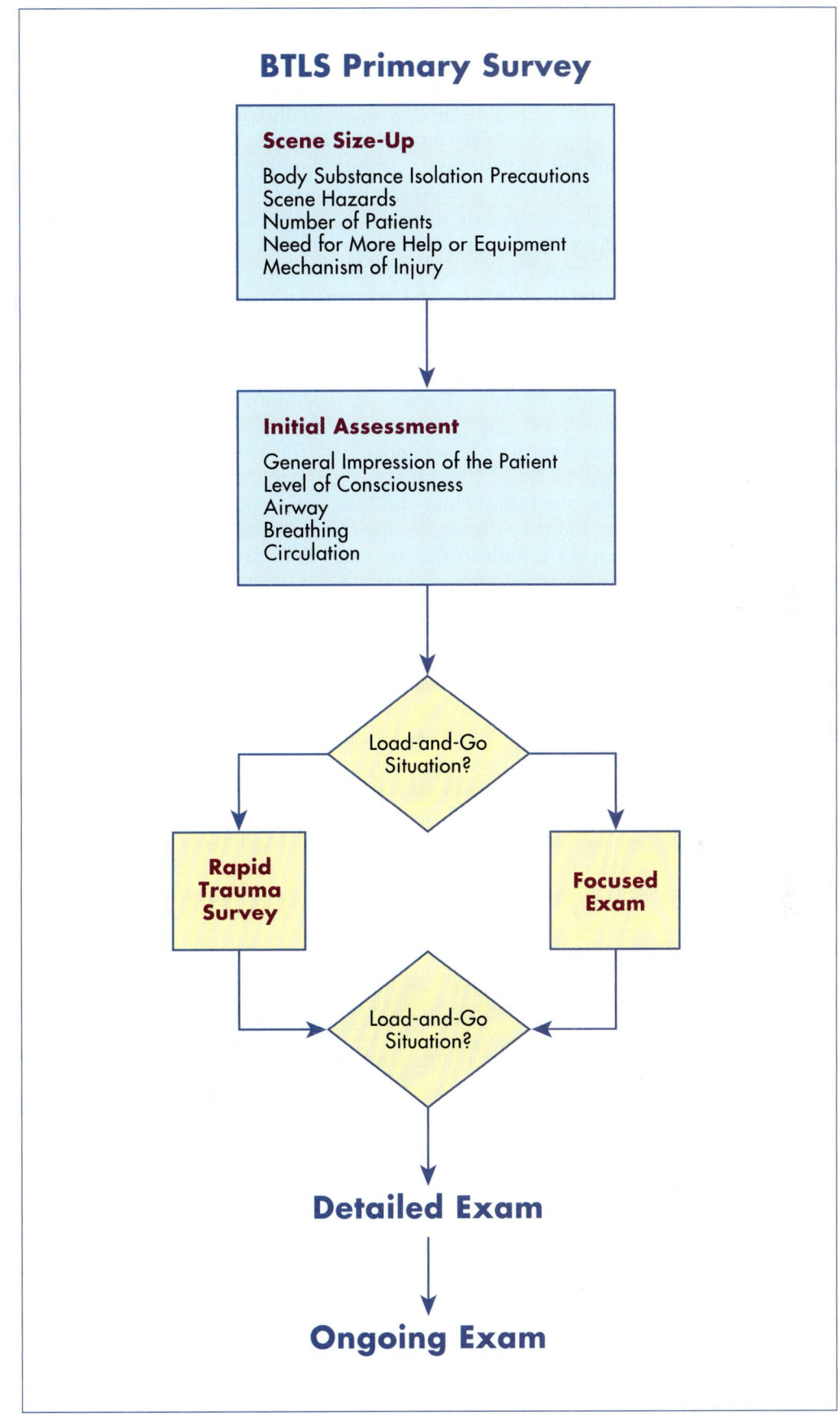

FIGURE 15-2 Steps in the assessment and management of the trauma patient. This is the same for both children and adults.

AIRWAY WITH C-SPINE STABILIZATION AND INITIAL LEVEL OF CONSCIOUSNESS

This aspect of assessment is easier in the child than in the adult. It is true that the child's tongue is large, the tissue is soft, and the airway is easy to obstruct, but other characteristics make it easier to manage the child's airway. For example, neonates are obligatory nose breathers, so just opening the mouth or clearing the nose with a bulb syringe can be lifesaving. To use the bulb syringe, collapse the bulb end of the syringe, put the point end in the nose of the child, and release the bulb. Remove the syringe from the nose; recollapse the bulb to empty the mucus, blood, or vomit, and repeat. The bulb syringe can be used to remove secretions from the posterior pharynx of infants as well.

Be sure to stabilize the neck in a neutral position with your hands. Do not take time to apply a cervical collar until you have finished the BTLS Primary Survey. Recognize the signs of airway obstruction in children: apnea, stridor, or "gurgling" respiration. So that the neck does not have to be moved, the jaw thrust should be the first airway maneuver in the unconscious child who has sustained trauma. In small children, the occiput is so big that it will flex the neck and may occlude the airway when the child is lying flat. It is often necessary to place a pad underneath the torso to keep the neck in a neutral position (see Figure 15-3 and Chapter 9). Hyperextension of the neck also may cause airway occlusion. For the unconscious child, an oral airway is very helpful to get the tongue out of the way and keep the airway open (see Chapter 5). If a tooth is loose, be sure to remove it from the mouth so that the child does not choke on it. The oral airway can stimulate a gag reflex, which is very sensitive in the conscious child, thus limiting the use of this airway to unconscious children with no gag reflex. Nasopharyngeal airways are too small to work predictably in children; do not use them. Give ventilation instructions as soon as you complete your evaluation of breathing.

Check the neck for signs of injury (bruises, marks, lacerations), carotid pulse, and distended neck veins, and feel for a deviated trachea. What appears to be minor blunt trauma to the neck can be life-threatening. A deviated trachea is difficult to detect in a small child, but has the same significance as in adults. Make a mental note of the child's initial level of consciousness as you begin your survey. Although a sleeping preschool child can look unconscious, remember that most children will not sleep through the arrival of emergency vehicles. Ask the parents to awaken the child to get an initial assessment of their airway and level of consciousness. Following a traumatic event, a decreased level of consciousness may suggest hypoxia, shock, head trauma, or seizure.

FIGURE 15-3 Most children require padding under their back and shoulders to keep the c-spine in a neutral position. *(Courtesy of Bob Page, NREMT-P)*

ASSESSMENT OF BREATHING

Assess the child for breathing difficulty. Count the child's respiratory rate. Most children breathe fast when they are having trouble and then, when they can no longer compensate, they have periods of apnea or a very slow respiratory rate. Note whether the child is "working" to breathe, demonstrated by retractions, flaring, or grunting. Look at the chest rise, listen for air going in and out, and feel the air coming out of the nose. If there is no movement, you must breathe for the child. If ventilation is inadequate, you must assist the child. When performing mouth-to-mouth ventilation for a small child, you may cover both the child's nose and mouth with your mouth. If the face mask does not fit well when performing bag-valve mask ventilation, try turning the mask upside down for a better seal. Pay attention to your hand placement (see Figure 15-4). Your large hands can easily obstruct the airway or injure the child's eyes. Give the breaths slowly at low pressure, less than 20 cm H_2O, to keep from inflating the stomach or causing a pneumothorax. The rates are 40 per minute for a child less than a year of age, 20 per minute for greater than 1 year of age, and 15 per minute for an adolescent. Most important, watch for chest rise. If the chest is rising, air is getting into the lungs. Check air entry on both sides of the chest with your stethoscope. *Gentle* cricoid pressure (Sellick maneuver, see Chapter 3) is useful and recommended in a child. Some self-inflatable bag-valve masks have a pop-off valve at about 40 cm H_2O pressure. The pressure generated by these devices is more than adequate most of the time. However, lungs are sometimes stiff from a near-drowning, bronchospasm, or aspiration, and more pressure is needed. Be familiar with your equipment. Make sure that your bag-valve mask does not have a pop-off valve.

As you package a child, you will often have to improvise. Tape and straps can restrict the child's chest movement, so assess ventilation frequently en route. Any child with a significant injury should receive supplemental oxygen (as close to 100% oxygen as possible), even if there seems to be no difficulty breathing. Injury, fear, and crying all increase oxygen demands on tissues. Children with any type of injury are likely to vomit; be prepared. Remember to give ventilation instructions to your teammate before moving to assessment of circulation.

ASSESSMENT OF CIRCULATION

Early shock is more difficult to diagnose in a child than an adult. Persistent tachycardia is the most reliable indicator of shock in a child. As pulses may be difficult to find and judge in a child, practice feeling them on most of your pediatric runs and on your children. In a child, the brachial pulse is usually easy to feel, whereas the carotid is not.

FIGURE 15-4   Bag-valve mask ventilation in a child.

Feeling a dorsalis pedis pulse causes less anxiety and may be easier to find than a femoral pulse. A weak rapid pulse with a rate over 130 is usually a sign of shock in all children except neonates (see Table 15-2). Decreased tissue perfusion may be manifested by prolonged capillary refill and cool extremities. Capillary refill may be used along with other methods to assess the circulation, but do not depend on it alone to diagnose shock. Although currently controversial, capillary refill should still be included as part of the Initial Assessment for shock in a child. To test capillary refill, compress the nailbed, the entire foot, or the skin over the sternum for 2 seconds and release to see how quickly the blood returns. Skin color should return to the precompressed state within 2 seconds. If it does not, the child has vasoconstriction, which can be a sign of shock.

Individual variances may make some of the signs of shock normal for a particular child. Tachycardia may occur because of fear or fever. Mottling may be normal in an infant less than 6 months of age, but it also may be a sign of poor circulation, so note it. Extremities may be cold because of nervousness, cold weather, or poor perfusion. Capillary refill may be prolonged in a child that is cold. In general, a child should be carefully evaluated and assumed to have signs of shock if there is persistent tachycardia or signs of poor peripheral perfusion (prolonged capillary refill or cool extremities).

The child's level of consciousness is also a useful indicator of circulatory status, yet note that circulation can be poor even though the child appears awake. As mentioned earlier, if the child is able to focus on their parent, or is consolable by the parent or a member of the EMS team, there is enough circulation to allow the child's brain to be working.

Low blood pressure is a sign of late shock, but measuring blood pressure in a frightened child can be time-consuming, especially for the inexperienced. To make it easier and more reliable to obtain blood pressure in an emergency, practice taking it at every opportunity. The rule of thumb for cuff size is to use the largest one that will fit snugly on the patient's arm. If there is too much noise, you can perform a blood pressure by palpation. Find the radial pulse, pump up the blood pressure cuff until you no longer feel the pulse, and allow air to leak slowly while observing the dial on the blood pressure cuff. Record the pressure at which you first feel the pulse and label it "p" for palpation. This will be a systolic blood pressure only and will be slightly lower than a blood pressure that can be auscultated. A systolic blood pressure less than 80 in children, and less than 70 in young infants, is a sign of shock.

Shock may be secondary to occult bleeding in the abdomen, chest, or in a femur fracture. Also, although we teach that patients don't go into shock from intracranial blood loss, this can happen in the young infant. Thus, if you see an infant in shock with no obvious source of bleeding, consider intracranial blood loss.

The antishock garment (MAST or PASG) is no longer recommended for treatment of shock except in special circumstances (see Chapter 7). Remember, older children wearing tight-fitting pants are already wearing a form of antishock garment. Cutting these off, like deflating traditional antishock garments, may produce a drop in perfusion. Thus, in children with signs of shock, it is wise to delay cutting off tight pants until after you have arrived at the hospital.

Table 15-2 **Ranges for Vital Signs.**

AGE	WEIGHT (KG)	RESPIRATIONS	PULSE	SYSTOLIC BLOOD PRESSURE (MMHG)
Newborn	3–4	30–50	120–160	>60
6 mo.–1 yr.	8–10	30–40	120–140	70–80
2–4 yr.	12–16	20–30	100–110	80–95
5–8 yr.	18–26	14–20	90–100	90–100
8–12 yr.	26–50	12–20	80–100	100–110
>12 yr.	>50	12–16	80–100	100–120

CONTROL OF BLEEDING

Obvious bleeding sources must be controlled to maintain circulation. Remember, the child's blood volume is about 80 to 90 cc per kilogram, so a 10-kg child has less than 1 L of blood. Three or four lacerations can cause a 200-cc blood loss, which is about 20% of the child's total volume. Therefore, pay closer attention to blood loss in a child than you do in an adult. Use pressure firm enough to control arterial bleeding if necessary. If you ask the parent or a bystander to help hold pressure, monitor them to be sure they are applying enough pressure to stop the bleeding. Use a bandage tight enough to control venous bleeding, not one that will just soak up the blood so that you do not see it. Elevating an injured extremity also can help to control bleeding.

DECISION: IS THERE A CRITICAL TRAUMA SITUATION PRESENT?

If you have found a critical trauma situation, the child needs rapid transport. Log-roll the child onto a pediatric spineboard and go. Remember to use a pad under the torso to align the neck in a neutral position. Appropriately sized rigid cervical collars are useful, especially in children over one year of age, and can help remind the patient and the providers not to move the head. Do not depend on the cervical collar alone; immobilize the head with tape and a head immobilizer. Children are portable and they can (and should) be transported rapidly. *There are very few procedures that should be done in the field.* Minutes count, especially in children. On-scene times of less than 5 minutes are desirable. Administer 100% oxygen to all critical pediatric patients. Assist ventilation if necessary. Not all emergency departments have the equipment or personnel to handle pediatric emergencies. Transfer arrangements for more severe problems should be worked out in advance so that when the injury occurs, confusion will be minimized and time will be saved. See Table 15-3 for a partial list of mechanisms of injury that are criteria for transport to an emergency department approved for pediatrics or a pediatric trauma center. These, plus pediatric burns, near-drowning, and head injuries with loss

Table 15-3 Suggested Criteria for Transfer to an Emergency Department Approved for Pediatrics or a Pediatric Trauma Center.

CRITERIA
Obstructed airway
Need for an airway intervention
Respiratory distress
Shock
Altered mental status
Dilated pupil
Glasgow Coma Score <13
Pediatric Trauma Score <8
Mechanism of injury (less reliable indicators) associated with severe injuries:
1. Fall from a height of 15 feet or more
2. An accident with fatalities
3. Ejected from an automobile in a MVC
4. In a MVC, the engine entered the passenger compartment
5. Hit by a car as a pedestrian or bicyclist
6. Fractures in more than one extremity
7. Significant injury to more than one organ system

of consciousness, should go to facilities qualified to handle major pediatric trauma. Call ahead so that the emergency department can have the necessary equipment and personnel ready. Perform Detailed Exams and Ongoing Exams en route if there is time.

If, after completing the Primary Assessment, you find no critical trauma situation, place the child on a backboard and do a methodical Detailed Exam.

DETAILED EXAM

As in adults, record accurate vital signs, take a SAMPLE history, and perform a complete head-to-toes exam, including a more detailed neurological exam. During your neurological exam make a notation of whether the child is consolable or distractible. Finish bandaging and splinting, and transport the child while continuously monitoring. Notify Medical Direction. Calculate the Glasgow Coma Score (GCS) and Pediatric Trauma Score during transport (Tables 15-4 and 15-5).

Table 15-4   Glasgow Coma Score.

		>1 YEAR	<1 YEAR	
EYES OPENING	4	Spontaneously	Spontaneously	
	3	To verbal command	To shout	
	2	To pain	To pain	
	1	No response	No response	
		>1 YEAR	<1 YEAR	
BEST MOTOR RESPONSE	6	Obeys		
	5	Localizes pain	Localizes pain	
	4	Flexion–withdrawal	Flexion–normal	
	3	Flexion–abnormal (decorticate rigidity)	Flexion–abnormal (decorticate rigidity)	
	2	Extension (decerebrate rigidity)	Extension (decerebrate rigidity)	
	1	No response	No response	
		>5 YEARS	2–5 YEARS	0–23 MONTHS
BEST VERBAL RESPONSE	5	Oriented and converses	Appropriate words and phrases	Smiles, coos, cries appropriately
	4	Disoriented and converses	Inappropriate words	Cries
	3	Inappropriate words	Cries and/or screams	Inappropriate crying and/or screaming
	2	Incomprehensible sounds	Grunts	Grunts
	1	No response	No response	No response

Table 15-5 **Pediatric Trauma Score**

Score	+2	+1	-1
Weight	>44 lb (>20 kg)	22–44 lb (10–20 kg)	<22 lb (<10 kg)
Airway	Normal	Oral or nasal airway	Intubated tracheostomy invasive airway
Blood pressure	Pulse at wrist >90 mmHg	Carotid or femoral pulse palpable 50–90 mmHg	No palpable pulse <50 mmHg
Level of consciousness	Completely awake	Obtunded or any loss of consciousness	Comatose
Open wound	None	Minor	Major or penetrating
Fractures	None	Closed fracture	Open or multiple fractures

INJURIES

HEAD INJURY

Head injuries are the most common cause of death in pediatric patients. The head is the primary focus of injury in the child because the child's head is proportionately larger than the adult's. The force of impact does some damage to the brain, but much of the brain damage from head injuries comes after impact, from preventable causes. To avoid this, you must do three things:

1. *Give oxygen.* Head injury increases brain cell metabolic rate and decreases blood flow in at least part of the brain.
2. *Keep blood pressure up.* Blood must get to the brain to carry oxygen, so systolic pressure must be at least 80 mmHg in the preschool child and 90 mmHg in older children. Be alert to recognize early signs of shock (tachycardia and poor perfusion).
3. *Be prepared to prevent aspiration.* Head injury patients frequently vomit. The Sellick maneuver should be used during bag-valve mask ventilation and any intubation attempts. Suction should be readily assessable for any child with a head injury.

Changing level of consciousness is the best indicator of head trauma. A child entering the emergency department with a GCS of 10 that has come down from 13 will be approached very differently from the child who has a GCS of 10 that has come up from 7. Assessments using vague words like "semiconscious" are not helpful. Instead, note specific points such as whether the child is distractible, consolable, reaches for the parent, or reacts to pain or voice. Assessment of pupils is as important in the child as in the adult. Note also whether the eyes are moving both left and right or whether they remain in one position. Do not move the head to determine this!

Children with head injury often fare much better than adults with the same degree of injury. Children with head trauma and low GCS may may do well if they receive aggressive medical management that focuses on maintenance of oxygenation, ventilation, and perfusion of the brain. Pediatric patients, similar to adults, should not be hyperventilated unless they have evidence of the cerebral herniation syndrome (see Chapter 8). Children with certain types of head injuries, such as epidural hematoma, may need immediate surgical intervention to give the brain the maximum chance of complete healing. Transport children with serious head injuries to a trauma center equipped to provide definitive care.

CHEST INJURY

Children generally give visible signs of respiratory distress, such as tachypnea, grunting, nasal flaring, and retractions. Be aware that children's normal respiratory rates are higher than adults' (Table 15-2). A child breathing faster than 40, or an infant faster than 60, usually has respiratory distress and would benefit from supplemental oxygen. A few grunts are not significant, but persistent grunting indicates a need for ventilatory assistance. A child in respiratory distress often breathes with her nose like a rabbit, which is called flaring. Retractions relate to caving in of the suprasternal, intercostal, or subcostal areas with inspiration. Retractions suggest the child is straining to breathe. If any of these signs are persistent, they should alert you that something is wrong with the respiratory system (pneumo/hemothorax, foreign body, pulmonary contusion).

Children with blunt chest injury are at risk for pneumothorax. Because the chest is small, a difference in breath sounds from side to side may be more subtle than in the adult. You may not be able to tell a difference, even by listening carefully. It is also difficult to diagnose tension pneumothorax in young children who usually have short, fat necks that mask both neck vein distension and tracheal deviation. If a tension pneumothorax develops, the heart and trachea should eventually shift away from the side of the pneumothorax. To help detect a shift of a child's heart, place an "X" over the point of maximum impulse (PMI) of the heart. Repeatedly check the location of the PMI.

Children in the preadolescent age group have highly elastic chest walls. Rib fractures, flail chest, pericardial tamponade, and aortic rupture are, therefore, seldom seen in this group. However, pulmonary contusion is common. If a child does have rib fractures or a flail chest, he has sustained a significant force to his chest and should be assumed to have internal injuries.

ABDOMINAL INJURY

The second leading cause of traumatic death in most pediatric centers is internal bleeding secondary to rupture of the liver and/or spleen. In children the liver and spleen both protrude below the ribs, exposing the organs to blunt trauma. This poor protection and the relatively large size of the liver and spleen in children allow these organs to be easily torn. Abdominal injuries are difficult to diagnose in the field. A child may have a severe abdominal injury with minimal signs of trauma. Any child with seat belt marks or bruises to his abdomen should be assumed to have internal injuries. If a child has blunt injury to the chest or abdomen, be prepared to treat for shock. The capsule of a child's liver and spleen are thicker than an adult's; therefore, bleeding is often contained within the organ. If a child with blunt trauma is in shock with no obvious source of bleeding, your decision should be to load-and-go. Any child who has been crying or suffered an abdominal injury will develop gastric distention and a tendency to vomit; be prepared.

SPINAL INJURY

Although children have short necks, big heads, and loose ligaments, C-spine injuries are uncommon before adolescence. Cervical spine injuries do occur, however, and you should immobilize all children with a potential spinal injury. A C-collar is not necessary if the head is properly immobilized in a padded device. Again, try to make a game of packaging the child. You can promise you will give him a ride in the ambulance as a reward after you get him all wrapped up and ready. Use a parent or other familiar person, if possible. Be sure your packaging does not restrict chest movement. As mentioned before, children up to about 8 years of age will need a pad under the torso to keep the neck in a neutral position.

CHILD RESTRAINT SEATS

A child in a wreck while properly restrained is much less likely to have a serious injury than an unrestrained passenger. If the child is in a car seat, he can usually be transported without being removed from the device. Assess the child as you would other trauma patients. Place padding around the child's head, and tape the head directly to the car seat. This method of transportation should only be used after a complete assessment that has revealed NO injury to the child. If the child has evidence of any serious injuries, he should be removed from the car seat and packaged. Some new-model cars have built-in infant restraint seats. These seats cannot be removed, so the child who is restrained in one of these will have to be extricated and placed on a pediatric immobilization device.

PITFALLS

1. Children require special equipment. Without this equipment, you cannot provide the pediatric patient with adequate care. See essential equipment in Table 15-1.

2. Because of strong compensatory mechanisms, children can look surprisingly good in early shock. When they deteriorate, they often "crash." If the mechanism of injury or the assessment suggests the possibility of hemorrhagic shock, load and go.

3. You are the only one to see the scene of the injury. Be alert to signs of child abuse.

SUMMARY

To provide good trauma care for children, you must have the proper equipment, know how to interact with frightened parents, know the normal vital signs for various ages (or have them posted in your trauma box), and be familiar with the injuries that are more common in children. Fortunately the assessment sequence is the same for children as for adults. If you perform your assessment well, you will obtain the information needed to make the right decisions in management. Focusing on assessment and management of the child's airway (with C-spine control), breathing, and circulation will result in the best possible outcome.

While assessment and management of the injured child are lifesaving skills, all of us involved in the care of the seriously injured child should be concerned also about prevention (see Appendix H). Car seats, bicycle helmets, seat belts, all-terrain vehicle injuries, water safety, scald burn injuries, firearm safety, and fire drills are within our area of concern. We should donate our time to teaching safety, and we should speak out for laws (infant seat restraints, seat belts, drunk driving) that save lives.

BIBLIOGRAPHY

1. Allhouse, M., T. Rouse, and M. Eichelberger. "Childhood Injury: A Current Perspective." *Pediatric Emergency Care,* Vol. 9, No. 3 (June 1993), p. 159.

2. American Academy of Pediatrics, Committee on Pediatric Emergency Medicine. *Emergency Medical Services for Children: The Role of the Primary Care Provider.* Elk Grove, IL: The Academy, 1992.

3. American Academy of Pediatrics, Joint Task Force on Advanced Pediatric Life Support. *APLS: The Pediatric Emergency Medicine Course,* 2nd ed. Elk Grove, IL: The Academy, 1993.

4. Dietrich, A., S. Shaner, and J. Campbell. *Pediatric Basic Trauma Life Support.* Oakbrook Terrace, IL: Basic Trauma Life Support International, 1998.

5. Nypaver, M., and D. Treloar. "Neutral Cervical Spine Positioning in Children." *Annals of Emergency Medicine,* Vol. 23 (February 1994), pp. 208–211.

6. Pigula, F. A., S. Wald, S. Shackford, and others. "The Effect of Hypotension and Hypoxia on Children with Severe Head Injuries." *Journal of Pediatric Surgery,* Vol. 28 (1993), pp. 310–316.

7. Schriger, D. L., and L. J. Baraff. "Capillary Refill—Is It a Useful Predictor of Hypovolemic States?" *Annals of Emergency Medicine,* Vol. 20 (June 1991), pp. 601–605.

CHAPTER 16

Trauma in the Elderly

Leah J. Heimbach, R.N., NREMT-P, J.D.
Jere F. Baldwin, M.D., F.A.C.E.P.,
F.A.A.F.P.

OBJECTIVES

UPON COMPLETION OF THIS CHAPTER, YOU SHOULD BE ABLE TO:

1. Describe the changes that occur with aging, and explain how these changes can affect your assessment of the geriatric trauma patient.
2. Describe the assessment of the geriatric trauma patient.
3. Describe the management of the geriatric trauma patient.

By the twenty-first century, it is estimated that citizens over the age of 65 years will comprise one-fifth of the U.S. population. The geriatric population already comprises a significant number of the patients being transported by ambulance. In the United States, over 30% of all patients transported by ambulance are over the age of 65.

"Elderly" is often understood as being 65 years or older because retirement benefits are usually initiated at this point in life. However, chronological age is not the most reliable definition of "elderly." It is more appropriate to consider the biologic processes that change with time, for example, the fewer number of neurons, the decreased functioning of the kidneys, and the decreased elasticity of the skin and tissues.

As a group, geriatric patients tend to respond to injury less favorably than the younger adult population. Geriatric patients who are injured are more likely to experience fatal outcomes, even if the injury is of a relatively low severity. According to the National Safety Council, falls, thermal injury, and MVCs have been identified as common causes of traumatic death in the geriatric population.

Falls account for the majority of injuries in the geriatric population, the most common pathology being fractures of the hip, femur, and wrist and head injuries. MVCs account for approximately 25% of geriatric deaths although the elderly drive fewer miles. The geriatric population has a higher incidence of collision than other age groups, second only to that group under the age of 25. Eight percent of deaths are attributable to thermal injuries. These injuries include inhalation, contact with the heat source resulting in scalding and flame burns, and electrical injury.

Little has been written on the response of the geriatric patient to trauma. By gaining an understanding of the normal physiologic changes involved in the aging process, you will be better prepared to provide optimum care to the geriatric trauma victim.

This chapter addresses these processes, highlights illnesses to which the geriatric patient is susceptible, and shows how these processes and illnesses make it difficult to predict the physiological response to trauma in the geriatric patient.

PATHOPHYSIOLOGY OF AGING

Aging is a gradual process whereby changes in bodily functions may occur. These changes are in part responsible for the greater risk of injury in the geriatric population.

AIRWAY: Changes in airway structures of the geriatric patient may include tooth decay, gum disease, and use of a dental prosthesis. Caps, bridges, dentures, and fillings all present potential airway obstructions in the geriatric trauma patient.

RESPIRATORY SYSTEM: Changes in the respiratory system begin to appear in the early adult years and increase markedly after the age of 60. Circulation to the pulmonary system decreases 30%, reducing the amount of carbon dioxide and oxygen exchanged at the alveolar level. There is a decrease in chest wall movement and in the flexibility of the muscles of the chest wall. These changes cause a decreased inhalation time resulting in rapid breathing. There is a decreased vital capacity (or decrease in the amount of air exchanged per breath) because of an increased residual volume (volume of air in the lungs after deep exhalation). Overall breathing capacity and maximal work rate may also decrease. If there is a history of cigarette smoking, or a history of working in an area with pollutants, these changes in breathing are even more significant.

CARDIOVASCULAR SYSTEM: Circulation is reduced due to changes in the heart and the blood vessels. Cardiac output and stroke volume may decrease, and the conduction system may degenerate. The ability of the valves of the heart to operate efficiently may decline. These changes may predispose the patient to congestive heart failure and pulmonary edema. Arteriosclerosis occurs with increasing frequency in the course of the aging process, resulting in an increased peripheral vascular resistance (and perhaps systolic hypertension). There may be a normally higher blood pressure in the elderly. Thus a significant change may occur in a patient when the normal blood pressure of 160 drops to 120 as a result of trauma. There may be a decreased blood flow to the periphery, making the capillary refill an inaccurate indicator of shock.

NEUROLOGICAL AND SENSORY FUNCTION: Several changes occur in the brain with age. The brain shrinks, and the outermost meningeal layer, the dura mater, remains tightly adherent to the skull. This creates a space or an increased distance between the brain and the skull. Instead of protecting the brain during impact, this space allows an increased incidence of subdural hematoma following trauma. There is also a hardening, narrowing, and loss of elasticity of some arteries in the brain. A deceleration injury may cause blood vessel rupture and potential bleeding inside the skull. There is decreased blood flow to the brain. The patient may experience a slowing of sensory responses such as pain perception and decreases in hearing, eyesight, or in other sensory perceptions. Many older patients may have a higher pain tolerance from living with conditions such as arthritis, or from being on analgesic medications chronically. This can result in their failure to identify areas in which they have been injured. Other signs of decreased cerebral circulation due to the aging process may include confusion, irritability, forgetfulness, altered sleep patterns, and mental dysfunctions such as loss of memory and regressive behavior. There may be a decrease in the ability, or even an absence in the ability, to compensate for shock.

THERMOREGULATION: Mechanisms to maintain normal body temperature may not function properly. The geriatric patient may not be able to respond to an infection with a fever, or the patient may not be able to maintain a normal temperature in the face of injury. The geriatric patient with a broken hip who has been lying on the floor in a room where the temperature is 64 degrees Fahrenheit can experience hypothermia.

RENAL SYSTEM: A decrease in the number of functioning nephrons in the kidneys of the geriatric patient can result in a decrease in filtration and a reduced ability to excrete urine and drugs.

MUSCULOSKELETAL SYSTEM: The geriatric patient may exhibit signs of changes in posture. There may be a decrease in total height due to the narrowing of the vertebral discs. There may be slight flexion of the knees and hips. There may be decreased muscle strength. This may result in a kyphotic deformity of the spine, resulting in the "s" curvature of the spine often seen in the stooped elderly. The geriatric patient may also have advanced osteoporosis—which is a thinning of the bone resulting in a decrease in the density of bone. This renders the bone more susceptible to fractures. Finally, there may be a weakening in the strength of the muscle and bone from the decrease in physical activity; this will also render the geriatric patient more susceptible to fractures with only a slight fall.

GASTROINTESTINAL SYSTEM: Saliva production, esophageal motility, and gastric secretion may decrease. This may result in decreased ability to absorb nutrients. The liver may be enlarged because of disease processes or may be failing due to disease or malnutrition. This may result in a decreased ability to metabolize medications.

IMMUNE SYSTEM: As the aging process continues, the geriatric patient may be less able to fight off infection. The patient in a poor nutritional state will thus be more susceptible to infection from open wounds, IV access sites, and lung and kidney infections. The geriatric trauma patient who is not otherwise severely injured may die from sepsis from an impaired immune system.

OTHER CHANGES: The total body water and total number of body cells may be decreased, and there is an increase in the proportion of the body weight as fat. There may be a loss in the capacity of the systems to adjust to illness or injury.

MEDICATIONS: Many geriatric patients take several medications that can interfere with their ability to compensate after sustaining trauma. Anticoagulants may increase bleeding time. Antihypertensives and peripheral vasodilators can interfere with the body's ability to vasoconstrict blood vessels in response to hypovolemia. Beta-blockers can inhibit the heart's ability to increase the rate of contraction even in hypovolemia shock.

A number of the aging processes contribute to the increased risk of injury to the geriatric patient. The changes that may increase susceptibility to injury include the following:

1. Slower reflexes
2. Failing eyesight
3. Hearing loss
4. Arthritis
5. Fragile skin and blood vessels
6. Fragile bones

Causative factors related to the aging process have been linked with specific injuries such as tripping over furniture and falling down stairs. Further investigation reveals that these falls are often related as much to a decrease in the function of special senses, such as loss in peripheral vision, as they are to syncope, postural instability, transient impairment of cerebrovascular perfusion, alcohol ingestion, or medication usage. Alterations in perception and delayed response to stressors may also contribute to injury in the geriatric patient. When treating the geriatric trauma patient, remember that the priorities are the same as for all trauma patients. However, you must give consideration to three important issues:

1. General organ systems may not function as effectively as those in the younger adult, especially the cardiovascular, pulmonary, and renal systems.
2. The geriatric patient also may have a chronic illness that may complicate the effectiveness of trauma care.
3. Bones may fracture more easily with less force.

ASSESSMENT AND MANAGEMENT OF THE ELDERLY TRAUMA PATIENT

Geriatric patient assessment, as with any assessment, must take into account priorities, interventions, and life-threatening conditions. However, *you must be acutely aware that geriatric patients can die from less severe injuries than younger patients*. In addition, it is often difficult to separate the effects of the aging process or of a chronic illness from the consequences of the injury. The chief complaint may seem trivial because the patient may not report truly important symptoms. You must search for important signs or symptoms. In the geriatric patient, it is not uncommon for the patient to suffer from more than one illness or injury at the same time. Remember that the elderly patient may not have the same response to pain, hypoxia, or hypovolemia as a young person. Don't underestimate the severity of the patient's condition.

You may have difficulty communicating with the patient. This could result from the patient's diminished senses, hearing or sight impairment, or depression. The geriatric patient nonetheless should not be approached in a condescending manner. Do not allow others to take over the reporting of events from the patient who is able and willing to communicate reliable information. Unfortunately, the patient may minimize or even deny symptoms out of fear of becoming dependent, bedridden, institutionalized, or even of losing a sense of self-sufficiency. It is important that you explain any actions, including removing any clothing, before initiating the physical assessment.

There are other considerations in assessing the geriatric trauma patient. Peripheral pulses may be difficult to evaluate. Older patients often wear many layers of clothing, which can impede physical assessment. You must also distinguish between signs and symptoms of a chronic disease and an acute problem, for instance:

1. The geriatric patient may have nonpathologic rales.
2. The loss of skin elasticity and the presence of mouth breathing may not necessarily represent dehydration.

3. Dependent edema may be secondary to venous insufficiency with varicose veins or inactivity rather than congestive heart failure.

Pay attention to deviation from expected ranges in vital signs and other physical assessment findings in the geriatric patient. An injury that is isolated and noncomplicated in the young adult may be debilitating in the older adult. This may be due to the patient's overall condition, lowered defenses, or inability to keep the effects of an injury localized.

When obtaining the past medical history, it is important to note what medications the patient may be taking. Medications may not only account for an abnormal pulse, but may also mask normal circulatory responses that would indicate deterioration in the circulatory system. The result can be a rapid decompensation without warning. Knowledge of the medications that the patient is taking can alert you that the patient's condition may be more unstable than that which is presented by current signs and symptoms. Antihypertensives, anticoagulants, beta-blockers, and hypoglycemic agents may profoundly influence the response of the geriatric patient to traumatic injury.

PRIMARY SURVEY

SCENE SIZE-UP: Survey the scene to decide if it is safe, to determine the number of patients, and to obtain the mechanism of injury. After the Primary Survey, it may be helpful to obtain further information and to verify the patient's history from reliable family members or neighbors. This is best done in an area where the patient is unable to overhear the conversation; otherwise it may suggest that the geriatric patient is less than a competent adult. Observe the surrounding area for indications that the patient is able to provide his own care, for signs of alcohol abuse or ingestion of multiple medications, and for signs of violence, abuse, or neglect. Abuse and/or neglect of the elderly is common. When your assessment of the patient and surroundings is suspicious for abuse or neglect, do not fail to notify the proper authorities. *Be sure to gather the patient's medications and bring them to the hospital.*

EVALUATE AIRWAY, C-SPINE CONTROL, AND INITIAL LEVEL OF CONSCIOUSNESS: As with any trauma patient, you must evaluate and provide an adequate airway and maintain C-spine control while assessing the initial level of consciousness. The initial level of consciousness has more significance with elderly patients than with younger patients. Subsequent health care providers may attribute a decreased level of consciousness to a preexisting condition rather than to the trauma. This is more likely to occur if you have not clearly indicated that the patient was clear, lucid, and cooperative at the scene.

If patients respond appropriately to the initial verbal statements, they have an open airway and are conscious. If they do not respond, gently open the airway with a modified jaw thrust while maintaining the neck in a neutral position. This position may be difficult to determine with certainty because of arthritis and kyphosis of the spine. It is important to recognize this and not to forcibly place the occiput flat on the backboard or ground. You should add padding to the spineboard to maintain the patient's usual spinal position.

The airway is likely to be partially obstructed. Clear the airway, being alert to possible teeth fragments due to decay and gum disease and dental devices such as caps, bridges, dentures, and fillings. Look, listen, and feel for movement of air. Ensure that the rate and volume of air exchange is adequate. The geriatric patient with unresolved airway difficulty or a decreased level of consciousness should be transported immediately. In such a case, frequently monitor the respiratory effort and level of consciousness.

BREATHING AND CIRCULATION: Place your face over the patient's mouth to look at the chest rise, to listen to the quality of the breath sounds from the mouth, and to feel the patient's breath against your ear. If the breathing is so fast that there is inadequate air exchange (greater than 24 breaths per minute), or if it is too slow (less than 12 breaths per minute), or if the volume of air being exchanged is inadequate, provide assisted ventilation with 100% supplemental oxygen. Check the rate and quality of the pulse at the wrist (check at the neck if there is no pulse at the wrist). Evaluate skin color and condition. Scan the patient for bleeding and control any bleeding with pressure.

RAPID TRAUMA SURVEY OR FOCUSED EXAM

The choice between the Rapid Trauma Survey and the Focused Exam depends on the mechanism of injury and/or the results of the Initial Assessment. If there is a dangerous generalized mechanism of injury (auto crash, fall from a height, etc.) or if the patient is unconscious, you should perform the BTLS Rapid Trauma Survey. If there is a danger-ous focused mechanism of injury suggesting an isolated injury (bullet wound of thigh, stab wound to the chest, etc.), you may perform the Focused Exam limited to the area of injury. If there is no significant mechanism of injury (dropped rock on toe) and the Initial Assessment was normal (alert with no history of loss of consciousness, breathing normally, radial pulse less than 120, not complaining of dyspnea or chest, abdominal, or pelvic pain), you may move directly to the Focused Exam based on the patient's chief complaint.

RAPID TRAUMA SURVEY

EXAMINE THE HEAD, NECK, CHEST, ABDOMEN, PELVIS, AND EXTREM-ITIES: Briefly assess the head and neck for injuries and to see if the neck veins are flat or distended and the trachea is in the midline. You may apply a rigid extrication collar at this time. Now look, feel, and listen to the chest. Look for both asymmetrical and para-doxical movement. Note if the ribs rise with respiration or if there is only diaphragmatic breathing. Look for signs of blunt trauma or open wounds. Feel for tenderness, instabil-ity, or crepitation (TIC). Now listen to see if breath sounds are present and equal bilat-erally. Make appropriate interventions for chest injuries. Remember that chest injuries are more likely to cause serious problems in older people with poor pulmonary reserve. Be especially alert to problems in patients with chronic lung disease. They usually have borderline hypoxia even when not injured. Briefly notice the heart sounds so you will have a baseline for changes such as development of muffled heart sounds. Rapidly expose and look at the abdomen (distention, contusions, penetrating wounds), and gently palpate the abdomen for tenderness, guarding, and rigidity. Check the pelvis and extremities for wounds, deformity, and TIC. Note whether the patient can move his fin-gers and toes before transferring to a backboard.

CRITICAL TRANSPORT DECISIONS: There are a few procedures that may be initiated on-scene, but do not delay transport. Examples of critical interventions that may be initiated at the scene are the following:

1. Provide airway management.
2. Assist ventilation.
3. Begin CPR.
4. Control major bleeding.
5. Seal sucking chest wounds.
6. Stabilize flail chest.
7. Decompress a tension pneumothorax.
8. Stabilize impaled objects.

Consider whether the time delay in initiating these procedures outweighs the risks of delaying transportation. As mentioned elsewhere, the chance of survival decreases with a corresponding increase in the length of scene time. The same indications for immediate transport apply for the elderly as for younger patients (see Chapter 2), but remember that you may not have as dramatic a response to injury in the elderly, so you should have a low threshold for early transport. If one of the critical conditions is pres-ent, immediately transfer the patient to a long backboard with appropriate padding,

FIGURE 16-1 Elderly patients often require padding under the shoulders and head to stabilize the spine.

apply oxygen, load the patient into the ambulance, and transport rapidly to the nearest appropriate emergency facility.

PACKAGING AND TRANSPORT: Package or prepare the elderly patient for transport as quickly and gently as possible. Take extra care when immobilizing the geriatric trauma patient. This includes padding void areas that may be exaggerated due to the aging process. The elderly patient with kyphosis will require padding under the shoulders and head to maintain the neck in its usual alignment (see Figure 16-1). Do not force the neck into a neutral position if it is painful to do so, or if the neck is obviously fused in a forward position. Remember to treat and transport the geriatric trauma patient, as you do all trauma patients, gently and quickly.

DETAILED EXAM AND ONGOING EXAMS: Perform a Detailed Exam on-scene if the patient is stable. If there is any question as to the patient's condition, you should transport and perform the Detailed Exam en route. Perform frequent Ongoing Exams. Frequently assess the patient's pulmonary status, including lung sounds and cardiac rhythm. All elderly patients should have cardiac monitoring and pulse oximetry, if available.

SUMMARY

You will be called upon to treat and transport an increasing number of geriatric trauma patients. Although the mechanisms of injury may be different from those of younger adults, the prioritized evaluation and treatment is the same. As a general rule elderly patients have more serious injuries and more complications than younger patients. The physiologic processes of aging and the frequent concurrent illnesses make evaluation and treatment more difficult. You must be aware of these differences to provide optimal care to the patient.

BIBLIOGRAPHY

1. Baker, S. P., B. O'Neil, M. Ginsburg, and others. *The Injury Fact Book.* New York: Oxford University Press, 1992.

2. Chadwick, B.A., and T. Heaton. *Statistical Handbook on the American Family.* Phoenix, AZ: Oryx Press, 1992.

3. Champion, H.R., S. Copes, D. Buyer, and others. "Major Trauma in Geriatric Patients." *American Journal of Public Health,* Vol. 79 (1989), p. 1278.

4. Diku, M., and K. Newton. "Geriatric Trauma." *Emergency Medicine Clinics of North America,* Vol. 16, No. 1 (Feb. 1998).

5. Fleisher, F., L. White, M. McMullen, and others. "The Geriatric Obstacle Course: A Training Session Designed to Help Prehospital Personnel Recognize Geriatric Stereotypes and Misconceptions." *Journal of Emergency Medicine,* Vol. 14, No. 4 (1996), pp. 439–444.

6. Gubler, K.D., R. Davis, T. Koepsell, and others. "Long-Term Survival of Elderly Trauma Patients." *Archives of Surgery,* Vol. 132 (September 1997).

CHAPTER 17

Trauma in Pregnancy

Ron W. Lee, M.D., M.B.A., F.A.C.E.P.
John E. Campbell, M.D., F.A.C.E.P.

OBJECTIVES

UPON COMPLETION OF THIS CHAPTER, YOU SHOULD BE ABLE TO:

1. State the twin goals of managing the pregnant trauma patient.

2. Describe physiological changes to the cardiopulmonary system during pregnancy and relate them to the following:
   a. Blood volume
   b. Cardiac output
   c. Stroke volume and heart rate
   d. Blood pressure
   e. Respiratory status

3. Describe the major physiological changes in the gastrointestinal and genitourinary systems during pregnancy.

4. Describe uterine response to maternal hypovolemia and relate its implications to assessment and management of the mother.

5. Predict potential injury to the mother and/or fetus based on the following mechanisms of injury:
   a. MVCs, including use of lap and shoulder restraints
   b. Penetrating abdominal injuries
   c. Falls, especially those resulting in pelvic fractures
   d. Burns

6. Compare and contrast evaluation and management of a pregnant to a nonpregnant trauma patient.

7. Identify transport considerations for a pregnant trauma patient.

The pregnant trauma patient represents a unique challenge for the prehospital provider. It is important to remember that the pregnant patient represents two patients with separate requirements, those of the mother and those of the fetus. Therefore, any intervention must have the twin goals of supporting the mother and identifying the needs of the fetus. The pregnant patient is also often at risk for a higher incidence of accidental trauma. The increase in fainting spells, hyperventilation, and excess fatigue that are common in early pregnancy, as well as the changes in the physiological parameters of the pregnant patient, such as the loosening of the pelvic joints, all add to the risk of minor accidental trauma. It is estimated that accidental injury may complicate 6 to 7% of all pregnancies. The pregnant patient with minor injuries rarely represents a problem for the prehospital provider, and therefore our discussion will be centered on moderate to severe traumatic injuries.

PHYSIOLOGICAL CHANGES DURING PREGNANCY

To understand the unique aspects associated with trauma in pregnancy, it is important to recall certain physiological processes that are peculiar to pregnancy. During the first 3 months of pregnancy, the fetus is being formed. The fetus is very tiny, so there is little growth of the uterus during this period. After the third month of gestation the fetus and uterus grow rapidly, reaching the umbilicus by the fifth month and the epigastrium by the seventh month (see Figure 17-1). The cardiopulmonary changes that occur during pregnancy are significant (see Figures 17-2a and b). The cardiac output will increase by 20 to 30% during the first 10 weeks of gestation. This increase in cardiac output peaks at term and approximates 6 to 7 L/min. The average maternal heart beat will increase by 10 to 15 beats per minute, while the systolic and diastolic blood pressure will often lessen by 10 to 15 mmHg when compared to the nonpregnant patient.

The respiratory status of the patient undergoes significant changes because of the enlarging uterus that will elevate the diaphragm and decrease the overall volume of the thoracic cavity. There tends to be some flaring out of the rib margins to compensate for this decrease in capacity. There is also an increase in the amount of gas exchange occurring over each minute. This leads to a relative alkalosis and predisposes the patient to the hyperventilation syndrome. The pregnant patient also undergoes a change that is described as the "hypervolemia" of pregnancy. This represents an increase of both red blood cells and plasma, yielding an increase in the total blood volume of approximately 45 to 50%. However, since there is a greater increase in plasma over blood cells, the patient tends to manifest a relative anemia.

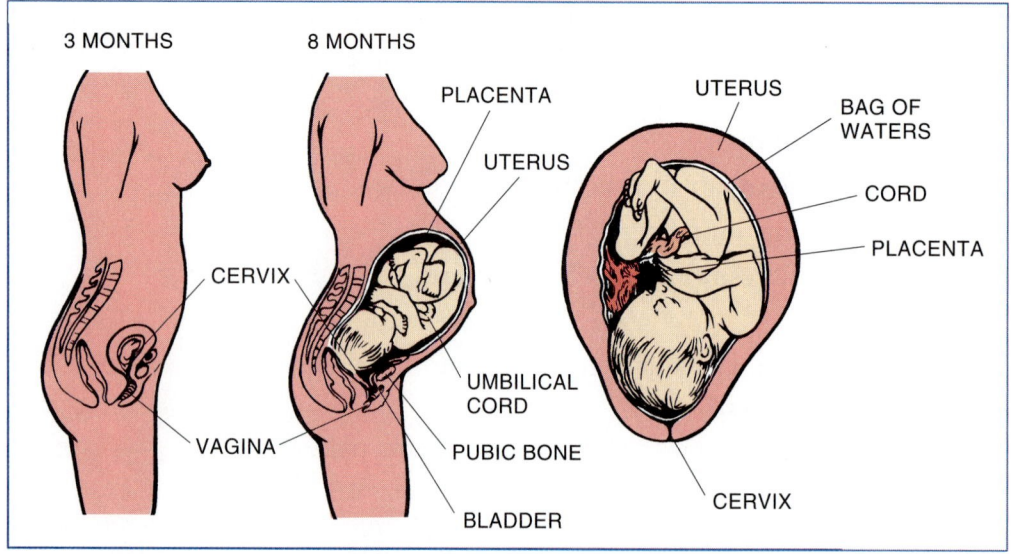

FIGURE 17-1   Anatomy of pregnancy: Uterus at 3 months and at 8 months gestation.

BLOOD VOLUME USUALLY INCREASES BY ABOUT 45%. DILUTION RESULTING FROM THE DISPROPORTIONATE INCREASE OF PLASMA VOLUME OVER THE RED CELL MASS "ANEMIA OF PREGNANCY."

CARDIAC OUTPUT INCREASES BY 1.0 TO 1.5 L/MIN DURING THE 1ST TRIMESTER, REACHES 6 TO 7 L/MIN BY THE LATE 2ND TRIMESTER, AND IS MAINTAINED ESSENTIALLY AT THIS LEVEL UNTIL DELIVERY.

THE STROKE VOLUME PROGRESSIVELY DECLINES TO TERM FOLLOWING A RISE EARLY IN PREGNANCY. HEART RATE, HOWEVER, INCREASES BY AN AVERAGE OF 10 TO 15 BEATS/MIN.

FIGURE 17-2A Physiological changes during pregnancy.

This enlargement in plasma volume is particularly important because the patient may lose 30 to 35% of the circulating blood volume before developing hypotension. This also means that if the injured pregnant patient has significant hypotension, she has already had a major loss of blood volume, and resuscitation will require large amounts of fluids (preferably blood).

The major physiological changes in the gastrointestinal system are secondary to the enlarging uterus, and lead to the following:

1. A compartmentalization of the organs within the abdomen. This compartmentalization now displaces most of the small bowels upward, while the uterus becomes the largest organ within the abdominal cavity. This is a major consideration when trying to identify organ systems that are injured from either penetrating or blunt trauma.

2. A general decrease in gastrointestinal motility, with a resulting delay in gastric emptying. This often places the injured pregnant patient at great risk for vomiting and aspiration.

The changes in the urinary system are many; however, the most significant is the displacement of the bladder anteriorly and superiorly, placing it in a position where penetrating or blunt trauma is more likely to do greater harm.

THE MEAN LEVEL OF BLOOD PRESSURE IS CHARACTERISTICALLY 10 TO 15 MMHG LOWER DURING PREGNANCY, THE DECLINE USUALLY APPARENT BY THE END OF THE 1ST TRIMESTER. WIDENED PULSE PRESSURE RESULTS FROM A PROPORTIONATELY GREATER REDUCTION IN THE DIASTOLIC COMPONENT.

PERISTALSIS IS SLOWED; THUS, THE STOMACH MAY STILL CONTAIN FOOD HOURS AFTER A MEAL. BE ALERT TO THE DANGER OF VOMITING AND ASPIRATION.

INJURY TO THE UTERUS OR PELVIS MAY CAUSE MASSIVE HEMORRHAGE.

FIGURE 17-2B Physiological changes during pregnancy *(continued)*.

The multiple changes in the reproductive system are significant in that the uterine blood flow, which is normally approximately 2% of the cardiac output, now increases to approximately 20%. It is important to realize that the vessels supplying the uterus are low-resistance vessels that vasoconstrict vigorously in response to the catecholamines produced in early shock. Therefore, under periods of stress there may be significant vasoconstriction with a reduction of blood flow to the uterus. Unfortunately, the uterus is not responsive to vasodilatation and cannot increase blood flow to the uterus in times of placental hypoperfusion. This means that very early in the shock syndrome, the pregnant patient will divert blood away from the fetus to save the mother. Thus the death of the fetus is more common if the mother has a period of hypotension.

RESPONSES TO HYPOVOLEMIA

Acute blood loss results in a decrease in circulating blood volume. The cardiac output decreases as the venous return falls. This hypovolemia causes the arterial blood pressure to fall, resulting in an inhibition of vagal tone and also the release of catecholamines.

The effect of this response is to produce vasoconstriction and tachycardia. This vasoconstriction profoundly affects the pregnant uterus. Uterine vasoconstriction leads to a reduction in uterine blood flow by 20 to 30%. This reduction in uterine blood flow may occur before any detectable change is noted in the blood pressure of the maternal system. The fetus reacts to this hypoperfusion by a drop in arterial blood pressure and a decrease in heart rate. The fetus now begins to suffer from reduced oxygen concentration in the maternal circulation. It is important to remember that some methods for oxygenation of the maternal patient in hemorrhagic shock may not always provide adequate oxygenation of the fetus. Therefore, it is important to give large amounts of supplemental oxygen to provide sufficient oxygen to the fetus, who suffers from both oxygen starvation and inadequate blood supply.

Another cause of hypotension in the pregnant patient results from the decreased venous return when the patient is in the supine position. The enlarging uterus can cause significant compression of the vena cava, which reduces venous return to the heart (see Figure 17-3). This effect is particularly evident after the twentieth week of gestation. The reduced venous return has been shown to lead to maternal hypotension, syncope, and fetal bradycardia. Therefore, you should transport all pregnant patients in the left lateral decubitus or decubent position. Do this only if it can be done without risk to the patient. If the type of patient trauma prevents this type of maneuver, you can prevent or alleviate the vena cava obstruction by one of the following methods:

1. Tilt or rotate the backboard 20 to 30 degrees to the left.
2. Manually displace the uterus to the left side during transport.

TYPES OF INJURIES

VEHICULAR COLLISIONS

A pregnant patient is subject to all types of accidental injuries, including MVCs, gunshot wounds, falls, and electrical and thermal injuries.

The most common cause of maternal injury is the blunt injury resulting from MVCs. A review of this type of injury indicates that when there is only minor damage to the vehicle, fewer than 1% of pregnant patients will sustain injury. As with nonpregnant patients, the probability of a major life-threatening injury is directly related to the damage inflicted on the vehicle. To best predict the severity of injury, you need to determine the answers to following questions:

1. How fast was the vehicle traveling at impact?
2. What was the position of the patient in the vehicle at the time of impact?
3. Were any restraints utilized?
4. Which body parts sustained the impact?
5. On what side of the vehicle did the impact occur in relation to the patient?

FIGURE 17-3 Venous return to the maternal heart may be decreased up to 30% because of uterine compression by the fetus. Transport the patient on her left side or tilt the backboard to the left.

Head injury is the most common cause of death in pregnant patients in MVCs. The other most common cause of death is internal injuries with uncontrolled hemorrhage. The old concern that an injury to the fetus is likely to occur with the seat belt connected was based on early data, which revealed that with the use of the *lap belt alone,* there was an increased incidence of injury to the uterus and fetus. However, the overall vehicular mortality for pregnant patients was less with the use of only the lap belt. The use of a *lap belt with shoulder restraint* decreases patient mortality and *has not shown any increase in uterine injuries.*

The most common cause of fetal death is maternal death. Fetal death with maternal survival occurs most often in abdominal trauma with placental separation or ruptured uterus (see Figure 17-4). In this case, the patient presents with vaginal bleeding, abdominal pain, and irritable uterus, and often some degree of hypotension.

Pregnant victims of MVCs have associated injuries, such as pelvic injuries, that often result in placental separation and concealed hemorrhage within the retroperitoneal area. The retroperitoneal area, because of its low-pressure venous system, can accommodate a loss of 4 or more liters of blood into that area with few clinical signs. Fetal skull fractures are much more common when maternal pelvic fractures occur.

PENETRATING INJURIES OF THE ABDOMEN

The most common type of penetrating injury to the pregnant patient is the gunshot wound. The probability of any abdominal organ being struck by a bullet is directly related to the size of the organ and the space it occupies within the peritoneal cavity. Therefore, in early pregnancy the likelihood of uterine injury or fetal injury is low. However, as the pregnancy progresses toward term, the chance for injury increases proportionately. The most common organs injured from gunshot wounds to the nonpregnant patient are the small bowel, liver, colon, and stomach, in decreasing order. The mortality and complication rates are related to the number of organs injured. About 19% of women who sustain gunshot wounds to the uterus will also have injuries to other organs. Fetal injuries from gunshot wounds to the uterus vary from 60 to 90%, with mortality of 40 to 70%. Fetal death is secondary to direct injury to the fetus or injuries to the membranes, cord, or placenta.

The second most common cause of penetrating abdominal wounds is the stab wound. Stab wounds to the abdomen have an associated mortality of approximately 1.4% in the nonpregnant individual. The enlarged uterus protects the pregnant patient from serious organ injury when lower abdominal stab injuries occur. However, due to

FIGURE 17-4 Blunt trauma to the uterus. Blunt trauma may cause separation of the placenta or rupture of the uterus. Massive bleeding may occur, but there may not be visible vaginal bleeding early.

compartmentalization, stab wounds to the upper abdomen often carry a higher incidence of visceral injury, especially to the small bowel. Fetal mortality in these injuries is related directly to maternal mortality, and when isolated fetal death occurs, it is usually secondary to either direct fetal injury or to prematurity.

FALLS

The incidence of significant injury to the pregnant patient resulting from a fall is proportional to the force of impact and the specific body part that sustains the impact. Injuries associated with pelvic fractures manifest an increase in placental separation and fetal fractures of the skull and long bones. The incidence of falls increases with the progression of the pregnancy. This is secondary to the loosening of ligaments from the hormone relaxin and the added weight gain that alters the patient's center of gravity. These falls may appear minor; however, many cases of minor trauma have resulted in fetomaternal hemorrhage or placental separation. These patients benefit from evaluation and monitoring in an emergency department.

BURNS

The overall mortality and morbidity resulting from thermal injuries to the pregnant patient is not markedly different from the nonpregnant individual. However, it is important to remember that the fluid requirement for the pregnant patient is greater than that of the nonpregnant individual. Fetal mortality increases when the maternal surface burn exceeds 20%.

EVALUATION

The evaluation of the injured pregnant female does not differ from that of the nonpregnant patient. The priorities remain the same:

1. Secure the *airway* and stabilize the C-spine.
2. Assess *breathing*.
3. Assess *circulation*.
4. Stop the bleeding.
5. Determine transport decision and critical interventions.
6. Transport.
7. Perform Detailed Exam (may be done before transport if patient is stable).
8. Perform Ongoing Exam.

MANAGEMENT OF THE PREGNANT PATIENT

The management of most injuries to the pregnant patient are the same as discussed in other chapters. However, severe hemorrhagic shock can occur from injuries to the uterus because this very vascular organ can bleed profusely. Rapid transport for surgical treatment to stop the bleeding is the most important treatment. If your system uses the antishock garment, you may inflate the leg compartments if the patient is in severe shock (blood pressure <50 mmHg).

OXYGEN ADMINISTRATION AND PATIENT TRANSPORT

Oxygen requirements for women in late pregnancy have been reported to be 10 to 20% greater than normal. Maternal shock of *any degree* will cause vasoconstriction of the uterus, with a marked decrease in oxygenation of the fetus. *Any injured pregnant patient should receive high-flow oxygen immediately.*

The transport of any pregnant patient whose pregnancy is greater than 20 weeks should occur with the patient on her back, with the uterus displaced to the left to pre-

FIGURE 17-5 Pregnant patient packaged and turned on her left side.

vent inferior vena cava obstruction. If there is no danger of spinal injury, you can transport the patient on her left side. If there is a possibility of spinal injury, secure the patient appropriately to the long spineboard, but prop up the board slightly on the right side so that the uterus is tilting to the left (see Figure 17-5). An alternate method is to manually hold the uterus to the left side.

PITFALLS AND IMPORTANT POINTS

1. Do not mistake normal vital signs in pregnant patients as signs of shock. The pregnant patient has a normal resting pulse that is 10 to 15 beats faster than usual and the blood pressure is 10 to 15 mmHg lower than usual. However, it is also important to realize that a blood loss of 30 to 35% can occur in these patients before there is a significant change in blood pressure. Therefore, be especially alert to all signs of shock, and monitor the vital signs with frequent Ongoing Exams.

2. Trauma to the abdominal compartment can cause occult bleeding in either the intrauterine or retroperitoneal area. Keep in mind that gradual stretching of the abdominal wall during pregnancy, along with hormonal changes within the body, make the peritoneal surface less sensitive to irritable stimuli. Therefore, bleeding can occur intraperitoneally, and the signs of rebound, guarding, and rigidity may not be present.

3. You are treating two patients; however, the mortality of the fetus is related to the treatment provided to the mother. The goal of prehospital intervention is to maximize the chances of maternal survival, which will provide the fetus with the best chance for survival.

4. Hypoxemia of the fetus may go unnoticed in the injured pregnant patient. Treatment should include high-flow oxygen.

5. Transport must include appropriate spinal immobilization, extremity splints, and prevention of vena cava compression.

6. If the mother dies, continue CPR and notify the hospital to be prepared for immediate caesarean section.

SUMMARY

Management of the pregnant patient requires a knowledge of the physiological changes that occur during pregnancy. The pregnant patient requires very close observation for signs of shock, and all pregnant trauma patients should receive high-flow oxygen. Pregnant patients require special techniques in packaging and transport to prevent the vena cava compression syndrome.

BIBLIOGRAPHY

1. American College of Surgeons Committee on Trauma. "Trauma in Pregnancy." In *Advanced Trauma Life Support*. Chicago: The College, 1989.

2. Buchsbaum, H. J. *Trauma in Pregnancy*. Philadelphia: W. B. Saunders, 1979.

3. Maull, K. I., G. S. Rozycki, R. E. Pedigo, and others. "Female Reproductive System Trauma." In *Trauma*, eds. E. E. Moore, D. V. Feliciano, and K. L. Mattox, pp. 553–560. Norwalk, CT: Appleton-Lange, 1987.

CHAPTER 18

Patients Under the Influence of Alcohol or Drugs

Jonathan G. Newman, M.D., F.A.C.E.P., NREMT-P

OBJECTIVES

UPON COMPLETION OF THIS CHAPTER, YOU SHOULD BE ABLE TO:

1. List signs and symptoms of patients under the influence of alcohol and/or drugs.

2. Describe the five strategies you would use to best ensure cooperation during assessment and management of a patient under the influence of alcohol and/or drugs.

3. Describe situations in which you would restrain patients and tell how to handle an uncooperative patient.

4. List the special considerations for assessment and management of patients in whom substance abuse is suspected.

The relationship between alcohol and trauma is well documented. For instance, it is reported that car crashes involving alcohol result in injuries to about 500,000 people a year. The involvement of drugs in trauma has not been as well examined. However, substance abuse, which includes individuals who have abused alcohol, drugs, or both, has been associated with a number of traumatic events. The trauma caused by substance abuse often results from accidents, car crashes, suicides, homicides, and other violent crimes. Therefore, it would not be surprising to find that a number of your trauma patients are under the influence of alcohol or some other substance. This group of trauma patients often presents with unique challenges that can require some special patient management techniques along with good BTLS care.

A high index of suspicion, combined with the results of your physical exam, the history obtained from the patient or bystanders, and evidence at the scene, can clue you into whether your patient is under the influence of alcohol or drugs.

Table 18-1 includes some commonly abused drugs along with signs and symptoms of their use.

ASSESSMENT AND MANAGEMENT

While your Primary Survey and Detailed Exam should follow the BTLS guidelines that have been described in this book (see Chapter 2), there are some particular aspects to be aware of when conducting your exam.

When you suspect the patient has abused substances, pay particular attention to mental status, pupils, speech, and respirations, and note any needle marks you may discover. An altered mental status can be seen in every form of substance abuse. However,

Table 18-1 Commonly Abused Drugs with Their Associated Signs and Symptoms.

DRUG CATEGORY	COMMON NAMES	SIGNS AND SYMPTOMS OF USE OR ABUSE
Alcohol	Beer, whiskey, wine	Altered mental function, confusion, polyuria, slurred speech, coma, hypertension, hyperthermia, tachycardia
Amphetamines	Bennies, ice, speed, uppers, dexies	Excitement, hyperactivity, dilated pupils, hypertension, tachycardia, tremors, seizures, fever, paranoia, psychosis
Cocaine	Coke, crack, blow, rock	Same as amphetamines plus chest pain; lethal dysrhythmia
Hallucinogens	Acid, LSD, PCP	Hallucinations, dizziness, dilated pupils, nausea, rambling speech, psychosis, anxiety, panic
Marijuana	Grass, hash, pot, tea, weed	Euphoria, sleepiness, dilated pupils, dry mouth, increased appetite
Opiates	Heroin, horse, big H, Darvon, codeine, stuff, morphine, smack	Altered mental status, constricted pupils, bradycardia, hypotension, respiratory depression, hypothermia
Sedatives	Thorazine; barbiturates; benzodiazepines, e.g., Librium, Valium, Xanax, Ativan	Altered mental status, dilated pupils, bradycardia, hypotension, respiratory depression, hypothermia

remember that an altered level of consciousness is due to a head injury or shock until proven otherwise. Pupils are often constricted in patients who have abused opiates. Dilated pupils are common in patients exposed to amphetamines, cocaine, hallucinogens, and marijuana. Patients who use barbiturates will have pupils that are constricted early on; however, if high doses have been consumed, the pupils can eventually become fixed and dilated. Speech can be slurred when patients use alcohol or sedatives, and patients who are under the influence of hallucinogens may seem to ramble when they talk. Respiration can be significantly depressed with opiates and sedatives.

The history supplied by the patient or bystanders can also help to establish whether substance abuse is involved. Try to find out what was used, when it was taken, and how much was taken. However, be aware that patients often deny that they have used or abused any substance. If possible, inspect the patient's surroundings for clues that drugs or alcohol may have been used. Note any alcoholic beverage bottles, pill containers, injection equipment, smoking paraphernalia, or unusual odors.

Trauma patients under the influence of alcohol or drugs can challenge the provider not only by their traumatic injuries but by their attitudes as well. *The way in which you interact with patients who have abused substances can determine if the patient will be cooperative or uncooperative.* How you speak to these patients can be as important as what you are doing for them. Your interaction style, if offensive, can make patients uncooperative and lose them precious minutes of the golden hour. If your interactive style is positive and nonjudgmental, the patient is more likely to be cooperative and to allow all the appropriate medical interventions, thus decreasing on-scene time. As noted before, all the substances that are abused can cause an altered mental state. When interacting with patients you must be prepared to deal with euphoria, psychosis, paranoia, or confusion and disorientation. Some strategies to help you gain your patient's cooperation follow:

1. Identify yourself to patients and orient them to their surroundings. Tell them your name and your title, for example, "EMT, Paramedic." Ask them their name and how they would like to be addressed. Avoid using generic names like "Bub" or "Honey." With this patient population it may be necessary to orient them to place, date, and what is going on. These patients may need to be reoriented frequently.

2. Treat the patient in a respectful manner and avoid being judgmental. Often a lack of respect can be heard in the tone of your voice or how you say things, not just in what you say. Never forget that you are there to save lives; this includes *all patients.* You are not a police officer (don't gather or destroy evidence), and you are not there to pass judgment on the patient's worth to society.

3. Acknowledge the patient's concerns and feelings. The patient who is scared or confused may be more comfortable with what is taking place if you recognize and address these feelings. Be gentle but firm. Explain all treatment interventions before they are performed. Be honest. Backboards and extrication collars are uncomfortable.

4. Let your patients know what will be required of them. For instance, they may be confused and not realize that they need to hold still while you are trying to immobilize them.

5. Ask closed-ended questions when getting your history from the patient. These are questions that can be answered with a yes or no. These patients may only be able to concentrate for short periods of time, and they may ramble when asked open-ended questions that require a full answer. Consider getting as much of the history as you can from relatives, friends, or bystanders. This may help improve the reliability of what you discover. Get as much relevant history as you can, *but do not delay transport.*

THE UNCOOPERATIVE PATIENT

A small percentage of your patients may be uncooperative. You must be firm with these patients. Set limits to their behavior, and let them know when their behavior is inappropriate. Consider physical restraint only if you are not able to secure enough cooperation to provide adequate care for your patient. Often a show of force may be enough to convince an uncooperative patient to allow medical care to be provided. First check with your local jurisdiction to determine what protocol you must use when restraining patients against their will. Most municipalities allow police officers to place people in custody if they are a threat to themselves or others. Severely injured trauma patients who refuse or will not cooperate with care can be considered a threat to themselves. Once the decision has been made to restrain the patient, it must be carried out with care. Securely immobilizing a patient with cervical collar, cervical immobilization device, backboard, and straps will serve to restrain most patients. Caution must be taken not to worsen any current injuries or to inflict any new ones. There is often no good solution to this predicament. Restrained patients may struggle so hard that spinal immobilization is rendered ineffective. The Reeves sleeve is one of the few pieces of equipment that is very effective in providing both restraint and immobilization (see Figure 18-1). Crews should plan and practice procedures for restraining patients. The trauma scene is not the place to learn new skills. Reassess restrained patients often. A review of the literature notes two cases of drug impaired patients dying by asphyxiation during prehospital restraint.

The standard BTLS approach to patient care will work well, even with patients under the influence of alcohol or drugs. Ensure that the scene is safe, determine the number of injured, and discover the mechanism of injury. Use universal precautions. This patient population includes people who are at high risk for infection with hepatitis B, hepatitis C, and HIV. Follow the Primary Survey and Detailed Exam as recorded in Chapter 2. Remember to note any mental status changes that might be associated with substance abuse. When performing the Detailed Exam be sure to include the specific areas that can provide clues to substance abuse. As with all trauma patients, treatment includes the consideration of oxygen and cardiac monitoring. Table 18-2 lists some drug categories and associated specific treatments or areas to pay close attention to when substance abuse is suspected.

FIGURE 18-1   Reeves sleeve.

Table 18-2 Drug Categories and Specific Treatments to Consider or Areas to Assess Closely.

DRUG CATEGORY	SPECIFIC TREATMENTS AND AREAS TO ASSESS
Alcohol	Watch for hypothermia.
Amphetamines	Monitor for seizures and dysrhythmias.
Cocaine	Monitor for seizures and dysrhythmias.
Hallucinogens	Provide reassurance.
Marijuana	Provide reassurance.
Opiates	Watch for hypothermia, hypotension, and respiratory depression.
Sedatives	Watch for hypothermia, hypotension, and respiratory depression.

SUMMARY

Knowing the signs and symptoms of alcohol and drug abuse will allow you to recognize the patient who may be impaired from their use. Assessing the patient for signs and symptoms outlined in this section can help you confirm your suspicions. Determining that your patient has abused some substance will allow you to pay attention to specific areas for critical changes as well as provide lifesaving interventions that may be indicated for individual substances. The five interaction strategies for improving patient cooperation are very important when dealing with the patient under the influence of alcohol or drugs, but these strategies should also be used with all patients. Remember that the patient's safety is a primary concern. If you must restrain a patient for his or her safety, do so in a preplanned manner that is most sensitive to your patient's needs.

BIBLIOGRAPHY

1. Bassuk, E., S. Fox, and K. Pendergast. *Behavioral Emergencies: A Field Guide for Paramedics,* p. 82. Boston: Little, Brown, 1983.

2. Bledsoe, B., R. Porter, and B. Shade. *Paramedic Emergency Care,* pp. 795–800. Upper Saddle River, NJ: Prentice Hall, 1991.

3. Caroline, N. *Emergency Care in the Streets,* 4th ed., pp. 628–637. Boston: Little, Brown, 1991.

4. Hafen, B., and K. Frandsen. *Psychological Emergencies and Crisis Interventions: A Comprehensive Guide for Emergency Personnel,* pp. 256–280. Englewood, CO: Morton, 1985.

CHAPTER 19

Blood and Body Fluid Precautions in the Prehospital Setting

Howard Werman, M.D., F.A.C.E.P.
Richard N. Nelson, M.D., F.A.C.E.P.

OBJECTIVES

UPON COMPLETION OF THIS CHAPTER, YOU SHOULD BE ABLE TO:

1. State the three viral illnesses that EMS providers are most likely to contract from exposure to contaminated blood or body fluids.

2. State the groups of people who are most likely to harbor the virus for the following illnesses:

   a. Hepatitis B

   b. Hepatitis C

   c. Acquired immunodeficiency syndrome and human immunodeficiency virus

3. Discuss the signs and symptoms of tuberculosis and describe protective measures to take when exposed to a patient with suspected tuberculosis.

4. Describe precautions EMS providers can take to prevent exposure to blood and body fluids.

5. Describe procedures for EMS providers to follow if they are accidentally exposed to contaminated blood or body fluids.

EMS personnel have always faced risks when carrying out their jobs. In the past, however, these risks have mostly involved highway hazards, fires, downed electrical wires, toxic substances, and scene security problems. Now you must assume you are also at risk of acquiring certain diseases from the patients you are treating. Fortunately, there are many precautions that may be taken to markedly reduce these risks. Additionally, measures can be taken to reduce the risk of acquiring these diseases following a potential exposure.

The spectrum of diseases to which you are potentially exposed is beyond the scope of this book. However, three types of viral infections are appropriate to discuss in conjunction with trauma management, since their modes of spread are primarily by contaminated blood and body fluids: hepatitis B, hepatitis C, and acquired immunodeficiency syndrome (AIDS).

HEPATITIS B

The term *viral hepatitis* is used to describe a group of infections involving the liver. At least five types of viruses have been described: hepatitis A, B, C, D, and E. Hepatitis A and E are spread primarily through contact with contaminated fecal material. Hepatitis D is transmitted through blood and body fluid exposure to patients already infected with hepatitis B. Because of their frequent contact with blood and needles, health care workers are considered at intermediate risk of becoming infected with the hepatitis B virus (HBV). Fortunately, hepatitis B is the one form of hepatitis for which there is an effective vaccine.

HBV is a major cause of acute and chronic hepatitis, cirrhosis, and liver cancer. An estimated 200,000 persons in the United States are infected each year; 12,000 of these are health care workers who acquire the disease through occupational exposure. Following acute infection, 5 to 10% of these patients continue to be chronic carriers of the virus (between 500,000 and 1,000,000 persons are carriers of the virus). These carriers are potentially infectious. HBV is spread by contact with contaminated blood or body fluids. Infection usually occurs from contaminated needle sticks or through sexual contact. It is estimated that 25% of health care workers who are exposed to a needlestick by HBV-contaminated blood will develop hepatitis B infection. Infection can also occur by contacting infectious secretions with skin lesions or mucosal surfaces. Routine testing of donor blood for HBV makes transmission from blood transfusion very rare.

Although HBV infection is uncommon in the general population, members of certain groups are considered much more likely to harbor the virus. High-risk groups are immigrants from areas where HBV is prevalent, institutionalized patients, intravenous drug users, male homosexuals, hemophiliacs, household contacts of HBV patients, and hemodialysis patients.

Two forms of protection are available to prevent infection following HBV exposure. The first, hepatitis B vaccine, produces active immunity against HBV infection. Persons receiving the vaccine are exposed to inactivated surface proteins from the virus and thus develop antibodies that prevent infection. The vaccine is safe and produces immunity in over 90% of persons vaccinated. In the United States the Occupational Safety and Health Administration (OSHA) requires that the vaccine be offered to any health care worker who is at risk of exposure to blood or contaminated body fluids. The second form of protection is hepatitis B immunoglobulin (HBIG). This preparation contains antibodies to HBV and provides temporary, passive protection against HBV. HBIG is used only when there has been a significant exposure to HBV in an unimmunized person.

HEPATITIS C

Recently, the hepatitis C virus (HCV) has been identified. This virus is thought to be responsible for a majority of what had been identified as non-A, non-B hepatitis infections. Antibodies to the HCV have been used to identify patients with previous HCV infection, although antibodies may not be detected during the early phases of the disease.

HCV is thought to be the leading cause of hepatitis resulting from blood transfusions. Unfortunately, this accounts for only about 5 to 10% of all cases of HCV infection. In addition to being spread by blood transfusion, the virus also appears to be spread by sharing of intravenous needles and sexual contact, much like HBV. Health care workers can acquire infection though needlesticks with contaminated needles; the likelihood of becoming infected with HCV after a single needlestick is estimated at 10%.

HCV infection tends to be less severe than HBV during the initial infection. However, there appears to be a greater likelihood of becoming a chronic carrier of the HCV following infection, placing the health care worker at an increasing risk of exposure. Liver failure and cirrhosis occur in 10 to 20% of chronic HCV carriers.

There is currently no available vaccine to protect against HCV infection. Evidence suggests that there is no protective effect provided by administering immune globulin following exposure to HCV.

ACQUIRED IMMUNODEFICIENCY SYNDROME AND HUMAN IMMUNODEFICIENCY VIRUS INFECTION

The acquired immunodeficiency syndrome is the most serious infectious complication caused by the human immunodeficiency virus (HIV). Patients with HIV infection develop a defect in their immune system. This predisposes the AIDS patient to a variety of unusual infections that are not generally seen in healthy patients of similar age. The disease has a uniformly high mortality, and its incidence is increasing. Although only 1% of the U.S. population is infected with the virus, studies of patients randomly tested in hospital emergency departments show that 2 to 9% of patients have evidence of HIV infection. At present, there is no effective vaccination or cure for the disease.

Patients infected with HIV can present with a wide spectrum of clinical manifestations. Most commonly, patients with HIV infection are asymptomatic carriers. Any patient who carries HIV, whether he manifests symptoms of AIDS or is asymptomatic, can transmit the virus. HIV appears to be transmitted in a manner similar to HBV. Although the virus has been cultured from a variety of body fluids, only blood, semen, and vaginal secretions have been implicated in the transmission of the virus. *There is no evidence to suggest that the HIV is transmitted by casual contact.* Transmission to health care workers has been documented only after accidental parenteral exposure (needlestick) or exposure of mucous membranes and open wounds to large amounts of *infected blood*.

HIV appears to be different from the hepatitis B virus in two ways:

1. The HIV virus appears to be easily inactivated by common sterilization methods such as U.S. Environmental Protection Agency–approved disinfectants, diluted household bleach, and alcohol.
2. HIV is transmitted far less efficiently than HBV. Several studies have shown that there is a seroconversion rate (demonstrating antibodies to HIV) of less than one in 300 health care workers who experience an accidental parenteral exposure and less than one in 1,000 who experience a mucous membrane exposure.

Several groups have been identified as having a high risk of HIV infection. These include male homosexuals or bisexuals, intravenous drug abusers, patients who have received blood transfusions or pooled-plasma products (e.g., hemophiliacs), and heterosexual contacts of HIV carriers. However, because of the difficulty in identifying HIV-infected patients, all contacts with blood and/or body fluids should be considered a potential HIV exposure.

There is currently no available vaccine to protect against HIV infection. Anti-retroviral drug regimens, though not a cure, have been shown to prolong the life of AIDS patients. Recently, anti-retroviral agents have been shown in some studies to reduce the risk of HIV transmission in health care workers immediately following a significant exposure to HIV-infected blood or body fluids. The decision to administer such agents should be based on the nature of the exposure, the likelihood that the patient is infected with HIV, and the duration of time following exposure (see Figure 19-1). In general, hollow needle exposures are more significant than solid instruments (such as a scalpel). Those studies that have shown a benefit in using these agents suggest that the drug effectiveness declines 2 hours after exposure.

TUBERCULOSIS

From 1985 to 1993, the incidence of active tuberculosis increased significantly to over 25,000 cases in the United States; it has been declining in the last several years. It is estimated that there are still 10 million cases of inactive tuberculosis in the United States. This has been the result of an increase in cases among persons infected with HIV and an increase in immigration of people from areas where tuberculosis infection is endemic (Asia, Latin America, the Caribbean, Africa). Risk factors for tuberculosis include homeless patients, certain immigrant populations, patients at risk for HIV infection, and persons who live in congregate settings (correction facilities, nursing homes, homeless shelters).

Tuberculosis is caused by a bacteria, *Mycobacterium tuberculosis,* that is spread from an infected person to susceptible persons through the air, especially by coughing or sneezing. Tuberculosis is spread only by persons with active infection of the lung or throat. It is estimated that up to 5% of health care workers will test positive for tuberculosis when working in high prevalence environments. Like HIV infection, most cases are asymptomatic and may persist for years. Clinical manifestations of the disease become apparent only when the patient's immune system fails to keep the bacteria in check. The bacteria then begins to infect the lungs and may spread to other portions of the body, particularly the kidneys, spine, or brain. Symptoms of the disease are most prominent in the lungs and include a bad cough that lasts longer than 2 weeks, pain in the chest, or coughing up bloody sputum. Other symptoms of tuberculosis are weakness or fatigue, weight loss, loss of appetite, fever, chills, or night sweats.

Treatment of tuberculosis includes antibiotic agents. These agents can be employed during the latent phase, when no symptoms are present, or may be used during acute infection. During the latent phase, isoniazid (INH) or rifampin is used for a period of 6 months to eradicate the infection. Three to four antibiotic agents are used when acute infection is confirmed. Some strains of the bacteria, however, have emerged that are resistant to many of the agents currently used to treat the disease.

Since 1990, the U.S. Center for Disease Control and Prevention has recommended the use of particulate respirators to prevent transmission of the bacteria to health care workers. High-efficiency particulate air filters (HEPA) are most effective in preventing transmission. Health care workers should receive tuberculin skin testing prior to employment and periodically thereafter to ensure that tuberculosis has not been acquired. Bacille Calmette-Guérin vaccination is effective in up to 80% of cases and should be considered for health care workers who work in areas with a high prevalence of drug-resistant tuberculosis. However, the vaccine makes the tuberculin skin test results unreliable.

PRECAUTIONS FOR PREVENTION OF HEPATITIS B, HEPATITIS C, AND HIV TRANSMISSION

Universal precautions refers to treating everyone (including yourself) as if they are infectious. Your goal is to prevent the spread of infection from you to the patient and from the patient to you. In today's environment, you must use the following precautions for each and every patient:

A. GENERAL CONSIDERATIONS

1. You should be knowledgeable about infection from hepatitis B, hepatitis C, and HIV. You should understand their etiologies, epidemiologies, and routes of transmission.

FIGURE 19-1   Risk assessment for anti-HIV therapy following blood and body fluid exposure.

2. If you have open or weeping lesions, take special precautions to prevent exposure of these areas to blood or body fluids. If these lesions cannot be adequately protected, avoid invasive procedures, other direct patient care activities, or handling of equipment used for patient care.

3. Perform routine handwashing before and after all patient contacts. Wash hands as soon as possible following exposure to blood or body fluids.

4. Become immunized against the hepatitis B virus.

B. PERSONAL PROTECTION DURING PATIENT EXPOSURES

1. Wear gloves if exposure to blood or other body fluids is anticipated. This precaution should be taken when performing an invasive procedure or handling any item soiled with blood or body fluid. Almost all trauma patients are risks for blood or body fluid exposure.

2. Disposable gowns, masks, and eye coverings are necessary only when extensive contact with blood or body fluids is anticipated. These precautions are advised when spraying or airborne spread of blood or body fluids is likely (e.g., blind insertion airway device insertion, vaginal deliveries, and major trauma).

3. Wear a HEPA mask when treating any patient with respiratory complaints to prevent the possible transmission of respiratory infection (such as tuberculosis).

4. Direct mouth-to-mouth ventilation of patients during CPR is to be discouraged. Use disposable mouthpieces when mouth-to-mouth ventilation is indicated.

C. HANDLING OF ITEMS EXPOSED TO BLOOD OR BODY FLUIDS

1. Consider any sharp instrument potentially infective after patient use. Place disposable syringes, needles, scalpel blades, and other sharp objects directly in puncture-resistant containers. Needles should *not* be recapped, bent, or otherwise manipulated following use. It is strongly recommended that you consider using recently developed exposure-proof parenteral injection sets.

2. Any disposable equipment such as masks, gowns, gloves, mouthpieces, and airways that have been contaminated by blood or body fluids should be collected in an impervious plastic bag. These plastic bags should then be disposed of in proper waste containers available in the hospital emergency departments or other health care locations.

3. Wash, with a low-sudsing detergent with a neutral pH, any surface spills on nondisposable equipment that does not usually come in contact with skin or mucous membranes. The equipment should then be wet down or soaked for 10 minutes in a 1:10 dilution of household bleach (or 70% isopropyl alcohol). Do not use bleach on metal objects because it can cause corrosion.

4. Wash, using a low-sudsing detergent with a neutral pH, nondisposable medical devices that will frequently contact skin or mucous membranes. Then soak them for 30 minutes or more in 2% alkaline glutaraldehyde (e.g., Cidex) or similar solution.

D. PROCEDURE AFTER ACCIDENTAL EXPOSURE TO BLOOD OR BODY FLUIDS

1. Thoroughly wash or irrigate the exposed area immediately following an exposure to blood or contaminated body fluids.

2. Notify the receiving facility of the possible exposure at the time of the incident. Ask the facility to cooperate in determining the serologic status of the source of the blood or contaminated body fluid. In some areas, informed consent need not be obtained to determine serologic status of the source.

3. Write a report of the incident as soon as possible. The minimum information that should be recorded on the report is included in Figure 19-2. The written ambulance report may be used to supplement, but not replace, the incident report. A copy of the report should be forwarded to the EMS coordinator, the EMS medical director, and the infection control committee (or equivalent body) of the receiving institution.

REPORT OF EXPOSURE TO BLOOD OR BODY FLUID

NAME OF EMS PERSONNEL _____

NAME OF EMS SERVICE _____

ADDRESS OF EMS SERVICE _____

_____

PHONE NUMBER (HOME) _____ (WORK) _____

DATE OF EXPOSURE _____ TIME OF EXPOSURE _____

NAME OF PATIENT _____

HOSPITAL ID NUMBER _____

PATIENT ADDRESS _____

_____

_____

PHONE NUMBER (WORK) _____ (HOME) _____

ROUTE OF EXPOSURE:

(   ) Parenteral exposure (needlestick or sharp instrument)

(   ) Mucous membrane

(   ) Open skin

(   ) Intact skin

(   ) Other _____

TYPE OF FLUID:

(   ) blood   (   ) emesis   (   ) saliva

(   ) stool   (   ) urine   (   ) other _____

SOURCE OF EXPOSURE:

HIV: (   ) Yes   (   ) No   (   ) Unknown

Hepatitis B: (   ) No   (   ) Acute   (   ) Chronic Carrier   (   ) Unknown

Hepatitis C: (   ) No   (   ) Acute   (   ) Chronic Carrier   (   ) Unknown

Tuberculosis: (   ) No   (   ) Yes

FIGURE 19-2   Sample Report Form.

RISK FACTORS:

( ) Homosexual   ( ) IV Drug Abuser

( ) Hemophilia   ( ) Dialysis Patient

( ) Sexual Contact of the Above

( ) Other _____

HIV Test: ( ) Pos.   ( ) Neg.   ( ) Unknown

Date of Test: _____

HBsAg: ( ) Pos.   ( ) Neg.   ( ) Unknown

Date of Test: _____

PERSONNEL DATA:

HBV Vaccine: ( ) No   ( ) Yes   TB skin test: ( ) No   ( ) Yes

Date Completed: _____

Doses: _____

HIV Test: ( ) Pos.   ( ) Neg.   ( ) Unknown

Date of Test: _____

HBsAg: ( ) Pos.   ( ) Neg.   ( ) Unknown

Date of Test: _____

HBsAb: ( ) Pos.   ( ) Neg.   ( ) Unknown

Date of Test: _____

Description of Circumstances Surrounding the Exposure, Including Measures
Taken After Exposure: _____

_____

_____

_____

INSTITUTION NOTIFIED: _____

PHYSICIAN OR RESPONSIBLE PERSON: _____

DATE OF NOTIFICATION: _____ TIME OF NOTIFICATION: _____

NAME OF EXPOSED PERSONNEL _____ DATE _____

SIGNATURE _____

FIGURE 19-2   Sample Report Form *(continued)*.

4. Any personnel who has had a significant exposure (e.g., needlestick or mucous membrane or open lesion contact with blood or contaminated secretions) should undergo HIV serology determination at the time of the incident. Repeat testing should be done at 1 month, 3 months, and 6 months for HIV and at 6 months for HCV following the exposure. If the individual has not already been immunized, hepatitis B vaccine should be administered. The administration of HBIG or IG should be determined by the serologic testing of both the source (where possible) and the exposed health care provider as well as by the assessment of the risk of the exposure.

5. In the case in which an EMS provider is found to have a positive HBV, HCV, or HIV serology, restrictions on patient care activities should be determined by the EMS coordinator and EMS medical director.

SUMMARY

Like most health care workers, you are at risk of exposure to many contagious diseases. Because of the presence of blood and contaminated secretions in many trauma victims, you must take extra precautions to avoid exposure to the viruses that cause hepatitis B, hepatitis C, and AIDS and to the bacteria that cause tuberculosis. Knowledge of the modes of exposure, as well as adherence to barrier precautions, will reduce your risk of contracting any of these infections. In the United States, the recent standards released by OSHA make adherence to these precautions mandatory for health care workers at risk for exposure to contaminated blood and body fluids.

BIBLIOGRAPHY

1. Fontanarosa, P. B. "Occupational Considerations for the Prehospital Care Provider." *Emergency Medical Clinician,* Vol. 8 (1990), pp. 119–134.

2. Friedland, L. R. "Universal Precautions and Safety Devices Which Reduce the Risk of Occupational Exposure to Blood-Borne Pathogens: A Review for Emergency Health Care Workers." *Pediatric Emergency Care,* Vol. 7 (1991), pp. 356–362.

3. Werman, H. A., and G. D. Kelen. "AIDS and Other HIV Infections." In *Emergency Medicine,* Vol. 1, eds. D. Schillinger and A. Harwood-Nus. New York: Churchill-Livingstone, 1989.

APPENDIX A

Optional Skills

Donna Hastings, EMT-P

OPTIONAL SKILL 1: ANTISHOCK GARMENT

OBJECTIVES

UPON COMPLETION OF THIS SKILL STATION, YOU SHOULD BE ABLE TO:

1. Recite the indications and contraindications for the use of the antishock garment.
2. Apply and inflate the antishock garment.
3. Deflate and remove the antishock garment.

Note: Antishock garments are also known as military antishock trousers (MAST) or pneumatic antishock garments (PASG).

INDICATIONS AND CONTRAINDICATIONS

INDICATIONS FOR USE OF THE ANTISHOCK TROUSERS IN TRAUMA PATIENTS

1. Shock secondary to hemorrhage that can be controlled
2. Neurogenic shock without evidence of other internal injuries
3. Isolated fractures of legs without evidence of other internal injuries (blow up to only air-splint pressures)
4. Systolic blood pressure less than 50 mmHg (controversial)

CONTRAINDICATIONS FOR USE OF ANTISHOCK TROUSERS

1. *Absolute:*
   a. Pulmonary edema
   b. Bleeding that cannot be controlled, such as penetrating chest or abdominal trauma
2. *Conditional:* Pregnancy—May use leg compartments

The National Association of EMS Physicians has developed a position paper on the use of antishock trousers in both medical and trauma situations. The reference for this position paper is recorded in the bibliography of Chapter 7.

TECHNIQUES

APPLICATION (see Figure A-1)

1. Evaluate the patient through at least the Primary Survey. Apply a blood pressure cuff to the patient's arm.
2. Have your partner unfold the trousers and lay them flat on a long backboard and place the backboard beside the patient.
3. Maintain mobility of the spine by log-rolling the patient (check the back quickly as you do this) onto the backboard. The top of the antishock garment should be just below the lowest rib.
4. Wrap the trousers around the left leg and fasten the Velcro strips.
5. Wrap the trousers around the right leg and fasten the Velcro strips.
6. Wrap the abdominal compartment around the abdomen and fasten the Velcro strips. Be sure the top of the garment is below the bottom ribs.
7. Attach the tubes from the foot pump to the connections on the trousers.

PROCEDURE FOR INFLATION OF TROUSERS

1. Recheck and record the vital signs.
2. Inflate the leg compartments while monitoring the blood pressure. If the blood pressure is not in the range 90 to 100 mmHg, inflate the abdominal compartment.
3. When the patient's blood pressure reaches 90 to 100 mmHg, turn the stopcocks to hold the pressure.
4. Remember, it is not the pressure in the trousers you are monitoring but the patient's blood pressure.
5. Continue monitoring the patient's blood pressure, adding pressure to the trousers as needed.

DEFLATION OF TROUSERS

Before deflation occurs, two large-bore IVs must be inserted and sufficient volume of fluids and/or blood given to replace the volume lost from hemorrhage. The antishock garment is usually deflated only at the hospital. The only reason to deflate them in the field is if they cause difficulty with breathing (pulmonary edema).

1. Record the patient's vital signs.
2. From Medical Direction, obtain permission to deflate the trousers.
3. Slowly deflate the abdominal compartment while monitoring the patient's blood pressure.
4. If the blood pressure drops 5 mmHg or more, you must stop deflation and infuse more fluid or blood until the vital signs stabilize again (this usually requires at least 200 cc).
5. Proceed from the abdominal compartment to the right leg and then left leg with your deflation, continuously monitoring the blood pressure and stopping to infuse fluid when a drop of 5 mmHg occurs.
6. If the patient experiences a sudden precipitous drop in blood pressure while you are deflating, stop and reinflate the garment.

APPLICATION OF ANTISHOCK TROUSERS TO A PATIENT REQUIRING A TRACTION SPLINT

1. Have your partner hold traction on the fractured leg.
2. Unfold the trousers and lay them flat on a long spineboard.
3. Log-roll the patient, holding traction on the injured leg and keeping the neck stabilized.
4. Slide the spineboard and the patient so that the top of the trousers is just below the lowest rib. If the patient is already on a spineboard, you may simply unfold the trousers and slide them under the patient while maintaining traction on the injured leg.

5. Wrap the trousers around the injured leg and fasten the Velcro strips.
6. Wrap the trousers around the other leg and fasten the Velcro strips.
7. Wrap the abdominal compartment around the abdomen and fasten the Velcro strips. Be sure that the top of the garment is below the bottom ribs.
8. Apply a traction splint (Thomas, Hare, or Sager) over the trousers. Attach the straps and apply traction.
9. Inflate the trousers in the usual sequence.

Adult garment and inflation pedal.

Pediatric garment.

1. Unfold the garment and lay it flat. It should be smoothed of wrinkles.

2. Log-roll the patient onto the garment, or slip it under him. The upper edge of the garment must be just below the rib cage.

3. Check for a distal pulse and enclose the left leg, securing the Velcro straps.

4. Check for a distal pulse and enclose the right leg, securing the Velcro straps.

5. Enclose the abdomen and pelvis, securing the Velcro straps.

6. Check the tubes leading to the compartments and the pump.

Note: Patient's clothing remains on for demonstration purposes. In actual use, clothing should be removed.

FIGURE A-1 Application of an antishock garment.

7. Open the stopcocks to the legs and close the abdominal compartment stopcock.

8. Use the foot pedal to inflate the lower compartments simultaneously. Inflate until air exhausts through the relief valves, the Velcro makes a crackling noise, or the patient's systolic blood pressure is stable at 90–100 mmHg.

9. Close the stopcocks.

10. Check the patient's blood pressure.

11. Check both lower extremities for a distal pulse.

12. If blood pressure is below 90 mmHg, open the abdominal stopcock and inflate abdominal compartment. Close stopcock.

FIGURE A-1 Application of an antishock garment *(continued)*.

OPTIONAL SKILL 2: ESOPHAGEAL GASTRIC TUBE AIRWAY

OBJECTIVES

UPON COMPLETION OF THIS SKILL STATION, YOU SHOULD BE ABLE TO:

1. Explain seven essential points about the use of this airway.
2. Correctly insert the esophageal gastric tube airway (EGTA).

Introduced in the early 1970s, blind insertion airway devices (BIADs) were designed for use by EMS personnel who were not trained to intubate the trachea. All of these devices (EOA, EGTA, PtL®, and Combitube®) are designed to be inserted into the pharynx without the need for a laryngoscope to visualize where the tube is going. All of these devices have a tube with an inflatable cuff that is designed to seal the esophagus, thus preventing vomiting and aspiration of stomach contents as well as preventing gastric distention during bag-valve mask or demand-valve mask ventilation. It was also thought that by sealing the esophagus more air would enter the lungs and ventilation would be improved. These devices have their own dangers and require careful evaluation to be sure that they are in the correct position. None of the BIADs are equal to the endotracheal tube, which has become the invasive airway of choice for advanced EMS providers.

Esophageal obturator airways (EOA) are designed to be inserted into the esophagus at a level beyond the carina. A cuff is then inflated to reduce the likelihood of gastric distension or regurgitation during bag-valve mask or demand-valve mask ventilation.

A more recent design, the esophageal gastric tube airway, has been introduced and should replace the older EOA. This design allows for the placement of a nasogastric tube through the lumen of the obturator for decompression of the stomach. In addition, ventilation occurs directly into the oropharynx rather than through the holes of the obturator.

You must remember seven essential points about the EGTA:

1. Use only in patients who are unresponsive and without protective reflexes.
2. Do *not* use in patients with upper airway or facial trauma in whom bleeding into the oropharynx is a problem. Do *not* use in any patient with injury to the esophagus (e.g., caustic ingestions) or in children who are below the age of 15 and of average height and weight.
3. You must ensure an adequate mask seal; this means appropriate lifting forward of the jaw, with every attempt to avoid movement of the head and neck.
4. Pay careful attention to proper placement. *Unrecognized intratracheal* placement is a lethal complication that produces complete airway obstruction. Such an occurrence is not always easy to detect, and the results are catastrophic. One of the great disadvantages of this airway is that you can determine correct placement only by auscultation and observation of chest movement—both may be quite unreliable in the prehospital setting.
5. You must insert gently and without force.
6. If the patient becomes conscious, you must remove the EGTA as it will cause retching and vomiting.
7. The EGTA is only recommended when endotracheal intubation is impossible or unsuccessful.

TECHNIQUE

The airway is relatively easily inserted and must never be forced. In the supine patient the following procedure is followed:

1. Ventilate with a mouth-to-mask or bag-valve mask and suction the pharynx before insertion of the airway.
2. After liberal lubrication, slide the airway, with mask attached, into the oropharynx while the tongue and jaw are pulled forward.
3. Advance the airway along the tongue and into the esophagus. Take care to observe the neck. Tenting of the skin in the area of the pyriform fossa or anterior displacement of the laryngeal prominence indicates that misplacement has occurred and indicates that you should reposition by pulling back and reinserting the airway.
4. Gently insert the airway so that the mask now rests easily on the face; then seal the mask firmly on the face as you pull the jaw forward to ensure a patent airway (see Figures A-2 and A-3).
5. Before inflating the cuff, attempt ventilation with a mouth-to-mask or bag-valve mask device. If you see the chest rise, hear breath sounds, and feel good compliance, inflate the cuff of the airway with 35 cc of air.
6. Following inflation, auscultate the lung fields again and feel the chest wall and observe for chest wall movement. The epigastrium should not distend.

If there is any doubt about placement of the airway, remove it and reinsert. If the patient becomes conscious, you must remove the EGTA. Extubation is likely to cause vomiting; be prepared to suction the pharynx and turn the backboard.

FIGURE A-2   Insertion of esophageal airway.

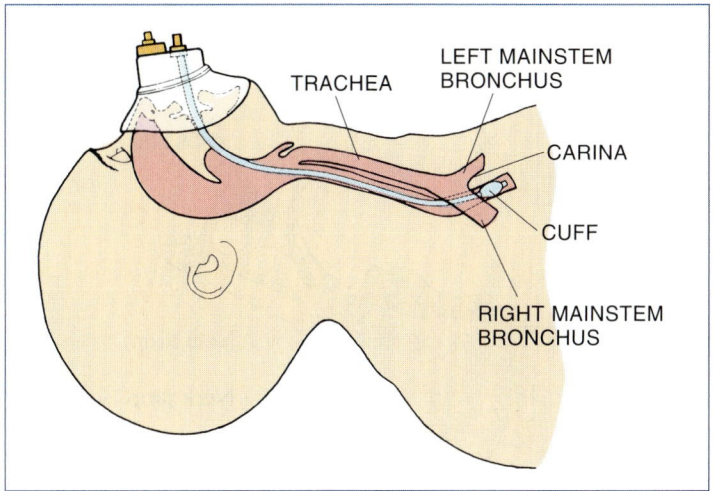

FIGURE A-3 Final position of EGTA.

OPTIONAL SKILL 3: PHARYNGOTRACHEAL LUMEN AIRWAY

OBJECTIVES

UPON COMPLETION OF THIS SKILL STATION, YOU SHOULD BE ABLE TO:

1. Explain the five essential points about use of this airway.
2. Correctly insert the pharyngotracheal lumen airway (PtL®).

Introduced in the early 1970s, blind insertion airway devices (BIADs) were designed for use by EMS personnel who were not trained to intubate the trachea. All of these devices (EOA, EGTA, PtL®, and Combitube®) are designed to be inserted into the pharynx without the need for a laryngoscope to visualize where the tube is going. All of these devices have a tube with an inflatable cuff that is designed to seal the esophagus, thus preventing vomiting and aspiration of stomach contents as well as preventing gastric distention during bag-valve mask or demand-valve mask ventilation. It was also thought that by sealing the esophagus more air would enter the lungs and ventilation would be improved. These devices have their own dangers and require careful evaluation to be sure that they are in the correct position. None of the BIADs are equal to the endotracheal tube, which has become the invasive airway of choice for advanced EMS providers.

The pharyngotracheal lumen airway is another airway developed for EMS providers who are not trained to perform endotracheal intubation. The PtL consists of a smaller-diameter long tube inside of a short large-diameter tube (see Figure A-4). The longer tube goes either into the trachea or the esophagus, while the shorter tube opens into the lower pharynx. Each tube has a cuff; the longer tube's cuff seals the esophagus or trachea, and the shorter tube's cuff seals the oropharynx so that there is no air leak when you ventilate the patient. You insert the PtL blindly into the pharynx, and then you must carefully determine whether the longer tube is in the esophagus or the trachea. If the long tube is in the trachea, you ventilate through it. If the tube is in the esophagus, you ventilate through the larger tube in the pharynx. The PtL has advantages over the EGTA

FIGURE A-4   Parts of the PtL® airway.

in that you don't require extra hands to keep a seal with a face mask and also the cuff in the pharynx prevents blood and mucous from entering the airway from above.

You must remember five essential points about the PtL:

1. Use only in patients who are unresponsive and without protective reflexes.
2. Do *not* use in any patient with injury to the esophagus (e.g., caustic ingestions) or in children who are below the age of 15 and of average height and weight.
3. Pay careful attention to proper placement. *Unrecognized intratracheal* placement of the long tube is a lethal complication that produces complete airway obstruction. Such an occurrence is not always easy to detect, and the results are catastrophic. Like the EGTA, one of the great disadvantages of this airway is that you can determine correct placement only by auscultation and observation of chest movement—both may be quite unreliable in the prehospital setting.
4. You must insert gently and without force.
5. If the patient regains consciousness, you must remove the PtL as it will cause retching and vomiting.

TECHNIQUE

The airway is relatively easily inserted and must never be forced. In the supine patient the following procedure is followed:

1. Ventilate with mouth-to-mask or bag-valve mask and suction the pharynx before insertion of the airway.
2. Prepare the airway by checking to be sure that both cuffs are fully deflated, that the long no. 3 tube (see Figure A-5) has a bend in the middle, and that the white cap is securely in place over the deflation port located under the no. 1 inflation valve.
3. After liberal lubrication, slide the airway into the oropharynx while the tongue and jaw are pulled forward.
4. Holding the PtL in your free hand so that it curves in the same direction as the natural curvature of the pharynx, advance the airway behind the tongue until the teeth strap contacts the lips and teeth. On very small patients you may have to withdraw the airway so that the teeth strap is up an inch from the teeth. Conversely, on very large patients you may have to insert the teeth strap into the mouth, past the teeth.

A

B

The PtL® airway inserted in the esophagus. Air and/or oxygen delivered into the short no. 2 tube passes into the lungs. An inflated cuff at the end of the long no. 3 tube seals the esophagus, while another inflated cuff seals the oropharynx and prevents air loss from the mouth and nose.

The PtL® airway inserted in the trachea. Air and/or oxygen is delivered into the long no. 3 tube after the stylet is removed. The inflated cuff at the end of the long tube keeps air from leaking from the trachea into the esophagus. The large cuff that is sealing the oropharynx serves as a secondary seal.

FIGURE A-5   The PtL® in place in (A) the esophagus or (B) the trachea.

5. Immediately inflate both cuffs. Make sure that the white cap is in place over the deflation port located under the inflation valve. Deliver a sustained ventilation into the inflation valve. You can detect failure of the cuffs to inflate properly by failure of the external pilot balloon to inflate or by hearing or feeling air escape from the patient's mouth and nose. This usually means that one of the cuffs is torn and that the airway must be removed and replaced. When you determine that the cuffs are inflating, continue inflation until you get a good seal.

6. Immediately determine whether the long no. 3 tube is in the esophagus or the trachea. First ventilate through the short no. 2 tube. If you see the chest rise, hear breath sounds, feel good compliance, and hear no breath sounds over the epigastrium, the long no. 3 tube is in the esophagus, and you should continue ventilating through the no. 2 tube.

7. If you do not see the chest rise, hear breath sounds, and feel good compliance when the no. 2 tube is ventilated, the no. 3 tube is probably in the trachea. In this case, remove the stylet from the no. 3 tube and ventilate through the no. 3 tube. If you see the chest rise, hear breath sounds, feel good compliance, and hear no breath sounds over the epigastrium, the no. 3 tube is in the trachea, and you should continue ventilating through the no. 3 tube.

8. When you are sure that the patient is being adequately ventilated, carry the neck strap over the patent's head and tighten it in place. Continually monitor the appearance of the pilot balloon during ventilation. Loss of pressure in the balloon signals a loss of pressure in the cuffs. If you suspect a cuff is leaking, increase pressure by blowing into the no. 1 inflation valve or replace the airway.

Like the EGTA, if the patient becomes conscious, you must remove the PtL. Remove the white cap from the deflation port to simultaneously deflate both cuffs. Extubation is likely to cause vomiting; be prepared to suction the pharynx and turn the backboard.

OPTIONAL SKILL 4: ESOPHAGEAL TRACHEAL COMBITUBE

OBJECTIVES

UPON COMPLETION OF THIS SKILL STATION, YOU SHOULD BE ABLE TO:

1. Explain the five essential points about use of this airway.
2. Correctly insert the Combitube®.

Introduced in the early 1970s, blind insertion airway devices (BIADs) were designed for use by EMS personnel who were not trained to intubate the trachea. All of these devices (EOA, EGTA, PtL®, and Combitube®) are designed to be inserted into the pharynx without the need for a laryngoscope to visualize where the tube is going. All of these devices have a tube with an inflatable cuff that is designed to seal the esophagus, thus preventing vomiting and aspiration of stomach contents as well as preventing gastric distention during bag-valve mask or demand-valve mask ventilation. It was also thought that by sealing the esophagus more air would enter the lungs and ventilation would be improved. These devices have their own dangers and require careful evaluation to be sure that they are in the correct position. None of the BIADs are equal to the endotracheal tube, which has become the invasive airway of choice for advanced EMS providers.

The Combitube is like the PtL airway in that it has a double lumen. However, in the Combitube the two lumens are separated by a partition rather than one being inside of the other (see Figure A-6). One tube is sealed at the distal end, and there are perforations in the area of the tube that would be in the pharynx. When the long tube is in the esophagus, the patient is ventilated through this short tube. The long tube is open at the distal end, and it has a cuff that is blown up to seal the esophagus or the trachea, depending on which it has entered. When inserted, if the long tube goes into the esophagus, the cuff is inflated and the patient is ventilated through the short tube. If the long tube goes into the trachea, the cuff is inflated and the patient is ventilated through the long tube. Like the PtL airway, this device has a pharyngeal balloon that seals the pharynx and prevents blood and mucous from entering the airway from above. The Combitube is somewhat quicker and easier to insert than the PtL airway but, as with the other BIADs, you must be sure that you are ventilating the lungs and not the stomach.

You must remember five essential points about the Combitube:

1. Use only in patients who are unresponsive and without protective reflexes.
2. Do not use in any patient with injury to the esophagus (e.g., caustic ingestions) or in children who are below the age of 15 and of average height and weight.
3. Pay careful attention to proper placement. Unrecognized intratracheal placement of the long tube is a lethal complication that produces complete airway obstruction. Such an occurrence is not always easy to detect, and the results are catastrophic. Like the EGTA and PtL, one of the great disadvantages of this airway is the fact that you can determine correct placement only by auscultation and observation of chest movement—both may be quite unreliable in the prehospital setting.
4. You must insert gently and without force.
5. If the patient regains consciousness, you must remove the Combitube as it will cause retching and vomiting.

TECHNIQUE

1. Insert the tube blindly, watching for the two black rings on the Combitube that are used for measuring the depth of insertion. These rings should be positioned between the teeth and the lips (see Figure A-6).
2. Use the large syringe to inflate the pharyngeal cuff with 100 cc of air. When inflated, the Combitube will seat itself in the posterior pharynx behind the hard palate.
3. Use the small syringe to fill the distal cuff with 10 to 15 cc of air.
4. The long tube will usually go into the esophagus. Ventilate through the esophageal connector. It is the external tube that is the longer of the two and is marked no. 1. As with the PtL airway, you must see the chest rise, hear breath sounds, feel good compliance, and hear no breath sounds over the epigastrium to be sure that the long tube is in the esophagus.
5. If you do not see the chest rise, hear breath sounds, feel good compliance, and you hear breath sounds over the epigastrium, the tube has been placed in the trachea. In this case, change the ventilator to the shorter tracheal connector, which is marked no. 2. Again you must check to see the chest rise, hear breath sounds, feel good compliance, and hear no breath sounds over the epigastrium in order to be sure that you are ventilating the lungs.

Like the EGTA and PtL, if the patient becomes conscious, you must remove the Combitube. Extubation is likely to cause vomiting; be prepared to suction the pharynx and turn the backboard.

FIGURE A-6 The Combitube® in place in the esophagus.

APPENDIX B

Radio Communications

Corey M. Slovis, M.D., F.A.C.P., F.A.C.E.P.

It is imperative that you provide your hospital base station physician with an accurate, succinct, on-scene assessment. This is an essential skill to develop. In general, the physician or nurse at the other end of the radio transmission will not be able to focus on more than 3 to 5 key bits of information. Thus, before beginning your call, you should spend a few moments thinking about what specifics of the history and physical exam need to be transmitted. The purpose of radio communication is not to give all of the available findings to the physician, but to transmit only that information needed for appropriate care in the field, or to ready the emergency department (ED) for patient arrival. If medications or procedures are being requested, then the radio report should focus on the information that justifies the request. Due to responsibilities to patients already in the ED, the physician receiving the call would like to spend a minimum of time on the radio.

When speaking over the radio, no matter how emergent the situation, you should speak clearly and avoid speaking rapidly in an emotional, high-pitched voice. However, using a slow monotone voice in reporting a cardiac arrest would be inappropriate as well. You should try to convey the urgency of the situation in a professional manner. The radio microphone should be held a few inches from your mouth to allow accurate voice transmission but not so far (greater than 6 inches) as to allow interference from other noises at the scene.

The following format for communications is designed to maximize the efficient transfer of information (see Tables B-1 and B-2, pp. 264 and 265). It may also be used for calls not involving trauma.

FOUR-PHASE COMMUNICATION POLICY

The BTLS communications policy is divided into four parts. The first of these phases is devoted to the EMS unit confirming radio contact with a specific hospital or base station.

PHASE 1: CONTACT PHASE

STEP 1—IDENTIFICATION: In attempting to establish radio contact, you should state what EMS service is calling, the unit's level of function (e.g., basic, paramedic), and the unit's identification number. For example, "This is county advanced unit 501 calling county hospital." It is important for you to identify your level of function so the physician knows which procedures and medications to consider. The EMS service should be identified, because different services operating in the same area may function with different protocols. The EMS unit's own identification number needs to be included for potential recontacting and for retrospective tape audit purposes. As different hospitals may have the same radio frequency, the specific facility being called should be stated by the caller each time contact is initiated.

STEP 2—FACILITY RESPONSE: The base station or receiving hospital should now respond by identifying the facility, which person is on the radio, and to what EMS unit they are responding. An example might be: "This is Dr. Thomas Smith at county hospital. Go ahead county advanced unit 501." By restating the EMS unit's service and number, confusion will be minimized when multiple units are involved with a single receiving facility. It is recommended that hospital-based radio operators identify themselves. This is important because the initial response is often not by a physician. It is just as important that physicians identify themselves so that you may record who is giving you orders.

PHASE II: IN-THE-FIELD REPORT

The second phase of communications is the most important. Here you should give all important Primary Survey information and request appropriate orders. This phase of communication is divided into the six steps that follow.

STEP 3—REIDENTIFICATION: Once contact has been confirmed, the in-the-field report begins by you reidentifying the EMS service, its level of function, and unit number. This information may not yet have been recorded or even heard by the physician who has probably just arrived at the radio console.

STEP 4—CHIEF COMPLAINT/ON-SCENE REPORT: After you have identified your level of function and unit number, the next sentence should provide the physician with the most complete picture of the patient possible. This sentence should include the patient's approximate age, sex, complaint, and/or mechanism of injury. Having information such as the victim's approximate age and sex allows the physician to get a mental picture of the patient. Similarly, by knowing the chief complaint and/or type of injury, the physician has an idea of the type of emergency call that he will be handling. An example of this part of communication might be: "We are on the scene with a 23-year-old female involved in a motor vehicle collision who is complaining of chest pain," or "We are on the scene with a 23-year-old female who has a gunshot wound to the chest." The patient's medications, additional complaints, or more complete description of injuries should not be given at this time.

STEP 5—LIFESAVING RESUSCITATION: If any emergency maneuvers or life-saving therapy has been performed during the Primary Survey, it should be reported next. Thus, if an airway maneuver has been performed or CPR started, it should be reported at this point. Examples of this include, "The patient's sucking chest wound has been sealed," or "We have begun CPR and defibrillated the patient." Results of a fingerstick glucose, if already performed on a comatose patient, should be reported during this phase.

STEP 6—VITAL SIGNS/PRIMARY SURVEY ABNORMALITIES: In the next sentence, you should give vital signs and/or Primary Survey abnormalities. In stable patients with a normal Primary Survey, a complete set of vital signs are blood pressure, pulse, respiratory rate, skin temperature (if pertinent), and oxygen saturation by pulse oximetry (if available—see Chapter 5). A typical communication might be: "The patient has a normal Primary Survey with vital signs of: blood pressure 130/90, pulse 90, respiration 16, and oxygen saturation of 98% on room air." If, however, there is an abnormal Primary Survey, a full set of vital signs does not always need to be reported. In this type of unstable patient, problems with airway, breathing, cardiovascular stability, and screening neurologic exam would be reported to the physician. In this so-called load-and-go type of call, unimportant physical findings, historical facts, or medication usage do not need to be reported at this time. A typical communication would be: "Primary Survey as follows: no palpable pulses present, respiration is 40, chest exam reveals a sucking chest wound; patient is confused and combative." Another example: "Blood pressure is 70 by palpation, pulse is 130 and weak, patient is very hot and dry. We found him in a warm enclosed room."

STEP 7—ESTIMATED TIME OF ARRIVAL: You should now state how much time it will take to get to the hospital from the present location. If you are en route, this should be reported. If, however, significant additional time is required to extricate or load the patient into the EMS vehicle, this should be specifically stated. Examples of the estimated time of arrival (ETA) phase of communication include: "We are en route to your location, our ETA is less than 4 minutes," or "We are still on-scene and will require 10 to 15 minutes before we begin transport to the hospital."

STEP 8—REQUEST FOR ORDERS: Before relinquishing radio control to the base station, you should state what orders are desired, that no orders are desired, or that the base station physician's help is needed to determine what to do for the patient. Examples of these respective situations include: "Requesting application of the PASG to maintain blood pressure," or "No orders requested," or "Base station, how do you advise?"

PHASE III: BASE STATION (HOSPITAL)-CONTROLLED ACTIVITY

In this phase of communication you are no longer in charge of the radio. You should now respond to the physician's approval or denial of orders. In other cases there may be talk back and forth between you and the physician.

STEP 9—PHYSICIAN'S RESPONSE: It is now up to the physician to determine how to proceed with management of the patient. The physician may merely agree with your request by stating, "Go ahead with your requested therapy" or might completely disagree, "Orders denied, transport the patient as soon a possible." With complicated patients, the physician may need more information than you have transmitted. This is not a criticism of the rescuer's radio abilities, but merely a need for the physician to obtain additional information. For example, "Are the patient's neck veins flat or distended?" Or "Does the patient seem to improve in the Trendelenburg position?" You should be prepared to answer routine questions readily and to perform requested maneuvers.

STEP 10—YOUR RESPONSE: You should confirm any given orders by repeating them. If the base station has given orders either that are incomplete or with which you disagree, it is now appropriate to give additional history or request an order. Examples of these problems include: "Be advised that the patient has a long history of cardiac problems and is on multiple medications," or "Base station, did you copy that the patient is hypotensive and that we are requesting use of the PASG?" If you cannot answer the questions, tell the physician. Examples of this type of exchange would be: "We don't have any available information on downtime," or "We are unable to attempt this, the patient is still trapped inside the vehicle."

PHASE IV: SIGN-OFF

The final phase of EMS–base station communications is the sign-off. You should make it very clear that the unit is leaving the medical frequency and returning to dispatch frequency.

STEP 11—EMS UNIT SIGN-OFF: You should now advise the base station that you are ending communications. Although everyone seems to favor a different phrase to end with, each EMS service should agree on a common sign-off phrase. The use of a time signal at the end of a comment is recommended but optional. Acceptable closings include: "Advanced unit 501 is clear," or "Unit 501 is out at 13:59 hours." Avoid using code numbers, as many physicians do not understand them or may use similar codes for different purposes; thus "Unit 501 is 10-8 your location code 3" is not recommended, nor is "501, 10-8, 1359."

STEP 12—BASE STATION CLOSING: The base station physician should similarly end communication with the same agreed-upon phrase: for example, "County hospital clear."

Keep a copy of Table B-1 by the EMS radio in the hospital. *You should try to concentrate on transmitting the most information with the least amount of words.*

Table B-1   **BTLS Communications Format.**

Phase 1: Establishing Contact

1. Initiation of call
   EMS service
   Level of function (basic, paramedic, etc.)
   Unit number
   Medical control facility being contacted

2. Receiving facility response
   Name of facility
   Name and title of radio operator
   Renaming of calling EMS service

Phase II: In-the-Field Report

3. Reidentification
   EMS service
   Level of function (basic, paramedic, etc.)
   Unit number

4. Chief complaint/on-scene report
   One brief sentence
   Includes age, sex, complaint, and/or mechanism of injury

5. Lifesaving resuscitation
   Patient's response to lifesaving maneuvers

6. Vital signs/primary survey abnormalities
   Vital signs in stable patient
   or
   Primary Survey in unstable patient

7. ETA
   State ETA

8. Request for orders
   State what is desired
   or
   State "no orders requested"

Phase III: Base Station (Hospital)-Controlled Activity

9. Physician response
   Agree or deny or state desired orders
   Request for additional history and/or information

10. Rescuer response
    Clarification or response to requested maneuver or therapy

Phase IV: Sign-Off

11. EMS unit sign-off

12. Base station sign-off

Table B-2   Do's and Don'ts of Successful Radio Communications.

Do's

Think about your report before making radio contact.

Be brief and concise.

Talk clearly.

Relate only the key points of the history—don't give every single fact you've learned about the patient.

State the patient's primary problem and what you are requesting early in the call.

Ask questions if you are unsure of the base station's reply.

Ask for clarification on therapies you think are wrong or dangerous.

Call your supervisor for "unresolvable" problems.

Don'ts

Don't make a speech.

Don't ramble.

Don't use jargon, codes, or abbreviations.

Don't significantly alter how you normally talk.

Don't assume anything.

Never give a therapy you think is dangerous.

Don't make unprofessional comments that will embarrass you when the tape is replayed.

Don't argue over the radio.

Documentation: The Written Report

Arlo F. Weltge, M.D., F.A.C.E.P.

With the recognition of the important and increasing role of the prehospital care provider has come deserved respect. However, with this recognition comes the expectation of a standard of care and resultant liability when the care does not meet that standard.

This appendix will show how to create a document that chronicles the medical care given, communicates medical information, and provides a permanent record that can be used as evidence that the standard of care was delivered.

THE WRITTEN REPORT

The EMS system written report can vary dramatically from being primarily a billing form to an excellent narrative medical record. In most EMS systems the written report usually will provide enough space for medical documentation to be adequate for the majority of transports, since most runs do not require much more than a simple transport.

It is important to use the system written report effectively. There should be enough space for a chief complaint, simple history and assessment, and space for other comments. All written reports should be filled out completely. Even though the transport may have been "simple," failure to document vital signs, to complete checkoff boxes for the history and physical, and to enter times, events, and other simple information may reflect poorly on the care delivered if the report is ever reviewed.

If the system report does not provide adequate space for a reasonable history and assessment, or if the case is more difficult, for example, requiring intervention or long transport times, or involving potential patient complications, it may be necessary to include a continuation sheet. The continuation sheet can be a simple form. It does require some basic information, including the patient's name, date, identification of the EMS system, and the run identification number. The report should be written at or near the time of the run, and the original must be signed and kept as a regular part of the system's medical records and attached to the regular written report. A simple continuation form is shown in Figure C-1.

A simple continuation sheet can be used for almost any situation or problem. The written, or narrative, report, using the continuation sheet, requires much more effort, however, since there are not a host of fill-in-the-blank or checkoff boxes to use when writing the report. To document a complex case adequately using the continuation sheet, you need to be familiar with the general form or sequence of a written narrative report. The form is dictated by convention (or otherwise known in the medical community as a generally agreed-upon habit or standard). Effective documentation requires using this convention as well as skill and practice.

The written report should be brief, yet, like the verbal report, relevant and focused. There are times when the clinical problem is confusing and the report must be more lengthy, but length does not necessarily reflect accuracy or relevancy. The report should document relevant events and discrepancies and should be written so another reader can reconstruct the events. The report should also justify the action, even if one's impression at the time was wrong. A "mistake" may have been entirely justified given the circumstances at the time, but that mistake can be justified only if the circumstances are clearly and honestly documented as part of the record.

The report contains the following information, but rarely will include all the information. In fact, it is more important to effectively treat the patient and document that treatment than it is to get all the information while the patient suffers because of lack of

THIS MUST BE ATTACHED TO CORRESPONDING EMS REPORT

DATE _____ HO NO: _____

NAME _____

ATTENDANT: _____

EMT REPORT:	TIME	B.P.	PULSE	RESP. RATE	TEMP.

SIGNATURE X

EMT CONTINUATION

P & S AMBULANCE TEXAS, INC.
7849 ALMEDA
HOUSTON, TEXAS 77054

WHITE - FINANCE, CANARY - HOSPITAL, PINK - SUPERVISOR

FIGURE C-1   Example of a continuation sheet.

treatment or delay in transport. It is reasonable to take brief notes and to fill out the written report at the hospital before returning to service. Care of the patient is the first goal.

1. *Run Call:* Note how the call was dispatched, particularly if there is discrepancy between the dispatch description and the actual findings. It is helpful, for example, to explain delays in transport if a call came in as a sick party when actually it was a motor vehicle accident with multiple victims. Document time whenever possible. The dispatch time is important because, realistically, it may be the last documented time until arrival at the hospital.

2. *Scene Description:* Document any scene hazards that delay or affect patient treatment or transport. It is easy to forget scene hazards, but delays may affect patient outcomes and the mention of scene hazards may help jog the memory of the run when reading the report at a later time.

   The mechanisms should be noted as well, and often this is most effectively done by stick figures (see Figure C-2). You are often the only source of the mechanism of injury for subsequent treatment providers. Clear, simple drawings of mechanisms are quick and easy, useful for communicating mechanism and suspicion of occult injuries, and can help jog the memory of the event at a later time.

3. *Chief Complaint:* Record age, sex, mechanism, chief complaint or injury, and time. These identifiers focus the thought process. If previously mentioned, mechanism does not have to be documented here.

4. *History of the Present Illness/Injury or Symptoms:* Record relevant positives and negatives. Document any relevant history that you obtain from the patient. If the history does not come from the patient but from another witness, note the source and the specific information from that person, especially when it conflicts with other history.

   Additional useful information includes the patient's recollection of the events immediately prior to the accident (e.g., did the patient faint first and then fall?), prior injuries to the same location (e.g., fractured the same leg last year), and any treatment given before your arrival (e.g., patient pulled from car by bystanders).

5. *Past Medical History:* Record previous illness, medications, recent surgery, allergies, and when the patient last ate. You are usually not responsible for getting a complete medical history. However, in acutely sick and injured victims, you may be the last person able to get this information before the patient loses consciousness. Again, treating the patient is the most important priority, but a little bit of useful information may save a lot of complications.

   Other information that can be useful may include relevant family history (any diseases that run in the family) and social history (use of alcohol, tobacco, or other drugs). This should be documented as the SAMPLE history:

   S—symptoms
   A—allergies
   M—medications
   P—past medical history (other illnesses)
   L—last meal
   E—events preceding accident

6. *Physical Exam:* Record appearance, vital signs, level of consciousness, Primary Survey, and Detailed Exam. A general statement of the appearance helps focus the reader on urgencies (e.g., the patient appeared alert and in no distress or appeared in extreme pain and was ashen and short of breath). The level of consciousness should be documented with the vital signs. This is best done using stimulus and response (responds to voice/pain with moan, decerebrate posturing). The best method is to note the stimulus that provokes a response by the AVPU method:

   A—alert
   V—responds to verbal stimuli
   P—responds to pain
   U—unresponsive

FIGURE C-2   Diagrams for mechanisms of injuries.

Document that a complete exam was done. Simply stating the body part (back, abdomen, upper extremity) with a zero or slash afterward can indicate that the part was examined and that there were no significant findings.

One of the easiest and best ways to document the exam in a seriously injured patient is to sequentially note the findings and procedures as one does the Primary Survey and Detailed Exam. It can be helpful to write "Primary Survey," note findings, describe the resuscitation, then start the rest of the exam with "Detailed Exam." By doing this, anyone reviewing the record can immediately recognize that you are oriented to trauma assessment, and by assumption, have performed an organized Primary Survey.

One picture is worth a thousand words and may aid the memory at a later date. Diagrams of injuries for locations or for severity (like cuts) should be simple yet contain enough detail to locate site of injury, that is, identify if it is right or left, volar (palmar) or dorsal, part of an extremity, or front or back trunk (see Figure C-3).

7. *Procedures (Indication, Procedure, Result):* Document the need, describe the procedure, and note the time and patient response when performing an invasive procedure. Any procedure potentially can have a harmful effect, sometimes delayed, so all procedures should be documented.

EXAMPLE

Properly Documented Prehospital Procedure

Patient was unconscious with no gag reflex. The respiratory rate was only 8 breaths per minute. An oral airway was inserted and the patient was ventilated with a bag-valve mask at a rate of 15 breaths per minute.

---

8. *Ongoing Exam (Recheck, Changes, Condition on Arrival):* Documenting the initial findings establishes a baseline, but Ongoing Exams during long transports, changes while the patient is still in your care, and condition on or just prior to arrival should be recorded as necessary to establish that decompensation did or did not occur while in your care. It is important to remember that as soon as the patient arrives, other people will perform an exam and record their findings. Any discrepancies or findings documented in their report will be presumed to have occurred while in your care unless documented by you as having existed prior to your intervention. The burden for documentation is then on you to show that complications did not occur while in transport but at the scene prior to your arrival. This is not to suggest that patients will not decompensate while in your care, but you should notice such decompensation and document that you responded to it.

9. *Impression:* Your impression may be included to summarize the significant findings. However, care must be taken not to overdiagnose. A tender forearm does not necessarily mean fracture any more than shortness of breath must mean a tension pneumothorax. Impressions should be as "generic" as possible, noting the actual finding, such as pain or bruising (not the diagnosis, such as fracture or pulmonary contusion), and should include relevant information such as distal pulse. Suspicions should be noted: Shortness of breath, decreased breath sounds on right, and tender right chest. Tender right forearm, possible fracture, sensation/pulse intact.

10. *Documenting the Priorities:* The detailed description is designed for the occasion when events allow time for gathering of the information and completion of the Detailed Exam. There are times when urgent priorities limit the evaluation to treating the immediate complications and the exam never gets past the Primary Survey. Care of the patient is the first priority. Often the best way to document

FIGURE C-3 Diagrams of injuries.

this is to describe the sequence as it occurs, using the Primary Survey and Detailed or Ongoing Exams.

EXAMPLE

Documenting the Priorities (Just the Facts)

Call: Single MVC.

Scene: One victim in roadway, car head-on into pole, patient through windshield supine in roadway.

Diagram: See Figure C-2.

Primary Assessment: Midtwenties, unresponsive male, ashen, grunting respiration with contusions to face, neck, and anterior chest. Absent radial pulse, rapid, thready carotid pulse, sucking wound right chest. Abdomen distended and tender, pelvis stable, extremities appeared to have no major injuries.

C-spine controlled manually, no change in respiration with jaw thrust, chest wound covered. Patient log-rolled onto long board, no obvious back injuries. Loaded and transported.

Ongoing Exam: Patient's right pupil fixed and dilated, left midposition. Respirations remained rapid and shallow. Patient given oxygen and ventilated by BVM. Arrived at city hospital in 3 minutes, patient still with rapid thready carotid pulse.

See Figure C-4.

SUMMARY OF THE NARRATIVE REPORT

1. Run call
2. Scene description
3. Chief complaint
4. History of the present illness/injury or symptoms
5. Past medical history
6. Physical exam
7. Procedures
8. Ongoing Exam
9. Impression
10. Documenting the priorities

CALL: INJURED PARTY 10:15 A.M.

SCENE: AUTO-PEDESTRIAN   DIAGRAM:
        SINGLE PATIENT KNOCKED DOWN (NOT THROWN
ANY DISTANCE) AND PULLED FROM THE STREET PRIOR
TO ARRIVAL BY BYSTANDERS. PATIENT LYING ON
SIDEWALK ON ARRIVAL.

CC: MID-TEEN MALE COMPLAINING OF PAIN IN THE HEAD AND NECK.

HISTORY:
    PATIENT: DENIES LOSS OF CONSCIOUSNESS. COMPLAINS OF HEAD AND NECK AND
LEFT HIP, BUT NO OTHER INJURIES. DENIES PAIN IN ARMS, LEGS, OR BACK.

    MOTHER: BRIGHT RED HAIR AND LIPSTICK – VERY EXCITED – STATES PATIENT IS
"ALLERGIC TO EVERYTHING," DID NOT SEE ACCIDENT.

    DRIVER: STATES PATIENT STEPPED OUT AND KNOCKED DOWN – NOT THROWN –
AND NOT KNOCKED OUT.

PMH: PATIENT: NO MEDICAL PROBLEMS, NO MEDICATIONS OR SURGERY, AND NEVER
BEEN HOSPITALIZED. THINKS HE IS ALLERGIC TO PENICILLIN AND CODEINE.

EXAM: ALERT MALE, SCARED BUT NOT CONFUSED.
        BP 110/70   P 98
HEAD — HEMATOMA RIGHT OCCIPUT, FACE NONTENDER PUPILS EQUAL REACTIVE
NECK — TENDER RIGHT SIDE C-COLLAR AND PLACED ON BACKBOARD
CHEST — NONTENDER BREATH SOUNDS EQUAL
ABD — NONTENDER SOFT
BACK — 0
UP/LOW EXT—00   + DISTAL PULSE AND MOVEMENT

PATIENT TRANSPORTED CODE I TO CITY GENERAL WITH C-COLLAR AND BACKBOARD.

10:25 EN ROUTE — ALERT REPT VS: BP 118/70   P 70

10:30 ARRIVED — PATIENT ALERT, VS UNCHANGED, MOVING ALL EXTREMITIES

IMPRESSION: AUTO-PEDESTRIAN WITH INJURIES HEAD AND LEFT HIP, AND PAIN IN
NECK. NO LOSS OF CONSCIOUSNESS.

FIGURE C-4   Example of a completed narrative report.

IMPROVING DOCUMENTATION SKILLS

Documentation reflects on the quality of clinical practice. Like clinical care, one can improve skills by practice as well as by observing the better qualities of others. Following are suggestions to help improve the quality of documentation.

Practice documentation with critique. Have somebody else try and reconstruct the events based on your narrative and evaluate what comments were useful and what comments were left out. Sometimes the most obvious events are the easiest to forget to document.

Read others' narrative reports and try to reconstruct the events.

Practice anticipating problems and criticisms. A fractured bone needs to have distal pulse and sensation checked and documented. Invasive procedures, complications, unusual events, or anticipated patient complaints can be noted and justification written. Many complications of invasive procedures, such as infections, may not be discovered for days or weeks. Anticipation of these delayed complications can be an important part of the documentation process.

Write to remind yourself. If there are specific events unique to this run or which will help you distinguish this run from other similar runs, note it in the record.

Be professional. People's lives depend on your care. Your records should reflect that you take your responsibility seriously. The medical record is not a place for humorous or derogatory comments. Use caution when describing the patient. Do not use words that could indicate your care was prejudiced by the patient's presentation. Words such as "the patient was hysterical" would be better written as "the patient was very excited and upset."

Be concise. Longer is not necessarily better. If it is of interest, write it down, but get to the point and write what is important.

Review your own records. Can you reconstruct the events and were complications anticipated? Would this record be a friend in court?

Practice quality care, including caring for the patient. A patient is a potential adversary or advocate. The excitement of the minute often results in a brusque attitude. Ask yourself if you would have been happy with the way you were treated if you had been the patient.

IMPORTANT POINTS ABOUT THE WRITTEN REPORT

The written report should be kept as a regular part of the patient's record and should be considered a legal document. There are some basic rules to follow:

1. Keep the report legible.
2. If there are blanks, fill them in. Empty boxes imply that the question was not asked. Open spaces imply that information might be added after the fact.
3. Never alter a medical record. If there is an error on the record, draw a single line through the error and make a note that it was an error and why.
4. The record should be written in a timely manner. Events fade and memory can be challenged. Write the chart as soon as possible after the event. If there is some delay, note the reason.
5. Always be honest on the chart. Never record observations not made. Never try to cover up actions. (We can't always be right, but we must always be honest.) The record, your primary source of support, may be discredited if any of your observations are shown not to be accurate.
6. Always make any changes or additions to the chart clearly distinguished, timed, and dated. Changes after the fact may be used against you if the appearance is that you were trying to alter the record in your favor. Such alterations give the appearance of lying.
7. What do you do if there is a complication or bad result and you did not record pertinent information on the run report? The best method is to sit down immediately and write, as accurately as possible, the sequence of events using whatever records are available and to the best of your memory. This is not as useful as a document transcribed at the time, but an accurate record even after the fact can be useful at a later date in reconstructing the events.

Trauma Care in the Cold

Jere F. Baldwin,* M.D., F.A.C.E.P., F.A.A.F.P.

One evening during the winter of 1998 it was reported that 24 of the United States and all of the Canadian provinces had temperatures below freezing. Thus, for many prehospital EMS providers, thought needs to be given to the application of BTLS in the cold environment. This appendix will address some of the problems encountered in applying the principles of BTLS in the cold. Although basic principles in the management of the hypothermic trauma patient (core temperature less than 95 degrees Fahrenheit or 35 degrees Celsius) are presented, this material does not pretend to be a treatise on hypothermia.

COLD WEATHER AND THE SIX STAGES OF AN AMBULANCE CALL

There are six stages of an ambulance call (see Figure D-1). The *predispatch stage* is the most important in the successful application of the principles of BTLS in the cold environment. Effective cold weather response is heavily dependent on adequate preparation before the emergency. EMS providers living in cold environments have already learned the importance of proper clothing, including hand and foot wear. Likewise, EMS systems operating in cold environments have already learned the importance of maintaining the rescue vehicle, which includes special tires and the use of engine warming blocks. EMS systems also must develop a system to keep their equipment at an appropriate temperature for immediate use. Obviously, the best solution is to keep the rescue vehicle in a heated garage.

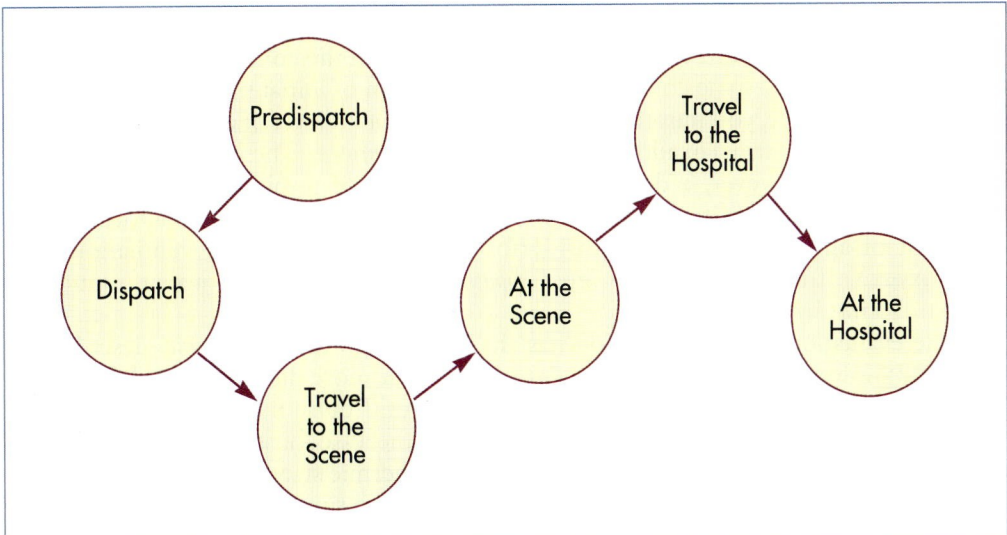

FIGURE D-1   Six stages of an ambulance call.

*Special warm thanks to Craig Lewis, David Akin, and Shiloh Lightfoot of Fairbanks, Alaska, for their invaluable assistance with this appendix.

The *travel to the scene stage* often takes on additional meaning in the winter. The shortest route, because of travel conditions, may not be the quickest or the safest. Several EMS systems have recognized that more than one mode of travel is needed. This may include any combination of helicopter, ambulance, snowmobile, or even dogsled.

The *travel to the hospital stage* may be long and arduous during winter rescue. The distances may be greater, the travel may be slower, and the vehicle more likely to break down or become stuck. Some EMS systems in North America have developed relay and backup systems for the patient. These relay systems facilitate the transfer of the patient to the nearest appropriate facility by the most appropriate mode of travel. The backup systems include a buddy system to ensure that there is someone aware of the location of the ambulance who can intervene in the event of a breakdown or a loss of communication.

SCENE SIZE-UP

On-scene trauma assessment in the cold environment starts with the *scene size-up*. The hazards may not be apparent; for example, the slippery walk or road underfoot or the hidden power line. The total number of victims may not be apparent; you must look for clues to more victims. A patient left in the cold is a fatal error. (It is easy to miss an unconscious, ejected patient at night or in poor visibility.) The essential equipment may need to be slightly different—hydraulic equipment does not work efficiently, batteries last 25% as long, flares last half as long. The phenomena of icy fog and the suspended vehicle exhaust from the rescue vehicles themselves cause decreased visibility. You must constantly reevaluate the safety of the scene, and you need the ability and backup equipment to react appropriately.

Determine the mechanism of injury. Look for clues to hypothermia. Even in a relatively warm 50 degree (10 degrees Celsius) environment, the patient could have hypothermia. Consider this possibility in the aged patient, the stroke victim, or the septic patient who has been lying on the bathroom floor for hours. Consider it with the intoxicated patient who has been lying at the foot of the basement stairs for hours. In the outside environment, wet clothing and the wind chill can cause rapid hypothermia in the trauma patient.

PRIMARY TRAUMA SURVEY

The BTLS Primary Trauma Survey is even more critical in the cold environment. Evaluation of the airway, C-spine control, and documentation of initial level of consciousness is the same. However, you must consider that the decreased level of consciousness could be a result of hypothermia in addition to any trauma or shock. The evaluation of breathing is the same; however, a decreased rate and depth of respiration may be due to hypothermia in addition to head injury or intoxication from alcohol or drugs. The treatment of an inadequate respiratory effort is the same: adequate ventilation with 100% oxygen. If the patient has *isolated hypothermia,* ventilate with *warm* humidified oxygen. Do not hyperventilate.

The evaluation of the circulation has the same importance that was described in Chapter 2; however, the cold environment may make it more difficult to evaluate. Note the rate and quality of the radial pulse. Check a carotid pulse if you can't feel a radial pulse. This may take longer than usual because of the vasoconstriction caused by the exposure or because the pulse is slowed by the hypothermic state. It is important not to start chest compressions on the hypothermic patient who simply has a slow weak pulse; the compressions could induce ventricular fibrillation. The examination of the skin color and condition may be nonproductive. Because of the peripheral vasoconstriction, the skin may be pale and cool even when the patient is not hypothermic. All cold patients (except those with spinal cord injuries) will have pale, cold extremities and delayed capillary refill.

The patient in a cold environment, especially the patient who is thought to be hypothermic, cannot be exposed for a complete examination of the chest, abdomen, pelvis, and extremities. Palpate the patient's chest with your bare hand (covered only with a latex glove) under all the layers of clothing. Palpate for tenderness, instability, and crepitation (TIC) as well as for deformity, abrasions, penetrations, paradoxical movement, burns, lacerations, and swelling. Feel for adequate and symmetric chest wall rise. Your hand is also also evaluating the patient's temperature. If the anterior chest underneath the clothing feels in any way cool, then the patient may be hypothermic. You may at this point decide that the patient is suffering from hypothermia in addition to the other injuries you may have found. *Handle the hypothermic patient very gently to prevent a lethal cardiac arrhythmia.* Even if the patient is hypothermic, you must complete the Primary Survey. Auscultate the lungs, and examine the neck, abdomen, pelvis, and extremities as best as you can. No more than 2 minutes should be spent doing the Primary Survey in the cold environment, in part to conserve body heat and to prevent further heat loss.

CRITICAL INTERVENTIONS AND TRANSPORT DECISION

When the Primary Survey is complete, you have enough information to decide if the patient is critical or stable. If you find that the patient falls into the load-and-go category outlined in Chapter 2, perform critical interventions and package the patient on a wooden or plastic backboard (not metal) and immediately load into an ambulance for transport. If the patient appears stable but is in a cold environment, or if it is cool but the victim is also wet, consider this a load-and-go situation. Gently transfer the patient to the warm ambulance for the Detailed Exam, additional critical care, and the Ongoing Exams. Close the ambulance door quickly to prevent any further heat loss from the vehicle so you can remove the patient's wet clothes soon after loading. At this point the baseline vital signs and further patient history can be obtained.

DETAILED EXAM

When the weather is cold, you should perform the Detailed Exam in the ambulance. Remove wet and cold clothing. Down clothing probably should not be cut off in the usual fashion since the heater in the ambulance will blow the feathers into the patient's wounds and the EMS equipment. Begin to rewarm the patient by both passive external rewarming with dry blankets in the warm ambulance and by core rewarming with warm (100 degrees Fahrenheit) humidified oxygen. This is usually an adequate method of rewarming for the patient with mild hypothermia (core temperature of 90 degrees Fahrenheit or greater). Do not massage or put hot compresses on the cold extremities. This may block the shivering reflex and may cause an "afterdrop" in core temperature. Rapid warming of the skin abolishes the vasoconstriction, allowing the cold blood in the extremities to return to the core causing a further lowering (afterdrop) of temperature. Perform the Detailed Exam as described in Chapter 2.

CRITICAL CARE AND ONGOING EXAM

Critical care is usually performed in the ambulance during transfer. Not only is this advantageous for the patient, but also your warm hands are better able to provide the care. Provide the patient with warm humidified oxygen in the ambulance; the plastic humidifier bottle can be filled with saline warmed to about 45 to 55 degrees Celsius (80–100 degrees Fahrenheit). But in 1999 there are no warming units that operate on the DC voltage of the ambulance. You can carry heated saline or water in a thermos. Perform frequent Ongoing Exams during transport. Especially watch the pulse, blood pressure, and the cardiac rhythm. The mildly hypothermic patient will often have muscle artifact (sometimes from the shivering), there may be sinus bradycardia, there may be a J or Osborne wave immediately after the QRS complex, or there may be atrial fibrillation. At 82.4 degrees Fahrenheit (28 degrees Celsius) core body temperature, there may be ventricular fibrillation that is unresponsive to defibrillation, and below 69.8 degrees (21 degrees Celsius) there may be asystole. The abdomen needs to be examined frequently. Your initial assessment may miss an abdominal catastrophe in the hypothermic patient. You should also frequently check and record the neurological exam.

CONTACTING MEDICAL DIRECTION

If your patient is hypothermic, it is extremely important to contact Medical Direction early. Even though it may take considerable time to arrive at the nearest appropriate medical facility, the facility needs time to assemble the proper trauma team or to arrange for more expeditious transfer to another facility. Medical Direction needs to know how long the patient was exposed to the cold and the patient's core body temperature. Remember that axillary and skin temperatures are not closely correlated with core body temperature in the cold environment. The oral temperature is inaccurate at temperatures below 96 degrees. A tympanic membrane thermometer is the most practical method to take an accurate core temperature in the ambulance.

SUMMARY

The application of the principles of BTLS in the cold is challenging and rewarding. You need a thorough understanding of the principles of BTLS and a knowledge of the conditions and limitations imposed by the cold environment. You also must always be aware that your patient may be hypothermic. The signs and symptoms of hypothermia are listed in Table D-1. This appendix has described how the presence of a cold environment and/or the existence of hypothermia changes the application of the BTLS principles.

BIBLIOGRAPHY

1. Auerback, P. S., and E. C. Geehr. *Management of Wilderness and Environmental Emergencies,* 2nd ed. St. Louis, MO: C. V. Mosby, 1989.
2. Hector, M. G. "Treatment of Accidental Hypothermia." *American Family Physician,* Vol. 45, No. 2 (1992), pp. 785–792.

Table D-1 Signs and Symptoms of Hypothermia.

NEUROMUSCULAR SYSTEM

Amnesia, dysarthria, poor judgement (34 degrees Celsius)
Loss of coordination, appearing "drunk" (33 degrees Celsius)
Shivering ceases (32 degrees Celsius)
Progressive decrease in level of consciousness (29 degrees Celsius)
Pupils dilated (29 degrees Celsius)
Loss of deep tendon reflexes (27 degrees Celsius)

GASTROINTESTINAL SYSTEM

Ileus

RESPIRATORY SYSTEM

Initial hyperventilation (34 degrees Celsius)
Progressive decrease in rate and depth of respiration (<34 degrees Celsius)
Noncardiac pulmonary edema (25 degrees Celsius)

CARDIOVASCULAR SYSTEM

Sinus bradycardia
Atrial fibrillation (30 degrees Celsius)
Progressive decrease in blood pressure (29 degrees Celsius)
Progressive decrease in pulse (29 degrees Celsius)
Ventricular irritability (28 degrees Celsius)
Hypotension (24 degrees Celsius)

KIDNEYS, BLOOD, ELECTROLYTES

Cold diuresis leading to hypovolemia and hemoconcentration
Lactic acidosis and hyperglycemia

Role of the Air Medical Helicopter

Russell B. Bieniek, M.D., F.A.C.E.P.
Pam Kirkpatrick, R.N.

Air medical helicopters were used extensively to transport injured servicemen during the military conflicts of Korea and Vietnam. On October 12, 1972, Flight for Life, the first hospital-based civilian air medical helicopter service, went into operation at St. Anthony Hospital in Denver, Colorado. In the years following this, similar programs were established at multiple hospitals and various other organizations across the United States and throughout the world. In 1998, according to the Association of Air Medical Services' (AAMS) database, there were over 200 air medical helicopter programs, transporting approximately 300,000 patients per year by both their U.S. members and a limited number of international members. The structure and role of these air medical programs vary tremendously, as does their integration with the local EMS system and involvement in trauma care.

The sponsoring agency and organizational structure of an air medical service encompass a wide range of models. They may be military or other government service—federal, state, or local; they may be independent or work in cooperation with local medical care providers to provide rescue and/or transportation of injured patients. The crews may be on call and/or the helicopter may need to be reconfigured or additional equipment may need to be brought on board. The far end of the spectrum is the fully dedicated medical helicopter that flies only critically injured or ill patients and whose interior is specifically designed and configured, always medically staffed and consistently available for a medical mission.

The role may be one of primary interfacility transport (hospital to hospital), scene transport (field to hospital), or as is most frequently the case, a combination of the two with varying percentages of each type. The involvement that an air medical service may have in the local EMS community may depend on its percentage of scene involvement.

The type of patient a service transports is usually a mixture of clinical classes, including neonatal, pediatric, cardiac, maternal, medical, and trauma. The service may transport all patients, they may limit their transports to specific types of patients, or they may have specific teams that accompany each clinical class of patients. The medical crew on board also varies with the specific program. An industry survey in 1997 revealed that 94% of medical helicopter programs utilize two medical attendants and 6% utilize one. The credentials of crewmembers vary widely, ranging from an EMT-B to a physician. The most common configuration for a two-attendant crew consists of a nurse and a paramedic. The makeup of the crew also may be determined by the type of medical mission to which the helicopter is dedicated.

If an air medical service is available in your region, it is important that you become acquainted with them and know in advance the type of cases for which you will utilize them. You also will need to know how to access them and how to involve them in your system to help improve patient care.

Multiple factors influence the availability of an air medical helicopter. These include scheduled maintenance, mechanical factors, weather, and being committed on a previous mission. This resource can be very beneficial to the EMS service and the patient, but there shouldn't be dependence on it. They may not be able to respond or have to cancel en route. Contingency plans must always be in place.

Regarding safety, there needs to be prior education and training with the air medical service. This education would entail learning proper communications between ground and air, picking and describing a safe landing zone, and coordinating unloading and loading of the aircraft. In the uncommon, but possible, event of an aircraft accident, correct knowledge of the helicopter's equipment and access could be vital to crew and ground personnel. Safety must always be the first concern, as in your BTLS training: "Is the scene safe?"

THE AIR MEDICAL HELICOPTER AND THE TRAUMA PATIENT

Caring for the trauma patient can be extremely challenging; however, it is quite rewarding to you and the patient if all the components are in place and things are done properly. As an established component and resource to an EMS service, the air medical helicopter can improve patient outcome by providing assistance in two areas. The first is speed of transportation; the second is the introduction of a higher level of clinical expertise, equipment, or procedures at the scene or en route to the hospital.

Helicopters obviously are able to transport patients quicker than ground units over long distances. This involves their ability to travel at high speeds and in a straight line. They also do not have to fight road conditions, either environmental or traffic. This decreases the exposure of the general public or the caregivers themselves to the potential dangers of an ambulance rushing through busy streets with other traffic and pedestrians.

In many areas of the United States the only care available at an accident scene is BLS. An air medical helicopter would then be able to provide ALS assessment and care at the scene and en route to the hospital. Often, even in areas where ALS is available, the air medical crew may be able to provide additional critical care expertise, skills, and/or equipment. Some of these may include, but are not be limited to, needle or surgical cricothyroidotomy, needle or tube thoracostomy, intraosseus needle insertion, pericardiocentesis, and various medications for such things as sedation and chemical paralysis of the head-injured patient for control of the airway and to assist in controlling increased intracranial pressure. Additional equipment might include pulse oximetry, end-tidal CO_2 monitors, positive pressure ventilators, and Doppler-assisted blood pressure monitoring devices, to mention a few. Many services also carry packed red blood cells to use in the field. The air medical service personnel also usually handle a higher volume of critically injured trauma patients than the average provider in a rural ground system, so they may exhibit greater familiarity and comfort in working with these patients.

For interfacility transports, the patient is evaluated by the nursing and physician staff at the referring hospital, who determine whether the patient requires additional evaluation and/or treatment at a facility with more resources available to handle the serious trauma patient. The air medical helicopter provides the vehicle, crew, and speed necessary to provide a continuum of the critical care environment en route during transport.

BTLS AND THE AIR MEDICAL HELICOPTER

BTLS provides a common language that can be used through the continuum of care for the seriously injured trauma patient. This requires coordinated education and training in a region and possibly could be an educational program offered by the air medical service. Trauma patients would then be assessed rapidly, accurately, and completely in the field by the prehospital providers, and the decision scheme that is developed for the region on utilizing the air medical service could be partly based on the results of this assessment, other specific trauma scores, types of injuries, and mechanism of injury. The air medical service would then understand the assessment and initial treatment that was done prior to their arrival, and the report could be accomplished quickly. The helicopter medical crew can then quickly do their BTLS assessment and begin transport with further treatments if necessary.

You must constantly evaluate your skills at doing a rapid assessment of the trauma patient. When you turn your patient over to another service, such as an air medical service for transport, you will not get immediate feedback on the outcome of the patient, as you do when you deliver the patient to the hospital yourself. The air medical service may serve as a link between you and the hospital to help obtain this important information. When cases are reviewed, the BTLS assessment and initial management can be used as a standard to compare with the actual care given.

SUMMARY

Air medical helicopter services are one of many special tools available to you and the hospital. As with all tools there needs to be initial and continued education and training to ensure proper and safe usage. This will improve the utilization of resources in your service area and help achieve everyone's common goal of maximizing patient outcome.

BIBLIOGRAPHY

1. Walters, E. "Program Profile, 20 Years of Service." *Journal of Air Medical Transport,* Vol. 11, No. 9 (1992).
2. Association of Air Medical Services (AAMS) Database, 110 N. Royal St., Ste. 307, Alexandria, VA 22314 (1998).
3. "1997 Medical Crew Survey." *AirMed,* Vol. 5 (1997).

Trauma Scoring in the Prehospital Care Setting

Leah J. Heimbach, R.N., NREMT-P, J.D.

Trauma scoring systems consist of assigning a numerical rating or score to various clinical signs, such as vital signs or response to pain. They are used to assess the severity of injury and are especially valuable in assessment of the trauma patient with multiple injuries. Trauma scoring systems have important uses in trauma systems at all levels, including the hospital setting and the prehospital setting and in overall health care system analysis. There are several methods of scoring severity of injury in trauma patients, including the Glasgow Coma Score and the Revised Trauma Score (see Tables F-1 and F-2).

In the hospital setting, trauma scoring systems have several uses, including the following:

1. Standardizing triage between health care facilities (deciding when it is appropriate to transfer a patient to a trauma center)
2. Allocating medical resources
3. Evaluating the health care facility's overall effectiveness in providing patient care
4. Conducting audits (making sure that patients who are predicted to survive their traumatic event actually do survive)
5. Predicting morbidity and mortality of patients based on a particular trauma score

Although prehospital care providers should never delay transport to complete a trauma score, trauma scoring systems can provide an objective and standardized way for you to triage patients appropriately (including whether a patient should go to a trauma center) and to communicate injury severity, using a common language, to other members of the health care team. Trauma scores recorded in the field are also useful in the analysis and research of EMS systems. This analysis can then be used to develop protocols for prehospital care to meet the needs of a specific EMS region. The BTLS patient assessment includes a neurological assessment, using the AVPU method (alert, responds to verbal stimulus, responds to painful stimulus, and unresponsive), and identifies parameters to determine whether the patient is a load-and-go. Communicating this information along with a list of the patient's injuries to the receiving hospital will allow the hospital personnel to gather the necessary resources to optimize care.

Table F-1 **Glasgow Coma Score.**

EYE OPENING	POINTS	VERBAL RESPONSE	POINTS	MOTOR RESPONSE	POINTS
Spontaneous	4	Oriented	5	Obeys commands	6
To voice	3	Confused	4	Localizes pain	5
To pain	2	Inappropriate words	3	Withdraws	4
None	1	Incomprehensible sounds	2	Abnormal flexion	3*
		Silent	1	Abnormal extension	2**
				No movement	1

*Decorticate posturing to pain
**Decerebrate posturing to pain

Table F-2 **Revised Trauma Score.**

Score	Score	Contribution to Revised Trauma
Total Glasgow Coma Score (see Table F-1)	13–15	4
	9–12	3
	6–8	2
	4–5	1
	3	0
Systolic blood pressure (mmHg)	>89	4
	76–89	3
	50–75	2
	1–49	1
	None	0
Respirations (per minute)	10–29	4
	>29	3
	6–9	2
	1–5	1
	None	0

Note: If total score is 11 or less, the patient should be taken to a trauma center.

The use of trauma scores in the prehospital setting can be confusing at a time when patient assessment, injury management, and communication to the receiving hospital need to be concise. It is recommended that you report the following information to the receiving facility:

1. Age, sex, and chief complaint
2. Mechanism of injury
3. Level of consciousness
4. What parameters led to the load-and-go decision
5. A list of the patient's injuries
6. What treatment was rendered
7. The patient's response to treatment

Many EMS regions will require the use of some type of trauma score system in the prehospital setting to facilitate patient care and/or to promote prehospital research. An example of the Revised Trauma Score is shown in Table F-2. An example of the Pediatric Glasgow Coma Score and Pediatric Trauma Score is shown in Tables F-3 and F-4.

BIBLIOGRAPHY

1. Champion, H. R., and others. "A Revision of the Trauma Score." *Journal of Trauma,* Vol. 29 (1989), p. 623.
2. Tepas, T. A. "Pediatric Trauma Score." *Journal of Pediatric Surgery,* Vol. 22 (1987), p. 14.

Table F-3   Pediatric Glasgow Coma Score.

		>1 YEAR	<1 YEAR	
EYES OPENING	4	Spontaneously	Spontaneously	
	3	To verbal command	To shout	
	2	To pain	To pain	
	1	No response	No response	
		>1 YEAR	**<1 YEAR**	
BEST MOTOR RESPONSE	6	Obeys		
	5	Localizes pain	Localizes pain	
	4	Flexion–withdrawal	Flexion–normal	
	3	Flexion–abnormal (decorticate rigidity)	Flexion–abnormal (decorticate rigidity)	
	2	Extension (decerebrate rigidity)	Extension (decerebrate rigidity)	
	1	No response	No response	
		>5 YEARS	**2–5 YEARS**	**0–23 MONTHS**
BEST VERBAL RESPONSE	5	Oriented and converses	Appropriate words and phrases	Smiles, coos, cries appropriately
	4	Disoriented and converses	Inappropriate words	Cries
	3	Inappropriate words	Cries and/or screams	Inappropriate crying and/or screaming
	2	Incomprehensible sounds	Grunts	Grunts
	1	No response	No response	No response

Table F-4   Pediatric Trauma Score.

SCORE	+2	+1	−1
Weight	>44 lb (>20 kg)	22–44 lb (10–20 kg)	<22 lb (<10 kg)
Airway	Normal	Oral or nasal airway	Intubated Tracheostomy Invasive airway
Blood pressure	Pulse at wrist >90 mmHg	Carotid or femoral pulse palpable 50–90 mmHg	No palpable pulse <50 mmHg
Level of consciousness	Completely awake	Obtunded or any loss of consciousness	Comatose
Open wound	None	Minor	Major or penetrating
Fractures	None	Closed fracture	Open or multiple fractures

Drowning, Barotrauma, and Decompression Injury

James H. Creel Jr., M.D., F.A.C.E.P.
John E. Campbell, M.D., F.A.C.E.P.

DROWNING

Approximately 7,000 people drown annually, making drowning the third leading cause of accidental death in the United States. Freshwater drownings are more common than saltwater drownings, and there are more immersion accidents in pools than in lakes, ponds, and rivers. The peak incidence occurs in the warm months and most commonly involves teenagers and children under the age of 4.

Drowning is death from suffocation after submersion in the water. There are two basic mechanisms:

1. Breath holding, which leads to aspiration of water and wet lungs
2. Laryngospasm with glottic closure and dry lungs

Both these mechanisms lead to profound hypoxia and death. With the aspiration of at least 22 cc per kilogram of seawater (which is hypertonic to the plasma), fluid is drawn into the alveoli from the circulation. Aspiration of at least 22 cc per kilogram of freshwater (which is hypotonic to the plasma) causes fluid to be absorbed across the alveoli into the circulation. These are of no concern in the prehospital phase. Survival of the victim depends on your rapid evaluation and management of the ABCs.

Initiate management as soon as possible. Be aware of surfing/diving mechanisms that indicate potential occult C-spine injury. Protect the cervical spine during rescue of the patient. In water, CPR is generally ineffective. Remove the patient to a stable surface as soon as possible; then initiate CPR and the appropriate protocol. In cases in which hypothermia is responsible for the near-drowning, it appears to provide the brain, heart, and lungs some degree of protection (diving reflex) by slowing the metabolism. Therefore, no one is dead until warm and dead; do not stop CPR.

BAROTRAUMA

Barotrauma refers to injuries due to the mechanical effects of pressure on the body. We all live "under pressure" since the weight of the air in which we live exerts force on our bodies. At sea level the weight of air pressing on the body equals 14.7 pounds per square inch (psi). Since solids and liquids are not compressible, they are not usually affected by pressure changes. The study of barotrauma is the study of the effect of pressure on gas-filled organs of the body. Gas-filled organs are ears, sinuses, upper and lower airways, stomach, and intestines.

To understand the effects of pressure changes, you must know some properties of gases. Boyle's law states that the volume of a gas is inversely proportional to the pressure applied to it. This simply means that if you double the pressure on a gas, the volume of the gas will decrease by one-half. If you halve the pressure on a gas, the volume will double. The pressure at sea level is called one atmosphere absolute (ATA). If you go up in an airplane (or climb a mountain), you have less atmosphere above you; thus the pressure decreases and the gas inside the body expands. Most commercial airliners fly at about

35,000 feet elevation (one-fifth ATA or gas volume five times normal) but are pressurized to a cabin pressure equal to 5,000 to 8,000 feet elevation (two-thirds to three-fourths ATA) so that gas expands to only about 1.2 to 1.4 times its original volume. Airline passengers notice no change except for "popping" of the ears as the expanding gas in the middle ears vents off through the eustachian tubes into the pharynx.

Water is much heavier than air. When one descends into salt water, there is a change of one atmosphere for every 33 feet of depth (34 ft for fresh water). This means that at 33 feet of depth the body is subjected to 2 ATA, and gas in the body has been compressed to one-half of its original volume. Because of the pressures involved, divers are exposed to certain potential injuries during both descent and ascent.

TRAUMA OF DESCENT: "MIDDLE EAR SQUEEZE"

Since there is a large pressure change during the first few feet of a dive, skin divers and snorkelers as well as scuba divers are subject to this type of injury. Let's say that a skin diver takes a breath and rapidly descends to a depth of 33 feet: All the gas in his body will decrease in volume by one-half. This includes gas in the lungs, intestines, stomach, sinuses, and middle ears. The elastic lungs, intestines, and stomach will simply decrease in size to match the volume of gas. Problems develop with the middle ears and sinuses if the pressure cannot be equalized. The sinuses (air pockets in the bones of the face and skull) each have an opening through which air from the pharynx can enter to equalize the pressure. If the openings are blocked, the skin diver will experience pain in the sinuses and may even develop bleeding and inflammation (barosinusitis). Other than the discomfort, this causes no serious problem. Each middle ear has an opening, the eustachian tube, through which air from the pharynx can enter to equalize pressure. If the eustachian tube is blocked (mucosal congestion from allergy, infection, etc.), the pressure will push in on the eardrum and cause intense pain. This begins to be noticeable at a depth of 4 to 5 feet. If the diver cannot equalize the middle ear pressure and yet continues to descend, the pressure will eventually rupture the eardrum and flood the middle ear with cold water (even the warm waters of the Caribbean are 20 degrees below body temperature). Cold water in the middle ear causes dizziness, nausea, vomiting, and disorientation ("twirly bends"). The result can be panic and drowning or near-drowning. The diver using a self-contained underwater breathing apparatus (scuba diver) who surfaces rapidly can develop air embolism or neurologic decompression sickness. Vomiting under water can cause aspiration and drowning.

Barotitis media (middle ear squeeze) requires no prehospital treatment. The pressure is relieved when the diver returns to the surface. If there is hearing loss or continued ear pain, the diver should see a physician for treatment of ruptured eardrum or bleeding into the middle ear. The conditions that you are more likely to have to manage are the near-drowning cases caused by the disorientation from water in the middle ears.

TRAUMA OF ASCENT

Injuries from expanding gas can occur as divers ascend. These injuries are much more common in scuba divers, since such injuries usually either require some time to develop (longer than a skin diver can hold his breath) or require the breathing of compressed air.

REVERSE MIDDLE EAR SQUEEZE

If a eustachian tube becomes blocked during a dive, the gas in the middle ear will expand and cause pain during ascent. If there is enough expansion, the eardrum can rupture, with all the symptoms and dangers mentioned previously.

GASTROINTESTINAL BAROTRAUMA

If the diver swallows air while breathing compressed air or if the diver has previously eaten gas-forming foods (e.g., beans), he may accumulate a significant amount of stomach or intestinal gas during a dive. If the diver was at a depth of 66 feet, the gas will expand to three times its original volume during ascent. If he is unable to expel this gas, he will develop abdominal pain and occasionally even collapse and develop a shock-like state.

PULMONARY OVERPRESSURIZATION SYNDROMES (BURST LUNG)

These occur only in divers who have been breathing compressed air. During a dive the lungs are completely filled with air, which is at a pressure equal to the depth at which the diver is swimming. If a diver panics and surfaces without exhaling, the rapidly expanding gas will overinflate the lungs and cause one of the three overpressurization syndromes listed below. Remember, the total volume of the lungs is about 6 L. An ascent from 33 feet would cause expansion to 12 L; 66 feet, 18 L; and 100 feet, 24 L. It is easy to see how delicate alveoli can be ruptured by this expansion. The expanding air will dissect into the interstitial space, pleural space, pulmonary venules, or a combination of the three.

1. *Air in the Interstitial Space:* This is the most common form of pulmonary overpressurization syndrome. As millions of tiny air bubbles escape into the interstitial tissue, they may dissect into the mediastinum and up into the subcutaneous tissue of the neck. Symptoms may develop immediately upon surfacing or may not develop for several hours. The diver may have increasing hoarseness, chest pain, subcutaneous emphysema in the neck, and difficulty breathing and swallowing. Any diver with these symptoms should get oxygen (no positive pressure ventilations unless the diver is apneic) and transport to the hospital. While interstitial air does not require treatment with a recompression chamber (hyperbaric chamber), these patients often develop air embolism or decompression sickness. They should be observed in a facility that is capable of providing recompression treatment if necessary.

2. *Air in the Pleural Space:* If the alveoli rupture into the pleural space, a pneumothorax and possibly a hemothorax will develop. The amount of pneumothorax will depend on how much air escaped into the pleural space and how far the diver surfaced after the air entered the pleural space. A 10% pneumothorax at 33 feet will be a 20% pneumothorax at the surface. A 20 to 30% pneumothorax at 33 feet may be a tension pneumothorax at the surface. The symptoms will be the same as for interstitial air except the diver will now have decreased breath sounds and hyperresonance to percussion on the affected side (may be on both sides). A tension pneumothorax will also have distended neck veins and shock (and possibly tracheal deviation—a rare sign). Give 100% oxygen and transport immediately.

3. *Air Embolism:* The most serious syndrome of overpressurization is pulmonary air embolism. If the overdistended alveoli rupture into the pulmonary venules, the millions of tiny air bubbles can return to the left side of the heart and then up the carotid arteries to the small arterioles of the brain. These bubbles, composed mostly of nitrogen, obstruct the arterioles and produce symptoms similar to a stroke. The symptoms produced depend on which vessels are obstructed. There will usually be loss of consciousness and focal neurological signs. The symptoms almost always occur immediately when the diver surfaces. This is a very important point in differentiating air embolism from decompression sickness (which usually takes hours to develop). The patient should be placed in Trendelenburg's position (30 degrees head down) on the left side, given 100% oxygen, and transported to a facility that can provide recompression treatment. The left-side, head-down position prevents further embolism of air to the brain and helps distend the vessels, thus allowing small bubbles to pass through and return to the lungs where they can be eliminated. This is one instance in which you should not hyperventilate or give positive pressure ventilations. Hyperventilation causes vasoconstriction, which will trap the bubbles. Positive pressure ventilation may force more air into the veins, worsening the injury (if the patient is not breathing, you must give positive pressure ventilation). This

patient must have immediate recompression in a recompression chamber no matter how much time has passed since the injury and no matter how far away the recompression chamber may be. In a recompression chamber, the pressure is raised to 6 ATA, which will decrease the size of the bubbles to one-sixth of their previous volume. This may allow them to pass through the capillaries back to the lungs to be expelled. Air embolism may rarely affect the coronary arteries, causing myocardial infarction, dysrhythmias, or cardiac arrest.

DECOMPRESSION ILLNESS

Decompression illness is caused by another property of gases. Henry's law states that the amount of gas dissolved in a liquid is directly proportional to the pressure applied. This means that twice as much gas would be dissolved in a liquid at 33 feet as at sea level. It also means that gas dissolved in a liquid at 33 feet will come out of solution as that liquid ascends. This is analogous to a sealed bottle of carbonated beverage that has no bubbles as long as it is sealed but bubbles the instant that the cap is removed and the pressure is released.

Nitrogen, which accounts for about 80% of the volume of inspired air, is an inert gas that dissolves in blood and fat. When a diver is under water, nitrogen dissolves in the blood and fat tissue. This nitrogen is released as he surfaces, so he must surface slowly enough to allow this nitrogen to be expelled through his lungs. The U.S. Navy has developed a set of tables of no-decompression limits that give general guidelines about how long one can stay at a certain depth without going through stage decompression during ascent. There are also standard air decompression tables for those dives that exceed the no-decompression limit. Theoretically, if one follows the recommendations of the tables, nitrogen bubbles will not form in the blood during ascent. This may not always be true because the tables were developed from a study of U.S. Navy divers, who are uniformly young, healthy, well-conditioned men who were diving in salt water. Today, there are 3 million recreational scuba divers and 300,000 new divers certified each year. Sport divers are not uniformly young, healthy, or conditioned. They are often older, poorly conditioned, and not always healthy. A special problem is obesity. Fat absorbs about five times as much nitrogen as blood or other tissue, so obese divers require longer decompression times or shorter dives. Sport divers should be very conservative when using diving tables, especially when diving in fresh water or in lakes above sea level. The greatest danger occurs when a diver who has been submerged for a significant period of time has a diving accident, panics, and surfaces rapidly. Nitrogen bubbles will form in his blood and tissue just as carbon dioxide bubbles form in champagne. This is a different injury from barotrauma or pulmonary overpressurization syndrome and may exist along with any of the barotrauma syndromes. It is frequently seen in divers in near-drowning situations. The symptoms are almost always delayed for minutes to hours after a dive. As a general rule, symptoms that develop within 10 minutes of surfacing are caused by air embolism until proved otherwise. Symptoms developing after 10 minutes are decompression illness until proved otherwise. A special case is the vacationing diver who is asymptomatic after a deep dive and then catches a plane home the same day. This diver may develop symptoms during flight since the cabin pressure is only two-thirds or three-fourths ATA. These symptoms may not appear until the diver has returned home far inland from the site of the dive. All emergency providers should have some knowledge of diving injuries.

TYPE I DECOMPRESSION ILLNESS

1. *Cutaneous ("skin bends")*: Millions of tiny nitrogen bubbles may form in the microvasculature of the skin. This causes a generalized itching rash that may be red and inflamed or mottled with a central purple discoloration. It is called "marbleized skin." This condition requires no treatment but may be an early sign of more serious

decompression sickness, so the patient must be observed. Give the patient 100% oxygen, and transport to a facility capable of recompression therapy.

2. *Musculoskeletal ("bends" or "pain-only bends"):* This is the most common presentation of decompression sickness. Over 85% of divers with decompression sickness will present with pain in the joints. The shoulders or knees are affected most commonly, but any joint may be affected. The pain is usually deep and aching, and there may be vague numbness around the affected joint. Characteristically, there are no physical findings and the pain may be eased by pressure such as inflating a blood pressure cuff. These patients require recompression therapy no matter how long it has been since the symptoms started and no matter how far the nearest recompression chamber may be.

TYPE II DECOMPRESSION ILLNESS

These syndromes are more serious and may be life-threatening. They are emergencies that require rapid diagnosis and treatment.

1. *Pulmonary ("chokes"):* Nitrogen bubbles forming in the vasculature of the lungs cause symptoms similar to the interstitial pulmonary overpressurization syndrome. The patient will develop cough, chest pain, difficulty breathing, and sometimes hemoptysis. These symptoms usually develop within an hour of surfacing (50%) but may be delayed for up to 6 hours and even rarely for 24 to 48 hours. Pulmonary overpressurization syndrome usually appears within a few minutes of surfacing. In either case the patient requires oxygen and recompression therapy. Here again, be careful of positive pressure ventilation, as it may cause gas bubble emboli to the brain.

2. *Neurologic:* Nitrogen bubbles in the nervous system may present with any symptom from personality changes to specific localized neurologic changes. By far the most common symptoms involve the lower spinal cord and often produce weakness or paralysis of the legs and urinary bladder. Bladder problems are so common that historically, urinary catheters were considered essential equipment for divers. These patients must have recompression therapy or irreversible paralysis will occur.

MANAGEMENT OF DIVING INJURIES

HISTORY

1. *Type of Diving and Equipment Used:* This is very important. Remember that skin divers and snorkelers cannot get overpressurization syndrome or decompression sickness, but all divers can drown. The treatment for near-drowning is very different from that for decompression sickness or air embolism.

2. *History of the Dive:* You need to know where the dive occurred, at what depth, how many dives, how long on the bottom, and any in-water decompression. This information is also needed for dives during the preceding 2 days.

3. *Past Medical History:* Pulmonary problems that predispose to air trapping (asthma or obstructive lung disease) are frequently associated with overpressurization syndrome.

4. *Exactly When the Symptoms First Occurred:* This may be helpful in differentiating air embolism and decompression illness.

5. *Complications of the Dive:* Did the diver run out of air? Was there an attack by marine animals? Did a diving accident occur?

6. *Travel After the Dive:* Traveling at higher altitudes may precipitate decompression sickness.

INITIAL MANAGEMENT

1. Follow standard patient assessment protocol: Primary Survey, critical interventions and transport decision, Detailed Exam, and Ongoing Exam.

2. If there is any chance of overpressurization syndrome or decompression illness, do not hyperventilate or give positive pressure ventilation. Positive pressure ventilation is indicated only for apneic patients.
3. Check for hypothermia (see Appendix D) in all diving accident victims.
4. Patients with air embolism or neurologic decompression sickness should be placed on their left side in the head-down position.
5. All diving accident patients should get 100% oxygen.
6. Shock and other injuries are treated by routine protocols.
7. If a recompression facility is needed and you need information about the one nearest to your facility, you may obtain assistance 24 hours a day through the National Diving Alert Network at Duke University: (919) 684-8111.

SUMMARY

No matter how far you may live from a large body of water, you may be called upon to manage a patient with near-drowning or diving injuries. When treating the near-drowning patient, the performance of the ABCs is most important in the prehospital phase, but don't forget the possibility of hypothermia. When treating barotrauma, you should not only follow the basic principles of BTLS, but also remember the importance of the history, patient positioning, the possibility of hypothermia, and the dangers of positive pressure ventilation.

BIBLIOGRAPHY

1. Jeppeson, S. *Open Water Sport Diving Manual,* 4th ed., pp. 2, 25–49. Englewood, CO: Jeppeson Sanderson, 1984.
2. Kizer, K. W. "Dysbarism." In *Emergency Medicine,* ed. J. E. Tintinalli, 3rd ed., pp. 678–688. New York: McGraw-Hill, 1992.

Injury Prevention and the Role of the EMS Provider

Janet M. Williams, M.D.
Jonathan M. Rubin, M.D.

THE INJURY EPIDEMIC

Every day prehospital health care providers serve the public by delivering quality emergency care. The BTLS curriculum has been developed to convey the principles of acute prehospital care of the injured patient. Well-trained prehospital care providers with BTLS skills save many lives of injured patients each year. Unfortunately, over 50% of trauma deaths occur immediately after the injury event. As a result, you often arrive at the scene only to find a patient who has died or is dying and for whom no life-saving measures can be taken. These cases illustrate the importance of recognizing injury as a preventable disease. Your role extends far beyond the acute care of the injured patient. The entire EMS community must become active in preventing injury from occurring in the first place.

Though underrecognized, injury is a major public health problem worldwide. In the United States injury is the single greatest killer between the ages of 1 and 44 and is responsible for more years of potential life lost than cancer and heart disease combined. In the United States alone, the cost of injury is estimated to be over $210 billion annually.

Injury has been misconceived by the public as being a result of an unavoidable "act of God," an "accident," due to "bad luck," or a result of a behavioral problem on the part of the injured individual. In reality, injuries are health problems that behave like classic infectious diseases. Injuries may be characterized by demographic distributions, seasonal variations, epidemic episodes, and risk factors. In addition, they are predictable and preventable. An analogy has been made between the cause of an injury and the cause of a disease such as malaria. Table H-1 illustrates how disease causation can be applied to both of these entities.

Traditionally, medical education programs have emphasized the treatment of acute injury and have neglected the concept of injury prevention and control. It is interesting that patients presenting with cardiac symptoms are nearly always asked if they have risk factors such as history of smoking, diabetes, hypertension, hypercholesterolemia, and family history of heart disease. In addition, these patients are counseled as to how to reduce their risk for heart disease. As health care providers, we have a responsibility to do the same for injured patients. Besides playing a vital role in the acute care of injured patients, prehospital care providers have a unique opportunity to assess risk factors for

Table H-1 **An Etiologic Comparison of Injury and a Classic Infectious Disease.**

DISEASE	HOST	AGENT	VECTOR/ VEHICLE	EXPOSURE EVENT
Malaria	Human	*P. vivax*	Mosquito	Mosquito bite
Injury (i.e., head injury)	Human	Kinetic energy	Motor vehicle	Crash

injury, to examine patients in the injury setting, to provide valuable injury information to other medical care providers, and to educate the public on injury prevention. In addition, prehospital care providers often see the "near-miss" patient who survives what could have been a fatal injury event. Such circumstances are an opportune time for prehospital care providers to give injury prevention advice.

WHAT IS AN INJURY?

Injury may be defined as any damage to the human body that results from acute exposure of physical energy or from an absence of vital entities such as heat and oxygen. There are five basic forms of injurious energy: thermal, mechanical, electrical, radiating, and chemical. Roughly three-fourths of all injuries are caused by exposure to mechanical or kinetic energy during incidents such as motor vehicle crashes, falls, and firearm discharges. Examples of injury resulting from a lack of heat or oxygen are frostbite and drowning. An individual's tolerance for injury depends on factors such as physical size, age, and presence of underlying disease.

Injury has also been defined as a disease that results from the interaction of three components of the epidemiology triangle: host, agent, and environment (see Figure H-1). The host refers to the human being or victim, the agent is the form of energy involved, and the environment provides the opportunity for the agent (energy) to be transmitted to the host.

The environment may be either protective and prevent injury or hostile and encourage injury (see Figure H-2).

The mechanism by which the agent or energy is transferred to the host is referred to as the vector. For example, during a motor vehicle crash, the automobile is the vector that may transmit physical (kinetic) energy to the host if the environment is permissive.

FIGURE H-1 The injury epidemiology triangle.

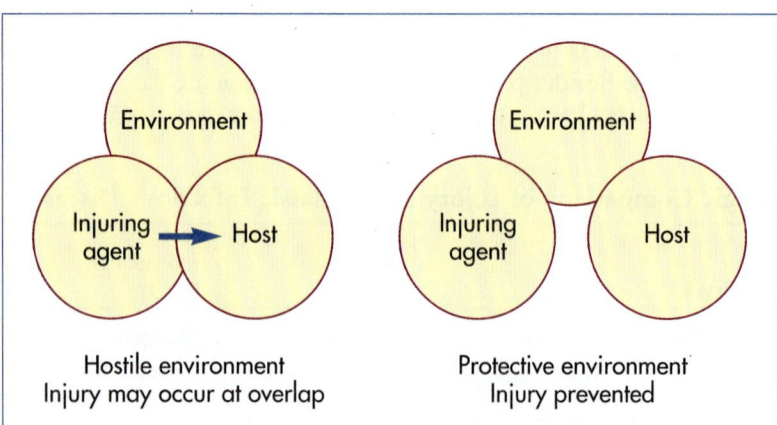

FIGURE H-2 The relationship of the environment, injuring agent, and host.

Injury may be classified as intentional or unintentional. Intentional injuries include those such as suicide, assault, and homicide. Unintentional injuries include those that are not deliberate or planned, such as falls, motor vehicle crashes, and burns. In some cases, it may be difficult to distinguish intentional from unintentional injury. Injury also may be categorized by the actual type of injury (such as fracture or head injury), by the mechanism or cause of injury (such as motor vehicle crash or fall), or by the population at risk (such as pediatric, black males, or the elderly).

THE INJURY PROCESS AND WHY INJURIES OCCUR

Injury results when the victim is exposed to energy in amounts that exceed the threshold of human tolerance. In most cases, energy is transmitted as the victim is attempting to perform a specific task or action. The performance of a task refers to how well the individual executes an action, and the task demand is the amount of skill that is required to successfully perform the task. Any time that an individual's performance is below the task demand for the action, there is potential for release of injurious energy (Figure H-3). For example, a drunk driver may lack the skills necessary to drive an automobile and ultimately crash. The crash results in the release of kinetic energy (motion), which may be transmitted to the driver, causing injury. In an unprotective environment, the energy is transmitted to the individual and results in an injury.

The environment may also protect the victim from injury in cases in which the road conditions are favorable, guard rails are present to prevent driving over an embankment, or the victim is restrained (Figure H-4).

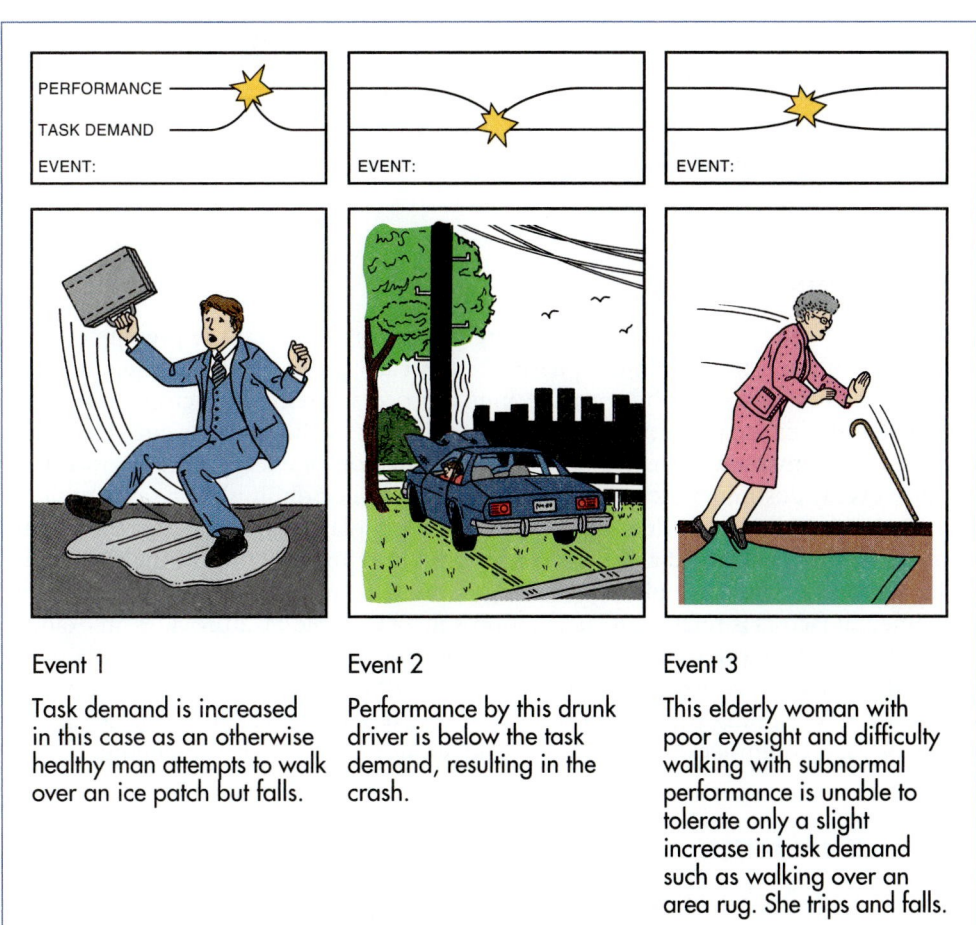

Event 1

Task demand is increased in this case as an otherwise healthy man attempts to walk over an ice patch but falls.

Event 2

Performance by this drunk driver is below the task demand, resulting in the crash.

Event 3

This elderly woman with poor eyesight and difficulty walking with subnormal performance is unable to tolerate only a slight increase in task demand such as walking over an area rug. She trips and falls.

FIGURE H-3   The relationship of performance and task demand in the injury process.

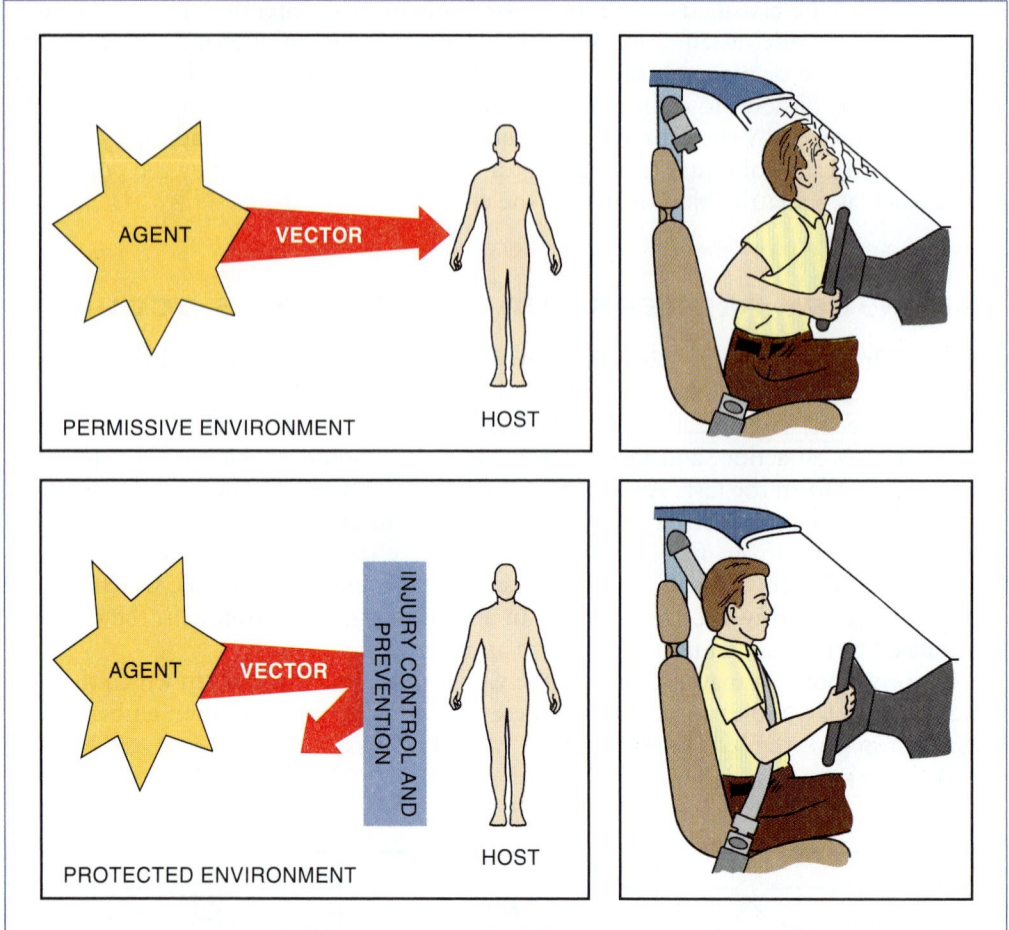

FIGURE H-4 The role of injury control and prevention in providing a protective environment.

ANALYZING INJURY EVENTS

An injury event can be analyzed by separating it into three phases: the preinjury phase, the injury event, and the postinjury phase. Within each phase, host, vehicle, and environmental factors may contribute to the injury process. Preinjury factors either contribute to or inhibit the potential release of energy prior to the injury event. The injury phase has factors that may enhance or inhibit transmission of energy to the host during the injury event. Postinjury factors tend to contribute to or diminish the severity of the injury once it has occurred. Prehospital care providers play a major role in the postinjury phase by providing rapid and high-quality care to injured victims in the field.

The analysis of the three phases of an injury event with respect to host, vehicle, and environmental factors is referred to as Haddon's matrix. Table H-2 provides an example of an analysis of a motor vehicle crash using Haddon's matrix. This tool is very useful for identifying factors contributing to the outcome of an injury event, broadening the discussion for developing prevention strategies, and revealing that most injuries are the product of a large number of causal factors and are not just random happenings.

WHAT IS INJURY PREVENTION AND CONTROL?

Perhaps the most important principle of injury prevention and control is that injury is a disease that is subject to prevention by modifying transmission of energy to the individual. The goal of primary injury prevention is to prevent injury from occurring in the first place. Examples include wearing a seat belt, helmet use by motorcyclists and bicyclists,

Table H-2 Haddon's Matrix.

	FACTORS			
PHASES	HOST	VEHICLE	PHYSICAL ENVIRONMENT	SOCIOCULTURAL ENVIRONMENT
Pre-event	Impaired capacity due to alcohol, age, poor vision, fatigue, inexperience, poor judgment	Defective parts (brakes, tires), poor maintenance, dirty windshield/windows, improper brake lights, ease of control, speed of travel	Narrow road shoulder, poor lighting, road curvature and gradient, road surface type, weather conditions, divided highway, visibility of hazards, signalization	Attitudes about alcohol, drunk driving laws, speed limits, injury prevention programs
Event	Tolerance of body to energy, injury threshold due to aging, chronic disease (osteo-porosis), etc., safety belt use	Placement hardness and sharpness of contact surfaces (dash, steering wheel), automatic restraints, vehicle size	Recovery areas, guard rails, fixed objects (trees, telephone poles), median barriers, embankments	Attitudes about seat belt use, enforcement of child safety seat laws
Postevent	Extent of injury sustained, knowledge of first aid, physical condition and age	Fuel system integrity (bursting gas tank), entrapment of victim	Access to EMS, quality of EMS care, availability of extrication equipment, rehabilitation programs	Training of EMS personnel, trauma system programs
Results	Physical and mental impairment	Cost of vehicle repair	Damage to environment	Legal costs, costs to society (loss of lives and income)

and the installation of smoke detectors. Strategies that attempt to minimize further injury or death after the initial trauma or injury event has occurred are called secondary injury prevention. Prehospital care providers practice secondary injury prevention, or acute care, by ensuring adequate airway, breathing, and circulation as well as C-spine immobilization and rapid transportation to the closest appropriate medical facility.

INJURY SURVEILLANCE

Injury surveillance data forms the foundation of injury control. Accurate and detailed data are needed to determine the incidence of specific injury events, the demographic distributions, the cause of an injury event, and injury risk factors, as well as other factors involved in injury. Prehospital data such as location of the injury site, mechanism of injury, host factors, agent factors, and environmental factors are required. Prehospital care providers are in a crucial position to document the mechanism of injury in great detail, including information such as the extent of damage to a motor vehicle (starred windshield or deformed steering wheel). Description of the location and conditions of the injury site also may be useful in identifying a dangerous section of road where motor vehicle crashes occur time and again or a hazardous area such as an unsafe play-ground where injuries occur frequently.

RISK FACTORS

Injuries are not random events. Some special populations, such as males, alcoholics, and certain age groups, are at higher risk for injury than others. A risk factor is a variable that makes an individual more likely to be injured. Injuries can be prevented by reducing or eliminating risk factors. An example of a host risk factor that may predispose an individual to injury is the use of drugs or alcohol while driving a motor vehicle. A high-risk group is defined as a subset of the population that has a higher incidence of injury. This group may be exposed to hazards more frequently, may be unable to avoid a hazard, or may have a lower injury threshold. Young males are one well-known group that is at higher risk for being involved in a motor vehicle crash than the general population.

PREVENTIVE INTERVENTIONS

Haddon's matrix can be used to identify the factors affecting the extent of injury during specific injury events. Some of the factors may be amenable to prevention strategies or interventions designed to reduce the incidence or severity of injury.

There are three types of interventions: educational, enforcement, and engineering. Interventions may also be classified as either active or passive. An active intervention requires a change in behavior by the individual in need of protection. Educational programs such as those that encourage seat belt use or installation of home smoke detectors are examples of active interventions that attempt to persuade individuals to alter their behavior for increased self-protection. These programs may increase public awareness but are often ignored by those who are at highest risk for injury such as the economically and educationally deprived. Laws against drunk driving and mandatory helmet use by motorcyclists are other examples of active interventions that are aimed at changing an individual's behavior. However, the introduction of a legal intervention does not necessarily imply that it will be enforced by the authorities or adhered to by the public. Unfortunately, alcohol continues to play a part in half of all fatal motor vehicle crashes despite laws against driving under the influence of alcohol. Active education and enforcement interventions are more effective when used together.

Passive interventions provide automatic protection and are generally more effective than active interventions since they do not rely on human behavior change. Modifications in the engineering and design of vehicles and the environment have been very effective in reducing the incidence and severity of injuries. The incorporation of air bags and softer dashboards into automobiles has significantly reduced the incidence and severity of motor vehicle–related injuries. Engineering improvements in road design also have been found to be effective countermeasures in preventing motor vehicle crashes.

DESIGNING INTERVENTIONS: When developing injury prevention programs, it is critical to recognize potential pitfalls for failure as well as ingredients for success. Many intervention programs are difficult to initiate, expensive to maintain, and require the use of limited community resources. The following suggestions will be helpful in selecting injury prevention activities:

1. Target efforts toward a problem that occurs frequently or results in severe injury in your community. In some regions, this may be house fires and, for others, motor vehicle crashes.
2. Address the problem injuries that have specific countermeasures that are known to be effective. Focus on limited, concrete solutions to specific injury events and avoid diffuse, general approaches. Examples of directed specific solutions include fire-safe cigarettes, smoke detectors for house fire prevention, and helmets for bicycle-related head injury prevention.
3. Make the intervention as simple as possible to increase public acceptance and minimize the chance of misuse.
4. Develop a critical mass of community awareness through broad-based grass-roots support, legislation, enforcement, and professional action. Prehospital care providers should take advantage of their connections with local and regional community leaders to build coalitions for effective prevention programs.
5. Promote institutionalization of programs that will last beyond the initial volunteer effort or temporary grant funding. Injury prevention programs should be designed to become a permanent component of prehospital care.

Table H-3 provides examples of injury-specific interventions that have been developed and found to be successful.

Table H-3 **Examples of Injury-Specific Interventions.**

INJURY EVENT	RISK FACTOR	EXAMPLES OF INJURY-SPECIFIC INTERVENTION
Drowning	2-year-old to 5-year-old males	Install fencing around pools at least one meter high with self-locking door; water motion alarm; swimming lessons; prominent "no diving" notices near shallow water; easy access to EMS
Bicycle	5-year-old to 12-year-old males	Encourage helmet use; use of safety reflectors; bicycle traffic lanes; rider education programs
Poisoning	1-year-old to 5-year-old children	Package medicines in childproof containers; install safety latches on storage cabinets
Falls	Elderly with poor vision and/or unstable gait	Remove throw rugs; use nightlights; hand rails on stairs; access to activate EMS

ROLE OF THE EMS PROVIDER IN INJURY PREVENTION AND CONTROL

There are four areas in which prehospital personnel can make an impact and prevent injuries in their community:

1. *Acute Care/Secondary Injury Prevention of the Injured Patient:* Medically trained personnel, such as BTLS providers, are the initial and vital link in the trauma care system. By providing prompt and appropriate care, many lives are saved each year.

2. *Community Education/Primary Injury Prevention:* As respected and credible members of the community, prehospital care providers have a unique opportunity to practice primary injury prevention since they interact directly with injured patients and their families. Less severely injured patients and their families and friends can be counseled about how the present and any future injury could be prevented. Examples include advising the public to wear helmets when riding bicycles, motorcycles, and all-terrain vehicles, as well as wearing seat belts and using child car seats in automobiles. By assessing the scene of the injury, prehospital personnel may identify specific injury prevention strategies for a given family, such as how to "childproof" a home or ways to make the home of an elderly person less risky for falls. As community spokespersons, prehospital care providers often interact with groups such as the local Parent Teachers Association and the Rotary Club. In doing so, community leaders will become more aware of the important concepts of injury prevention and work toward developing a safer community.

3. *Public Policy:* Seat belt and fire-safe cigarette legislation are two examples of regulations that have been instituted with the support of EMS personnel. Seat belt legislation has been very effective in increasing the number of people who wear seat belts and decreasing the number of highway deaths. For those states without seat belt laws, EMS personnel can be effective in encouraging the passage of such legislation. Similarly, it was prehospital care providers who found that the most common cause of fatal house fires is cigarette smoking. With their support, a fire-safe cigarette has been developed. Prehospital care providers may be the first to recognize a new

injury pattern or high-risk group for a specific injury. By reporting this type of information to local and state authorities, injury prevention strategies may be put into place by legislators in hopes of reducing fatal and serious injuries.

4. *Research/Injury Surveillance:* Accurate documentation of the circumstances surrounding injuries such as demographics, location, mechanism of injury, and associated risk factors is important in identifying problem injuries and designing and implementing prevention strategies. Providing reliable information to local community leaders, legislators, and physicians such as the location of the "dangerous intersection," the poorly supervised quarry, and the "unsafe" playground can lead to the development of effective injury prevention strategies and a safer community.

SUMMARY

Prehospital care providers are a vital link in the chain of the national injury control effort. Their interaction with the public is an opportunity to practice both primary and secondary injury prevention. As part of the medical community, EMS personnel provide information to emergency physicians and nurses, which is important in the acute care of injured victims as well as in injury control research. The injury epidemic can be addressed only through a concerted effort by the medical, community, and legislative organizations.

BIBLIOGRAPHY

1. American College of Emergency Physicians. *Guidelines for Trauma Care Systems.* Dallas, TX: The College, September 16, 1992.

2. Baker, S., B. O'Neill, M. J. Ginsburg, and G. Li. *The Injury Fact Book.* New York: Oxford University Press, 1992.

3. Centers for Disease Control and Prevention. *Injury Control in the 1990s: A National Plan for Action.* Atlanta, GA: The Centers, 1993.

4. Centers for Disease Control and Prevention. *Setting the National Agenda for Injury Control in the 1990s: Position Papers from the Third National Injury Control Conference.* Atlanta, GA: The Centers, 1992.

5. Committee on Trauma Research, Commission on Life Sciences, National Research Council, and the Institute of Medicine. *Injury in America: A Continuing Public Health Problem.* Washington, DC: National Academy Press, 1985.

6. Christoffel, T., and S. P. Teret. *Protecting the Public, Legal Issues in Injury Prevention.* New York: Oxford University Press, 1993.

7. Kaalbfleisch, J., and F. Rivera. "Principles in Injury Control: Lessons to Be Learned from Child Safety Seats." *Pediatric Emergency Care* (1989), pp. 131–134.

8. Martinez, R. "Injury Control: A Primer for Physicians." *Annals of Emergency Medicine,* Vol. 19 (1990), pp. 72–77.

9. The National Committee for Injury Prevention and Control. *Injury Prevention: Meeting the Challenge.* New York: Oxford University Press, 1989.

10. Wilson, M. H., and others. *Saving Children, A Guide to Injury Prevention.* New York: Oxford University Press, 1991.

Multicasualty Incidents and Triage

David Maatman, NREMT-P/IC
Roy Alson, Ph.D., M.D., F.A.C.E.P.
Jere Baldwin, M.D., F.A.C.E.P., F.A.A.F.P.
John T. Stevens, NREMT-P

OBJECTIVES

UPON COMPLETION OF THIS APPENDIX, YOU SHOULD
BE ABLE TO:

1. Compare and contrast the definitions of a Disaster and Multicasualty Incident.
2. Define span-of-control.
3. List the responsibilities of Medical Command, Triage Officer, Transport Officer, Treatment Officer, and Staging Officer.
4. Describe the Initial Assessment.
5. Identify Priority 1, 2, 3, and 4 patients

DEFINITIONS

Disaster: An event that overwhelms the ability of the system to respond. This definition is relative and is based on the availability of resources within the system and community.

ICS: Incident Command System. An organizational structure designed to improve safety and emergency response operations of all types and complexities.

MCI: Multicasualty Incident. An incident involving a large number of persons injured in which the EMS system is unable to manage the situation utilizing day-to-day procedures. An MCI may be classified as a disaster but not all disasters are MCIs.

Paper Plan Syndrome: Having a written MCI/Disaster Plan without training the individuals who would most likely activate and work it.

Span of Control: An effective management/supervision of subordinates. Usually limited to five subordinates per manager/supervisor.

Triage: To prioritize or sort injuries or the injured. Usually sorted into four categories, Priority 1, 2, 3, and 4 (Red, Yellow, Green, and Black).

INTRODUCTION

It is not uncommon for EMS to have more than one patient at a trauma scene; however, most day-to-day operational procedures are designed for the single patient incident. Safety, organization, and communication are paramount in all EMS activities. When faced with multiple patients this need is even greater. It is essential that these components are effective and that all entities of the emergency system are working from the same plan.

An effective and efficient way to obtain this unity is to have medical operations adopt an Incident Command System (ICS) as a template for organization. Primary functional components of a Medical Incident Command System (MICS) include Medical Command, Triage, Treatment, Transport, and Staging. Even with a single patient incident these four components exist; however, one person usually is responsible for the functions of all components. There is a Medical Command person in charge of the patient care (team leader), injuries are triaged (prioritized assessment), treatment is provided for the patient, a transport decision is made, and deployment of on-scene vehicles is determined from a point of safety, ingress, and egress (staging).

Designing and implementing an MICS, based on an ICS, will provide EMS with dependable, reproducible results when faced with multiple patient incidents. The MICS must be simple enough for new users but expandable enough to provide the necessary structure to manage large incidents.

INCIDENT COMMAND SYSTEM

ICS was developed in southern California in the early 1970s. The typical on-scene components of an ICS are Command, Fire Suppression, Rescue/Extrication, Law Enforcement, and Medical (Figure I-1).

The structured flexibility of an ICS enables it to be adapted to all types of emergency incidents: fire, rescue, law enforcement, and multicasualty incidents. Because of its modular design, the structure of the ICS can be expanded or compressed, depending on the changing conditions of an incident. It must be staffed and operated by qualified personnel from an emergency service agency.

If an on-scene incident command system is not immediately established, other rescuers will take independent actions, which will frequently be in conflict with each other. These independent actions (freelancing) may be dangerous and disruptive in an environment that requires organization and accountability. Without organization and accountability, chaos will occur and too many people will attempt to command the incident. If you do not control the situation, the situation will control you.

MEDICAL INCIDENT COMMAND

One sector of the on-scene ICS is Medical. The medical sector is broken down into manageable components (subfunctions or branches). The five primary components of an MICS are Medical Command, Triage, Treatment, Transport, and Staging (Figure I-2).

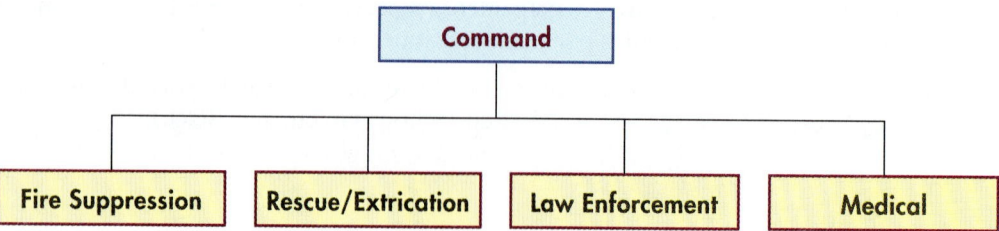

FIGURE I-1   On-scene incident command structure.

FIGURE I-2   Medical incident command.

It may not be necessary to have one person in each position, but it is necessary to ensure the function of each position is executed. At a scene with multiple patients, it may be necessary to have more than one person take on the function of these components. When considering the need to expand or condense the MICS, the best indicator is current or anticipated span-of-control. The general rule is to have one person supervise five subordinates. Some latitude may be given due to the complexity of the situation. A highly complex or difficult situation may require a span-of-control of 3:1, or a simple situation may allow up to 7:1.

All participants of an ICS need to know their responsibilities. Provided below are some ideas and suggestions in determining the responsibilities of the medical sector officers of an ICS.

MEDICAL COMMAND

1. Establishes liaisons with on-scene Incident Command
2. Establishes working MICS with appropriate sectors
3. Ensures that proper rescue/extrication services are activated
4. Ensures law enforcement involvement as necessary
5. Ensures that helicopter landing zone operations are coordinated
6. Determines the amount and types of additional medical resources and supplies
7. Ensures that area hospitals and Medical Direction are aware of the situation so they can prepare for casualties
8. Designates assistance officers and their location
9. Maintains an appropriate span-of-control
10. Works as a conduit of communications between subordinates and the Incident Commander

EMS STAGING OFFICER

1. Maintains a log of available units and medical supplies
2. Coordinates physical location of incoming resources (i.e., ambulances and helicopters)
3. Coordinates incoming personnel who wish to aid at the scene
4. Provides updates to Medical Command as necessary

TRIAGE OFFICER

1. Ensures proper utilization of the Initial Assessment triage system or other local protocol
2. Ensures that triage tags or other visual identification technique is properly completed and secured to the patient
3. Makes requests for additional resources though Medical Command
4. Provides updates to Medical Command as necessary

TREATMENT OFFICER

1. Establishes suitable treatment areas
2. Communicates resource needs to Medical Command
3. Assigns, supervises, and coordinates treatment of patients
4. Provides updates to Medical Command as necessary

TRANSPORT OFFICER

1. Ensures the organized transport of patients off-scene
2. Ensures an appropriate distribution of patients to all local hospitals to prevent hospital overloading
3. Completes a transportation log
4. Contacts receiving hospitals to advise them of the number of patients and condition (may be delegated to a communications officer)
5. Provides updates to Medical Command as necessary

TRIAGE

As a triage officer, you are to spend less than one minute doing an Initial Assessment to determine the priority of a patient. It cannot be overemphasized that the person doing the triage does NOT render any treatment to a patient. Treatment is to be done by the treatment sector of the MICS. A triage officer who allows himself to begin treatment of victims is no longer a triage officer, and the function of triage must be reassigned. Once the medical priority of a patient has been determined, using the BTLS Triage Decision Tree (Figure I-3), the triage officer should affix an appropriately completed triage tag (Figure I-4) or other visual identification technique to the victim and move on to the next victim to be assessed.

TYPICALLY PATIENTS ARE PRIORITIZED INTO FOUR CATEGORIES:

Priority 1: Red Tagged—Critical condition, unstable but salvageable (load-and-go)

Priority 2: Yellow Tagged—Serious condition, potentially unstable

Priority 3: Green Tagged—Stable condition, minor injuries, "walking wounded"

Priority 4: Black Tagged—Dead or alive but nonsalvageable*

INITIAL ASSESSMENT

Although there is a tendency to over triage, one must refrain from this because of its impact on the resources available to the EMS system. We need to be as accurate in our triage assessment as possible.

Three basic human systems need to be quickly evaluated to determine the patient's medical priority:

Respiratory system

Circulatory system

Neurological system (LOC)

By utilizing the BTLS Initial Assessment during the triage phase and the Rapid Trauma Assessment or the Focused Assessment in the treatment phase, we will be accurate in our assessment and make the best use of resources by providing the greatest amount of good to the greatest number of patients.

---

*Some EMS systems will group the "alive but nonsalvageable" patients in the Priority 1 category and work on them as long as resources are available and it does not take away from the needed resources for a salvageable patient.

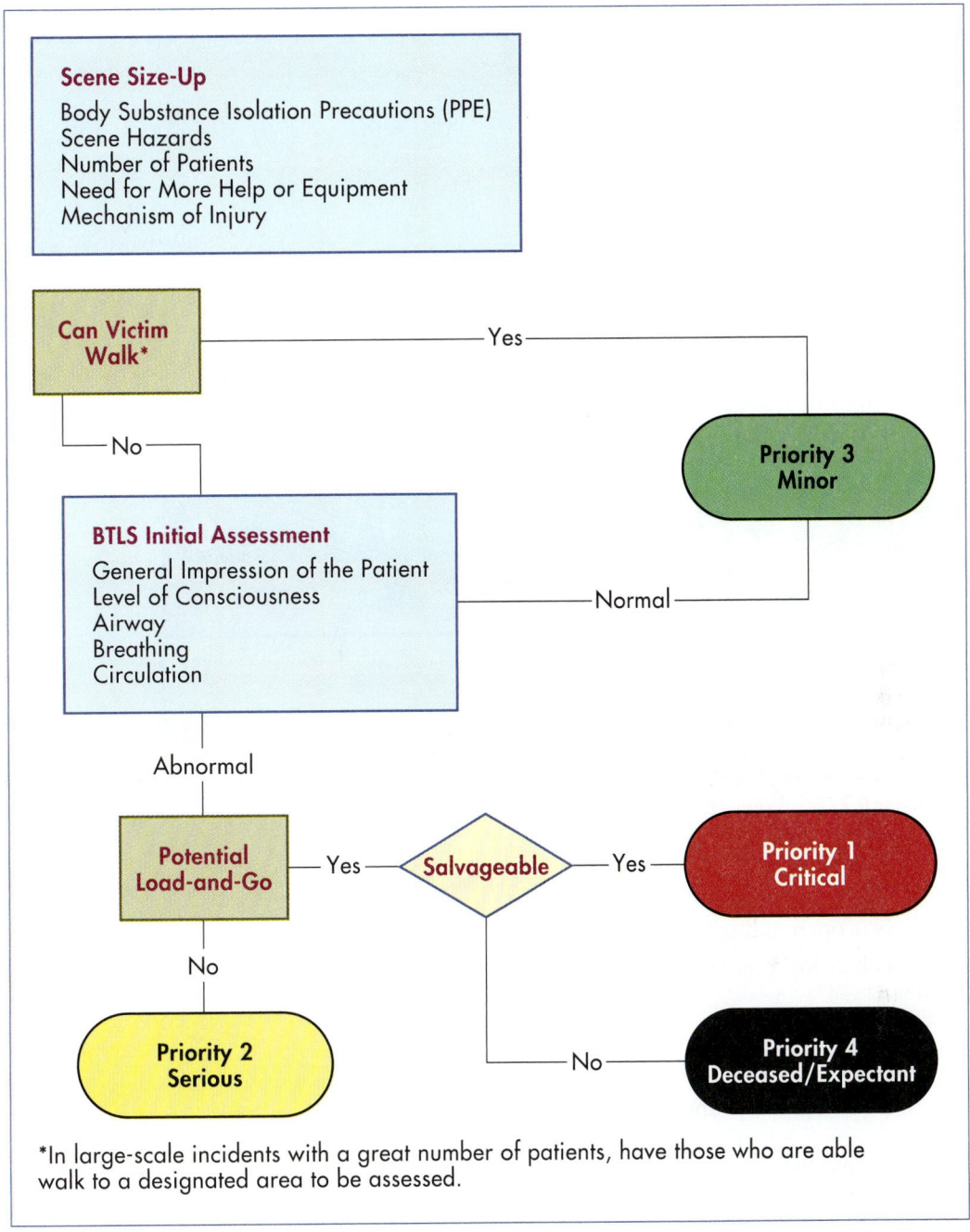

FIGURE I-3 BTLS Triage Decision Tree. This decision tree reflects the steps of initial triage. Subsequent and more detailed assessments should occur throughout patient care.

GENERAL IMPRESSION (Patient Overview)

Victim's approximate age?

What position is he in?

What is his activity (aware of surroundings, anxious, in distress)?

Is he perfusing (skin color)?

Are there any major injuries or bleeding?

LEVEL OF CONSCIOUSNESS

FIGURE I-4   Triage tag.

AIRWAY

Is it open and self maintained?

Is it compromised?

BREATHING

Is the victim breathing?

What is the rate and quality?

CIRCULATION

Is there a pulse?

What is the rate and quality?

Once the Initial Assessment has been completed and you have figured in a "survivability factor," you have a good idea how to prioritize the patient. An example of applying the survivability factor would be if you were presented with a geriatric patient and a pediatric patient with similar critical injuries and you only have enough resources for one. Which one do you choose and why? The decision should be based on objective evaluations rather than emotions.

SPECIAL CONSIDERATIONS

INJURED RESCUERS

Many ICSs provide a separate medical component at the scene of the incident for the care and treatment of the rescuers. Structurally this sector is part of the logistics component of a large ICS structure. In the event of illness or injury to one of our colleagues, we need to be assured that they will not fall into the triage system of the victims of the incident. We are obligated to take care of our own. This will enable our fallen colleague to return to duty quicker and help the overall operation by providing the remaining rescuers the peace of mind of knowing that their fellow rescuer has not been forgotten.

STANDARD OF CARE

When reviewing the care of a patient of an MCI, we have to consider the adverse circumstances EMS was operating under at the time of the incident. During normal day-to-day operations, standard protocols treat all patients for the worse case scenario and thus many patients are overtreated. When manpower and resources are available, it is prudent to provide such care. However, when working in an MCI or disaster environment the inefficient use of manpower and resources may be catastrophic. The guiding principle in triage and treatment of victims of an MCI is to do the greatest good for the greatest number of patients with the least depletion of available resources.

CRITIQUE AND DEBRIEFING

The management of all MCIs and disasters should be formally critiqued. Primary focus should be on what worked and what did not. An MCI/Disaster Plan is a dynamic document and modified when there is a problem. In addition to taking time to critique the incident, time must also be taken to provide Critical Incident Stress Debriefing (CISD) for the participants of an incident. The mental health of EMS professionals is as important as the physical health.

SUMMARY

The priorities of any incident, no matter how small or large, should be safety, organization, and then patient care. To provide the most effective and efficient patient care, one must approach it in a safe and organized fashion.

To have an effective MICS requires its use in day-to-day operations, including the routine, small emergencies. The rehearsal of the MICS on smaller situations will develop proficiency and allow for a smooth transition into the larger, more complex incidents. Activating the MICS only when an incident reaches a high level can result in a lack of familiarity with its use. Routine activation of the system develops confidence in its use for all levels of command and agencies involved. To avoid the paper plan syndrome, the regular implementation and review of an MCI/Disaster Plan is paramount to having successful operations.

A MICS is not a magic wand that will save lives by itself, nor will it replace common sense and good judgment required of experienced EMS professionals. Successful management of a situation still requires properly trained people who know what to do and how to do it. MICS properly utilized can increase the overall effectiveness of the participants by providing a proactive approach to management. If you don't manage the situation, the situation manages you. The key to effective performance in a leadership role is not necessarily rank but the understanding of the duties of that position and the ability to properly function at that level.

On large-scale incidents an operation may last for days or even weeks and will require additional resources. As part of the disaster plan, an ICS provides the structure for the necessary administrative, planning, financial and logistical support.

MCI CASE
SELF-REVIEW

SITUATION

A school bus is struck by a car. The bus rolled over with seven people on board. There is one person in the car.

LOCAL EMS RESOURCES

7 ground ambulances available

1 helicopter available

2 acute care hospitals in 30-mile radius (one designated Level I trauma center)

1 volunteer fire department with first aid training

RESPONSE TIMES

Volunteer fire department and first ambulance on scene 11 minutes from time of call.

Additional ambulances on scene 15–20 minutes after first arriving ambulance.

Helicopter on-scene 25 minutes after they have been requested.

Ground transport time to Level I trauma center 25 minutes, 20 minutes for other hospital.

TRIAGE

Review the following initial assessments of the victims. Determine what priority you would make them and discuss your decisions with others. It is not uncommon to have disagreement between EMS personnel. There may not be a single right answer.

A. 6 y/o Female, still inside bus
LOC—Unresponsive
Skin—Cool/Pale/Moist
Airway—Partial obstruction
Breathing—Agonal at 6/min.
Circulation—Radial pulses absent, carotid approximately 80/min.
Miscellaneous—Legs pinned under a seat

B. 8 y/o Male, still inside bus
LOC—A&O×3
Skin—Warm/Pale/Dry
Airway—Open, self-maintained
Breathing—24/min., nonlabored
Circulation—Radial pulses approximately 80/min.
Miscellaneous—Deformity to right femur and mangled right hand

C. 10 y/o Female, outside bus sitting against a tree
LOC—A&O×3
Skin—Warm/Normal/Dry
Airway—Open, self-maintained
Breathing—20/min., nonlabored
Circulation—Radial pulses approximately 130/min.
Miscellaneous—Pain right hip, crepitus on right side of pelvis

D. 7 y/o Male, sitting up inside bus, not pinned
LOC—A&O×3 but anxious
Skin—Warm/Pale/Dry
Airway—Open, self-maintained
Breathing—40/min. with gasping
Circulation—Radial pulses approximately 100/min.
Miscellaneous—Chest pain and unable to get his breath. Breath sounds clear.

E. 13 y/o Female, inside bus
LOC—Unresponsive
Skin—Cool/Pale
Airway—Extensive facial trauma, not self-maintained
Breathing—Absent
Circulation—Absent
Miscellaneous—Open head injury

F. 9 y/o Female, sitting next to "E" hysterical
LOC—Alert but hysterical
Skin—Cool/Pale/Dry
Airway—Open, self-maintained
Breathing—36/min., nonlabored
Circulation—Radial pulses approximately 120/min.
Miscellaneous—No obvious signs of injury

G. 55 y/o Female, restrained bus driver. She is trying to help the children
LOC—A&O×3
Skin—Warm/Normal/Dry
Airway—Open, self-maintained
Breathing—18/min., nonlabored
Circulation—Radial pulses approximately 90/min.
Miscellaneous—3-inch laceration on forehead with slow bleeding

H. 48 y/o Male, unrestrained driver of the car, strong smell of alcohol on patient
LOC—Alert but confused
Skin—Warm/Normal/Moist
Airway—Open, self-maintained—slurred speech
Breathing—16/min., nonlabored
Circulation—Radial pulses approximately 100/min.
Miscellaneous—Hematoma on forehead, pupils slow to respond

GLOSSARY

abruptio placenta   early separation of the placenta from the uterus.

acidosis   a condition caused by accumulation of acid or loss of base from the body.

adventitia   the layer of loose connective tissue forming the outermost coating of an organ.

aerobic   requiring oxygen.

air bag   a passive restraint system in automobiles and other vehicles.

alkalosis   a pathologic condition resulting from accumulation of base or loss of acid in the body.

anaerobic   lacking oxygen.

anoxia   absence of oxygen supply to the tissue.

asphyxia   a condition due to lack of oxygen; suffocation.

aspirate   taking foreign matter into the lungs during inhalation.

assessment   to evaluate the condition of a patient.

ATV   all-terrain vehicle.

AVPU   a description of the level of consciousness. AVPU stands for: A—alert, V—responds to verbal stimuli, P—responds to pain, U—unresponsive.

avulsion   an injury in which a piece of a structure is torn away.

axial loading   compression forces applied along the long axis of the body. *Example:* a fall in which a victim lands on his feet and force is transferred up his legs to his back, causing a compression fracture of a lumbar vertebra.

bag-valve mask   a system of artificial ventilation in which the oxygen inflow fills a bag that is attached to a mask by a one-way valve.

Battle's sign   swelling and discoloration behind the ear caused by a fracture of the base of the skull.

BIADs   blind insertion airway devices, such as the esophageal tracheal Combitube®.

BLS   burns, lacerations, swelling. Can also mean basic life support.

bronchospasm   contraction of the smooth muscle of the bronchi.

Broselow tape   a tape used to estimate the weight of a child by measuring her length.

BSI   body substance isolation. A procedure used to prevent being contaminated by a patient's body fluids. This usually entails gloves and possibly a gown and face shield.

BVM (bag-valve mask)   a system of artificial ventilation in which the oxygen inflow fills a bag that is attached to a mask by a one-way valve.

capillary blanch or refill   test for impairment of circulation: pressure on tip of the nail will cause the bed to turn white, if it does not turn pink again by the time it takes to say "capillary refill," the circulation is impaired. The test has been found to be unreliable for early shock.

carbonaceous sputum   sputum that is "sooty" or black.

carina   the lowest part of the trachea, where the trachea divides to form the two mainstem bronchi.

catecholamines   a group of chemicals of similar structure that act to increase heart rate and blood pressure.

C-collar (cervical collar)   a device to limit movement of the neck.

central cord syndrome   an injury to the spinal cord that produces more los of sensory and motor function in the arms than in the legs.

cerebral perfusion   blood flow to the brain.

C.N.S.   central nervous system; the brain and spinal cord.

compliance   the "give" or elasticity of the lungs and chest wall. This influences how easy it is for the patient to breath.

concussion   a jarring injury to the brain resulting in disturbance of brain function.

contracoup   an injury to the brain on the opposite side of the original blow.

contralateral   situated or affecting the opposite side.

contusion   bruising; the reaction of soft tissue to a direct blow.

constricted   to shrink or contract.

COPD   chronic obstructive pulmonary disease. The end result of asthma, chronic bronchitis, or emphysema.

copious   large amount.

coup   an injury to the brain on the same side as the original blow.

crepitation   feeling of crackling; the sensation of fragments of broken bones rubbing together.

CSIC cervical spinal immobilization collar.

Cushing's reflex a reflex whereby the body reacts to increased pressure on the brain by raising the blood pressure.

DCAP deformities, contusions, abrasions, penetrations.

DCAP-BTLS deformities, contusions, abrasions, penetrations, burns, tenderness, lacerations, swelling.

DCAPP deformities, contusions, abrasions, penetrations, paradoxical movement.

deceleration to come to a sudden stop, decreasing speed.

decubent position the position assumed when Lying down.

delivered volume the amount of air that you actually deliver to the lungs with each breath when you perform artificial or assisted ventilation.

denatured to destroy the usual nature of a substance.

dermis the inner layer of the skin, containing hair follicles, sweat glands, sebaceous glands, nerve endings, and blood vessels.

detailed exam a comprehensive head-to-toes exam to find additional injuries that may have been missed in the brief Primary Survey.

diaphoresis to perspire profusely.

diuretic an agent that promotes the excretion of urine.

doll's eyes oculocephalic reflex; a test of brain stem function that is never performed in the prehospital setting.

dura the tough fibrous membrane forming the outermost of the three coverings of the brain.

EGTA esophageal gastric tube airway; an improved esophageal obturator airway.

EMS emergency medical services.

endotracheal intubation the insertion of a tube into the trachea to assist or control ventilation.

EOA esophageal obturator airway.

epidermis the outermost layer of skin.

epidural outside the dura; between the dura and the skull.

ETA estimated time of arrival. An estimation of when you will arrive at the receiving hospital.

etiology the cause of a particular disease.

ET tube endotracheal tube.

evisceration the protruding of internal organs through a wound.

expeditious quick, speedy.

exsanguinate to bleed to death.

extrication removal of a patient from a dangerous position or situation.

FROPVD flow-restricted, oxygen-powered, ventilation device. An artificial ventilation device that provides 100% oxygen at a flow rate of 40 L/min at a maximum pressure of 50 ± 5 cm water.

full-thickness burn third degree burn.

gastric insufflation the filling of the stomach by air when performing positive pressure ventilation.

genioglossus muscle the muscle that pulls the tongue out of the mouth.

grunting a deep, guttural noise made in breathing; a sign of respiratory distress in small children.

GSC (Glasgow Coma Score) A method to measure the severity of injury of a head-injury patient.

Hare splint a type of traction splint.

Heimlich maneuver a method of dislodging food or other material from the throat of a choking victim.

hemiparesis partial paralysis affecting one side of the body.

hemoptysis to spit up blood or blood-stained sputum.

hemothorax the presence of blood in the chest cavity within the pleural space, outside the lung.

hypercarbia high blood carbon dioxide level.

hyperresonant giving an increased vibrant sound on percussion; tympanic.

hypertympany hyperresonant.

hyperventilation increased amount of air entering the lungs, >24 breaths per minute for an adult.

hypoventilation decreased amount of air entering the lungs, <12 breaths per minute or breathing that is too shallow.

hypovolemic shock hemorrhagic shock; shock caused by insufficient blood or fluid within the body.

hypoxia   a deficiency of oxygen reaching the tissues of the body.

ICP   intracranial pressure. The pressure inside the skull.

impaled object   a penetrating object that is still in place in a patient's body.

Initial Assessment   part of the Primary Survey. This is a rapid exam of airway, breathing and circulation. It is performed on all patients.

intra-abdominal   within the abdomen.

intracranial   within the skull.

intrathoractic   within the chest.

ipsilateral   situated on or affecting the same side.

JVD   jugular vein distention. Distended jugular veins in the neck.

kinematics   the phase of mechanics that deals with possible motions of the body.

labial angle   corner of the mouth.

laryngeal mask airway (LMA)   An invasive airway device to assist ventilation.

lateral decubitus position   position assumed when lying on one's side.

lesion   an injury or abnormal condition of a part.

LMA   laryngeal mask airway. An invasive airway device to assist ventilation.

LOC   level of consciousness.

MAP   mean arterial blood pressure.

MAST   military antishock trousers. Also called pneumatic antishock garment (PASG). A device that applies circumferential pressure to the legs and abdomen to raise the blood pressure in hypotensive patients.

MCI   multiple casualty incident. An emergency situation in which there are multiple injured patients.

mean arterial blood pressure   diastolic blood pressure plus 1/3 (systolic minus the diastolic blood pressure).

medial   toward the middle.

minute volume   the volume of air breathed in and out in 1 minute. This varies from 5 to 12 liters per minute.

mortality   frequency of death or death rate.

MVC   motor vehicle collision.

nasopharyngeal airway   an artificial airway positioned in the nasal cavity.

necrosis   the death of tissue.

neonate   newborn infant.

nonrebreather mask   an oxygen mask that allows the patient to breath oxygen at a concentration close to 100%

NP airway   nasopharyngeal airway. An artificial airway positioned in the nasal cavity.

occult injuries   injuries hidden or concealed from view.

oropharyngeal airway   an artificial airway positioned in the oral cavity to keep the tongue from occluding the airway

osteomyelitis   inflammation or infection or a bone or bones.

pallor   paleness, absence of skin color.

palpate   to examine by touch.

paradoxical motion   the motion of the injured segment of a flail chest, opposite to the normal motion of the chest wall.

parenchymal   the essential elements of an organ.

paresis   slight or incomplete paralysis.

paresthesia   abnormal sensation; a "tingling" sensation.

partial-thickness burn   a burn that does not injure the full thickness of the skin. A first degree burn involves only the epidermal layer. A second degree burn involves the epidermis and part of the dermis.

PASG   pneumatic antishock garment. Also called military antishock trousers (MAST). A device that applies circumferential pressure to the legs and abdomen to raise the blood pressure in hypotensive patients.

patent   open.

pathophysiology   the basic processes of the disease.

perfusion   the passage of blood or fluid through the vessels of an organ.

personal watercraft (PWC)   a small motorized watercraft that one or two persons can ride. Much like a motorcycle except it travels on water.

pia mater   innermost of the three layers of tissue that envelop the brain.

placenta previa   an abnormal location of the placenta, so that it covers the opening of the uterus (cervical os).

PMS pulse, motor, sensory. Description of the exam of an injured extremity

pneumothorax the presence of air within the chest cavity in the pleural space. but outside the lung (collapsed lung).

pocket mask a small face mask for performing assisted ventilation. It is made to be carried in the rescuer's pocket.

potential space a space that does not exist except under abnormal circumstances. *Example:* Normally the lungs completely fill the chest cavity so that the pleural space (between the lungs ar,d the chest wall) is only a potential space. If the pleural space contains blood it is a hemothorax.

PPE personal protection equipment such as gloves, face shields, and impervious gowns.

primary survey a brief exam to find immediately life-threatening conditions. It is made up of the Initial Assessment and either the Rapid Trauma Survey or the Focused Exam.

pulse oximeter a noninvasive device for measuring the arterial oxygen saturation in the peripheral circulation.

pulse pressure the sensation given by the heart contraction to the palpating finger on an artery.

raccoon's eyes swelling and discoloration around both eyes; a late sign of basilar skull fracture.

respiratory reserve lung tissue over and above the body's need to provide oxygenation for the body.

RTSS radio telephone switch station; a type of radio that accesses the telephone lines.

Sager splint a type of traction splint.

SAMPLE history the least amount of information needed on a trauma patient. S—symptoms, A—allergies, M—medications, P—past medical history, L—last oral intake (last meal), E—events preceding the injury.

scaphoid shaped like a boat. When used to describe the abdomen, scaphoid means sunken in.

scuba diver a diver who is able to remain under water by breathing compressed air from a breathing apparatus needing no connection with the surface. SCUBA stands for self-contained underwater breathing apparatus.

Sellick maneuver a maneuver (posterior pressure on the cricoid cartilage) to prevent gastric insufflation and vomiting.

sheering forces forces that occur in such a direction to cause tearing of an organ.

sibling brother or sister.

skin diver a diver who holds his breath when swimming under water. He uses no artificial breathing methods.

snoring to breathe in a hoarse, rough noise, usually with the mouth open.

snorkeler a diver who uses a short tube (snorkel) in order to float on the surface and observe underwater life. When diving, a snorkeler must hold her breath.

spontaneous pnemothorax collapsed lung caused by the rupture of a congenitally weak area on the surface of the lung.

stridor breathing that has a high-pitched, harsh noise; a sign of impending airway obstruction.

stroke volume the amount of blood pumped by the heart in one beat.

subcutaneous emphysema the presence of air in soft tissues, giving a very characteristic crackling sensation on palpation; the Rice Krispies feeling.

tachypnea adult respiratory rate of 24 or more breaths per minute.

tamponade compression of a part of the anatomy, as the compression of heart by pericardial fluid.

tension pneumothorax a condition in which air continuously leaks out of the lung into the pleural space, increasing pressure within the space with every breath the patient takes.

Thomas' splint a type of traction splint.

TlC Tenderness, Instability, Crepitation. An acronym for the description of the exam of a bony area.

tidal volume the amount of air that is inspired and expired during one respiratory cycle.

traction the action of drawing or pulling on an object.

trajectory the direction a missile takes in flight or after striking a body.

transected to cut transversely.

Trendelenburg position patient supine with lower body elevated about 30 degrees.

vallecula the space between the base of the tongue and the epiglottis.

vasomotor affecting the size of a blood vessel.

venous pressure pressure of the blood in the veins.

viscera any large interior organ in any one of the three great cavities of the body, especially the abdomen.

volatile a substance that evaporates rapidly at room temperature when exposed to air.

wheezing whistling sounds made in breathing; a sign of spasm or narrowing of the bronchi.

INDEX